T0419267

CANCER STEM CELLS

CANCER ETIOLOGY, DIAGNOSIS AND TREATMENTS

Additional books in this series can be found on Nova's website under the Series tab.

Additional E-books in this series can be found on Nova's website under the E-books tab.

CANCER STEM CELLS

MELISSA E. JORDAN
EDITOR

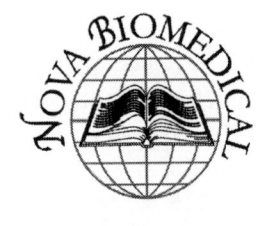

Nova Science Publishers, Inc.
New York

NOTICE TO THE READER

The Publisher has taken reasonable care in the preparation of this book, but makes no expressed or implied warranty of any kind and assumes no responsibility for any errors or omissions. No liability is assumed for incidental or consequential damages in connection with or arising out of information contained in this book. The Publisher shall not be liable for any special, consequential, or exemplary damages resulting, in whole or in part, from the readers' use of, or reliance upon, this material.

Independent verification should be sought for any data, advice or recommendations contained in this book. In addition, no responsibility is assumed by the publisher for any injury and/or damage to persons or property arising from any methods, products, instructions, ideas or otherwise contained in this publication.

This publication is designed to provide accurate and authoritative information with regard to the subject matter covered herein. It is sold with the clear understanding that the Publisher is not engaged in rendering legal or any other professional services. If legal or any other expert assistance is required, the services of a competent person should be sought. FROM A DECLARATION OF PARTICIPANTS JOINTLY ADOPTED BY A COMMITTEE OF THE AMERICAN BAR ASSOCIATION AND A COMMITTEE OF PUBLISHERS.

LIBRARY OF CONGRESS CATALOGING-IN-PUBLICATION DATA

Cancer stem cells / editors, Thomas Dittmar and Kurt S. Zanker.
    p. ; cm.
 Includes bibliographical references and index.
 ISBN 978-1-61668-971-1 (hardcover : alk. paper)
 1. Cancer cells. 2. Stem cells. I. Dittmar, Thomas. II. Zdnker, Kurt S.
 [DNLM: 1. Neoplastic Stem Cells. QZ 202 C215658 2010]
 RC269.7.C376 2010
 616.99'4042--dc22

           2010016707

Published by Nova Science Publishers, Inc. † New York

CONTENTS

PREFACE

Cancer stem cells (CSCs) are cancer cells that possess characteristics associated with normal stem cells, specifically the ability to give rise to all cell types found in a particular cancer sample. CSCs are therefore tumorigenic (tumor-forming), perhaps in contrast to other non-tumorigenic cancer cells. CSCs may generate tumors through the stem cell processes of self-renewal and differentiation into multiple cell types. This book presents new research on cancer stem cells including mesenchymal stem cells and their role in tumor progression; Wnt signaling in colon cancer stem cells; genetic and epigenetic alterations that drive leukemic stem cell self-renewal and others.

Chapter I - Acute myeloid leukemia has emerged as a paradigm for the concept of the cancer stem cell. This hypothesis presumes that the disease is maintained by a rare population of leukemia-initiating stem cells which have acquired genetic or epigenetic changes. It is most likely that a single (epi)genetic event will not be sufficient to cause leukemia, but that a number of sequential events are required. Similar to normal hematopoietic stem cells, both intrinsic as well as extrinsic factors that arise from the bone marrow niche, provide essential cues that regulate cell fate decisions such as leukemic stem cell self-renewal and differentiation. In this chapter, we will review the genetic and epigenetic abnormalities that underlie the process of leukemic transformation, and will discuss which events potentially co-operate to induce leukemia.

Chapter II - Of the many markers for cancer stem cells (CSCs) in lung cancer reported to date, the cell surface antigen CD133, nuclear β-catenin accumulation, the side population phenotype, and high aldehyde dehydrogenase (ALDH) activity seem to be most reliable. In this chapter, we review the results of studies on lung CSCs and discuss the significance of these markers from a biological, pathological, and clinical viewpoint. In addition, we present our own data, focusing primarily upon ALDH1A1. Twenty-seven lung cancer cell lines (nine small cell lung carcinoma (SCLC) cell lines and eighteen non-small cell lung carcinoma (NSCLC) cell lines) were examined for mRNA and protein expression and fractions of cells with activity. ALDH1A1 mRNA was strongly expressed in five cell lines, of which three were SCLC cell lines and two were NSCLC cell lines. Two of the SCLC cell lines consistently expressed the protein and had a large fraction of cells with ALDH activity, but the third did not. Both the NSCLC cell lines expressed the protein, but only one had a large fraction of cells with strong ALDH activity. In brief, the level of ALDH1A1 mRNA did not always parallel that of the protein in SCLC cell lines, while the level of ALDH1A1 protein did not necessarily parallel that of ALDH activity in NSCLC cell lines. The ALDH1A1 protein level or ALDH activity level was well associated with the mRNA level of CD133, which is the most commonly used marker for CSCs, in SCLC cell lines, but not in NSCLC cell lines, suggesting an abundance of CSC populations in SCLC compared to in NSCLC. From the current findings, the mechanism and pathway that regulate the expression of ALDH1A1 mRNA and its protein, and its enzymatic activity as well differ greatly between SCLC and NSCLC cells. We speculate that ALDH (its expression and activity) is only one of the factors determining the stemness of CSCs in lung cancers. In conclusion, the CSCs in SCLC and NSCLC differ distinctly in terms not only of their abundance but also of the regulatory mechanism of ALDH1A1 expression and activity, as well as its role in the maintenance/activation of stemness. Exploring the mechanism of ALDH's activation and its role in the maintenance of the stemness not only of CSCs but also of normal stem cells would provide a novel paradigm for stem cell biology.

Chapter III - Mesenchymal stem cells (MSCs) are adult stem cells that derive from the bone marrow. A major feature of these cells is their ability to differentiate into adipocytes, chondrocytes or osteocytes. They are also defined by the expression of certain markers, such as CD105, CD73 and CD90, and the lack of others (CD45, CD34, CD14, CD79a and HLA-DR). This expression profile makes them distinct from other bone-derived cells. Several functions have been attributed to MSCs. E.g., MSCs modulate immune responses by suppressing the activities of a number of immune cells. This function is thought to be important to prevent excessive inflammation in the wound healing process. MSCs are chemoattracted to wounds. Probably mistaking tumors for wounds, MSCs also enter solid tumors, where they modulate the activities of tumor cells by exposing them to a plethora of cyto- and chemokines. Recently, MSC-secreted CCL5 has been shown to trigger breast cancer cells to metastasize to lung. Moreover, MSCs are able to differentiate into carcinoma-associated fibroblasts (CAF) which are known to have tumor-promoting activity. This review will summarize the current knowledge on the functions of MSCs in tumor progression.

Chapter IV - Colorectal cancer is the second leading cause of cancer-related death in the United States. Among many gene mutations associated with colorectal cancer, mutation of APC (adenomatous polyposis coli) or β-catenin, which activates Wnt signaling, represents the initiation step of colon tumorigenesis. Wnt signaling is known to play multiple roles in early development and formation of human cancers. In addition, Wnt signaling also regulates the self-renewal and differentiation of adult stem cells. Recently, cancer stem cells have emerged as an exciting new concept in cancer research. However, many challenging questions have also arisen. What is the definition of a cancer stem cell? Where do such cells originate and what are the markers for these cells? What's the genetic and epigenetic machinery that regulate the homeostasis of this cell population? What is the mechanism underlying the process of cancer stem cell-involved tumorigenesis? In this review, we will discuss the development and trends in the field of cancer stem cell research, with emphasis on colon cancer stem cells. Since Wnt signaling is involved in both intestinal stem cells and colon cancers, we will first discuss the mechanisms of the Wnt signal transduction pathway, and then discuss the roles of Wnt signaling in normal intestine and in colon cancer. Finally, we will discuss the challenges and opportunities in colon cancer stem cell research.

Chapter V - The biology of stem cells and their properties have already been recognized as integral to tumour pathogenesis in several types of cancer. A role for stem cells has been demonstrated, so far, for the hematopoietic system diseases, as well as for several solid tumours such as breast, brain and lung cancer. There is a rising interest in the field of oncology in order to understand if cancer stem cells can play a key role also in the pathogenesis of head and neck tumours. It is likely that cancer stem cells are a minor population of tumour cells that possess the stem cell property of self-renewal. The evidence that the development of a tumour comes from a small number of cells with stem-like characteristic, could bring to the identification of therapies against these cellular targets, fundamental for maintenance and progression of the lesion. This new model for cancer will have significant implications for the way we will study and treat tumours.

Head and neck cancer is still the sixth most common cancer type worldwide. Disappointingly, despite significant advances in surgical and other treatments that enhance quality of life, survival rates have only moderately improved during the last 20 years.

Aim of this chapter is to discuss among this new model of cancerogenesis.

Chapter VI - Recent insights regarding the function of cancer stem cells are particularly intriguing when considered in the context of the metastatic cascade. As evidence for the direct involvement of cancer stem cells in initiating the growth of metastatic lesions is scant, this chapter will focus on known events in malignant transformation that are likely to involve or affect cancer stem cells, which may give rise to primary tumors of varying degrees of malignancy and metastatic potentials. The role of cancer stem cells in the later steps of the metastasis cascade will also be discussed. Finally, this chapter will explore potential characteristics vulnerabilities of cancer stem cells involved in metastasis, and speculate on how these weaknesses may be exploited to generate novel therapeutic and diagnostic approaches.

Chapter VII - Recent insights regarding the function of cancer stem cells are particularly intriguing when considered in the context of the metastatic cascade. As evidence for the direct involvement of cancer stem cells in initiating the growth of metastatic lesions is scant, this chapter will focus on known events in malignant transformation that are likely to involve or affect cancer stem cells, which may give rise to primary tumors of varying degrees of malignancy and metastatic potentials. The role of cancer stem cells in the later steps of the metastasis cascade will also be discussed. Finally, this chapter will explore potential characteristics vulnerabilities of cancer stem cells involved in metastasis, and speculate on how these weaknesses may be exploited to generate novel therapeutic and diagnostic approaches.

Chapter VIII - To examine the factors involving human carcinogenesis in order to design new strategies for prevention and treatment, a new approach from the current reductionalistic molecular oncological view will have to be made. In addition, this view must take into account both biological and cultural evolutionary factors that interact with the biology of the pathogenesis of cancer. An integrated hypothesist that links many incomplete hypotheses, such as the stem cell or de-differentiation theories of cancer, the multi-stage, multi-mechanism or "initiation/promotion/progression" theory, the mutation and epigenetic theories of carcinogenesis, and the "cancer stem cells" hypothesis, has been outlined. The emergence of somatic and germ-line stem cells during the biological evolution of the multi-cellular organism created new functions to regulate, homeostatically, phenotypes, such as growth control, differentiation, apoptosis, senescence and adaptive functions of terminally differentiated cells. The evidence supporting the stem cells as target cells for the initiation process was reviewed. The biological consequence of the initiation of an adult stem cell appears to be the inhibition of asymmetric cell division, or the blockage of "mortalization" of a normal "immortal" stem cell, not the "immortalization" of a normal, "mortal" cell. Promotion, functionally, is the clonal expansion of initiated stem cells by both mitogenesis and the inhibition of apoptosis. These promoting conditions occur during wound healing, compensatory hyperplasia after cell death, chronic inflammation, growth factors and by many dietary and environmental, non-mutagenic chemicals. All of these promoting conditions inhibit cell-cell communication, either by disruption of gap junctions in progenitor cells or by interfering with secreted negative growth regulator-receptor signalling in cells not having functional gap junctions, thereby releasing initiated stem cells from mitotic inhibition. Tumor promoters are characterized by threshold levels, exposing the initiated cells for regular and long periods of time in the absence of anti-promoters and having species, gender, cell-type specificities. The normal stem cell appears to give rise to the initiated stem cell which ultimately can accrue all the phenotypes of an invasive, metastatic "cancer stem cell". As the tumor grows, some of these cancer stem cells can partially differentiate to become cancer "non-stem cells". Finally, to understand how cultural evolution affects the human cancer patterns, domestication of certain animals helped to change dietary habits which can influence the carcinogenic process. These dietary factors can influence the adult stem cells, in utero and postnatally, so as to either increase or decrease the risk to cancer by altering the stem cell pools and by increasing or decreasing the promotion of the initiated stem cells. This might provide a mechanistic basis for the "Barker hypothesis".

In: Cancer Stem Cells
Editor: Melissa E. Jordan, pp. 1-30

ISBN: 978-1-61668-971-1
© 2010 Nova Science Publishers, Inc.

Chapter I

GENETIC AND EPIGENETIC ALTERATIONS THAT DRIVE LEUKEMIC STEM CELL SELF-RENEWAL

Vincent van den Boom[*], Sarah J. Horton[*] and Jan Jacob Schuringa[#]
University of Groningen, University Medical Center Groningen, Groningen,
The Netherlands.

ABSTRACT

Acute myeloid leukemia has emerged as a paradigm for the concept of the cancer stem cell. This hypothesis presumes that the disease is maintained by a rare population of leukemia-initiating stem cells which have acquired genetic or epigenetic changes. It is most likely that a single (epi)genetic event will not be sufficient to cause leukemia, but that a number of sequential events are required. Similar to normal hematopoietic stem cells, both intrinsic as well as extrinsic factors that arise from the bone marrow niche, provide essential cues that regulate cell fate decisions such as leukemic stem cell self-renewal and differentiation. In this chapter, we will review the genetic and epigenetic abnormalities that underlie the process of leukemic transformation, and will discuss which events potentially co-operate to induce leukemia.

INTRODUCTION

Acute myeloid leukemia (AML) arises from genetic defects in ·the hematopoietic stem cell (HSC). HSCs can undergo self-renewal divisions to ensure maintenance of the stem cell pool as well as generate large numbers of mature functional blood cells via migration, differentiation, proliferation and (anti-) apoptotic events. Complex processes such as self-

---

[*] These authors contributed equally.
[#] Correspondence concerning this article should be addressed to: Jan Jacob Schuringa, Tel: +31 50 3619391; Fax: +31 50 3614862; Email: j.schuringa@int.umcg.nl.

renewal and differentiation must be tightly controlled as a shift in the balance towards self-renewal severely impairs the hematopoietic process and might ultimately lead to the development of AML [1]. Thus a thorough understanding of the mechanisms involved in the regulation of self-renewal divisions of normal and leukemic stem cells are pivotal in tackling the highly malignant disorder of AML.

AML is in most cases a stem cell disease [2-4]. The malignant clone is hierarchically organized – strikingly similar to the normal hematopoietic system [5]- and consists of rare leukemic stem cells (LSC) that have the exclusive capacity to transfer disease into irradiated recipients. The more committed blast population within the leukemic clone lacks these properties. The most convincing evidence comes from transplantation studies in which the SCID leukemia-initiating cells (SL-IC) of all subtypes of AML, regardless of the heterogeneity in maturation characteristics of the leukemic blasts, resided exclusively in the immature $CD34^{+}/CD38^{-}$ compartment [2,4]. However, this finding was challenged recently by a study which demonstrated that most SL-ICs were present in the $CD34^{+}/CD38^{+}$ fraction of AML samples when the immune mediated clearance of anti-CD38 coated cells was prevented [6]. Thus a multipotent progenitor (MPP) rather than an HSC may serve as the cell of origin in some AMLs and this will be discussed in more detail in part I.

Leukemic transformation is regarded as a multistep process in which a number of sequential events ultimately induce the full spectrum of leukemia [7,8]. These transformation steps include chromosomal translocations such as t(8;21), inv(16) and t(15;17), as well as mutations in tyrosine kinase receptors (FLT3, C-KIT) or signal transduction molecules such as RAS, JAK2 and NPM1 (reviewed in [8,9]). Multiple events ultimately lead to enhanced self-renewal and differentiation defects of the LSC. A number of studies have indeed elegantly shown that oncogenes such as AML1-ETO and FLT3-ITDs do not result in leukemic transformation individually, but act synergistically when expressed within the same stem cell [7]. Furthermore, the fact that the incidence of AML increases with age (approximately half of AML patients are more than 65 years of age) further strengthens the notion that an accumulation of genetic and/or epigenetic alterations makes the stem cell compartment more prone to the development of AML. In this chapter we will review the current understanding of how genetic and epigenetic events might affect stem cell self-renewal properties and how these hits might collaborate in the process of leukemic transformation.

I. GENETIC ALTERATIONS IN LSCs THAT AFFECT SELF-RENEWAL AND/OR DIFFERENTIATION

Translocations

CBF Fusion Genes

The genes encoding the heterodimeric transcription factor complex AML1/CBFβ are among the most frequently mutated in human acute leukemia. CBFβ enhances the DNA binding capacity of AML1, whose target genes play critical roles in hematopoiesis. Conditional gene targeting studies in mice have demonstrated that while both subunits are essential for fetal HSC development, CBFβ but not AML1 is essential for the maintenance of adult HSCs [10]. The most common chromosomal rearrangements involving the *AML1/CBFβ* genes are the t(8;21)(q22;q22) translocation which generates the *AML1-ETO* fusion gene and inv(16)(p13q22) which generates the *CBFβ-MYH11* fusion gene. Various mouse models have been generated in an attempt to model disease induced by these fusion proteins. A myeloproliferative disorder resulted when AML1-ETO expression was targeted to the HSC compartment using the *SCA1* promoter (Table 1, [11]). However, other AML1-ETO models did not result in the development of AML unless the animals were treated with mutagenic agents [12].

Although AML1-ETO conditional knock-in mice did not develop AML, myeloid progenitors isolated from these mice displayed enhanced re-plating potential *in vitro* [13]. Furthermore, elevated numbers of HSCs and abnormal myeloid cells were observed in the bone marrow of mice transplanted with AML1-ETO retrovirally transduced murine HSCs [14]. Retroviral delivery of AML1-ETO to human $CD34^+$ cord blood cells resulted in HSC expansion in stromal co-culture assays and enhanced proliferation in cytokine driven liquid cultures. However, transplantation of these cultured cells into NOD/SCID mice did not result in leukemia [15-17]. Taken together these studies suggest that AML1-ETO expression promotes the self-renewal of HSCs but requires co-operating mutations to induce overt leukemia.

The mechanisms by which AML1-ETO promotes the self-renewal of HSCs remain unclear although up-regulation of survivin expression may be a contributing factor [18]. The finding that the *AML1-ETO* translocation can be detected in neonatal Guthrie card spots suggests that the translocation occurs *in utero* as the initiating event and results in the generation of a pre-leukemic clone. Secondary genetic or epigenetic events are then required for the development of clinically overt leukemia [19]. A recent report found that AML1-ETO expressing cells displayed an enhanced mutation rate *in vivo* and suggested that AML1-ETO may directly facilitate the acquisition of secondary events by suppressing endogenous DNA repair pathways [20].

In contrast to AML1-ETO, CBFβ-MYH11 conditional knock-in mice spontaneously developed AML in the absence of mutagen treatment [21]. Interestingly the genes *Plag1* or *Plag2*, which were previously shown to co-operate with CBFβ-MYH11 in AML development [22], were over-expressed in many of the AML samples in this conditional model. Retroviral over-expression of CBFβ-MYH11 increased the proliferative capacity of human $CD34^+$ CB cells but did not result in leukemia upon transplantation into NOD/SCID mice [23]. These studies suggest that like AML1-ETO, expression of CBFβ-MYH11 confers a pre-leukemic status to the cells by enhancing their self-renewal. Subsequent alterations which will be discussed later on are required for the transition to overt leukemia.

RARα Fusion Genes

The promyelocytic leukemia – retinoic acid receptor alpha (PML-RARα) fusion protein, which is expressed as a result of the t(15;17)(q22;q21) translocation, is found in > 95% of cases of acute promyelocytic leukemia (APL). Unlike other types of AML in which disease is thought to originate from an HSC, numerous studies suggest that APL arises from a committed progenitor. This theory is supported by the lack of PML-RARα expression in the HSC ($CD34^+CD38^-$) compartment isolated from APL patients [24] and the inability of these cells to transplant leukemia into NOD/SCID mice [2].

Table 1. Summary of the models for the most common genetic events in myeloid leukemia

	Translocations		
Gene	**Model**	**Phenotype**	**Ref.**
AML1-ETO	**Mouse** Transgenic-*Sca1*	Myeloproliferative disorder.	[11]
	Mouse Knock-in	Embryonic lethal. Abnormal myeloid cells in fetal liver with increased self-renewal potential.	[194]
	Mouse Conditional knock-in	Enhanced re-plating *in vitro*. AML upon ENU treatment.	[13]
	Mouse Retroviral transduction	Increased numbers of abnormal cells in the BM. No AML.	[14]
	Human (CD34$^+$ CB) Retroviral transduction	Long-term proliferation *in vitro*. No AML.	[15,17]
CBFβ-SMMHC	**Mouse** Knock-in	Embryonic lethal. Lack of definitive hematopoiesis.	[195]
	Mouse Knock-in chimera	Block in myeloid and lymphoid differentiation. AML after ENU treatment.	[196]
	Mouse Conditional knock-in	AML with median latency of 5 months.	[21]
	Human (CD34+ CB) Retroviral transduction	Increased proliferation *in vitro*. No leukemia.	[23]
PML-RARα	**Mouse** Transgenic- *hCathepsin G*	Myeloproliferative disorder, low frequency of APL with long latency.	[26,27]
	Mouse Transgenic-*hMRP8*	Low frequency of APL with long latency.	[25]
	Mouse Transgenic – *hCD11b*	Slight impairment in hematopoiesis. No leukemia.	[28]
	Mouse (lin$^-$ BM) Retroviral transduction	Short latency, high penetrance APL. Impaired neutrophil differentiation.	[30]
	Human (lin$^-$ PB) Retroviral transduction	Enhanced promyelocytic differentiation but subsequent block in vitro.	[29]
NUP98-Hoxa9	**Mouse** Transgenic - *hCathepsin G*	Myeloproliferative disorder, eventual progression to AML.	[197]
	Mouse (whole BM) Retroviral transduction	Myeloproliferative disorder, eventual progression to AML.	[35]
	Human (CD34$^+$ CB) Retroviral transduction	Increased proliferation and HSC self-renewal *in vitro* and *in vivo*.	[36]
MLL-AF9	**Mouse** Knock-in	AML within 6-9 months preceded by myeloproliferation. Small number of ALL cases.	[198,199]
	Mouse (cKit$^+$ BM) Retroviral transduction	Myeloid immortalisation *in vitro*, AML *in vivo*.	[42]
	Human (Lin$^-$ CB) Retroviral transduction	Enhanced proliferation *in vitro*. ALL upon transplantation into NOD/SCID mice.	[43]
	Human (CD34$^+$ CB) Retroviral transduction	Immortalisation *in vitro*. AML or ALL *in vivo*.	[44]
MLL-ENL	**Mouse** Translocator	Rapid AML within 4 months.	[48]
	Mouse (Lin$^-$ BM) Retroviral transduction	Myeloid immortalisation *in vitro*, AML *in vivo*.	[41]
Gene	**Model**	**Phenotype**	**Ref.**
BCR-ABL (p210)	**Human** (Lin$^-$ CB) Retroviral transduction	Enhanced proliferation in vitro. ALL in NOD/SCID mice.	[43]
	Mouse Transgenic - *metallothionein*	T, B or myeloid acute leukemia	[200,201]
	Mouse Transgenic - *Tec*	ALL in founder mice. CML in transgenic progeny.	[202]
	Mouse	Acute pre-B cell leukemia reversible upon	[203]

	Transgenic inducible (Tet-Off system)	tetracycline treatment.	
	Mouse Transgenic-*Sca1*	CML with longer latency (4-18 months). Progression to either myeloid or lymphoid blast crisis.	[59]
	Mouse (whole BM) Retroviral transduction	CML with short latency and high penetrance. T lymphoid lymphoma or CML in secondarys.	[56,57]
	Human (Lin⁻ CB) Retroviral transduction	Enhanced erythroid differentiation *in vitro*, myeloproliferative disease *in vivo*.	[58,204]
Point mutations / insertions			
CEBPα	**Mouse** N-terminal knock-in mutant (p42 deficient)	AML with complete penetrance. Latency 6 months – 1 year.	[74]
	Mouse Knock-in mutant chimeras	C-terminal mutant: Immature erythroid leukemia.	[75]
		N-terminal mutant: AML with shorter latency than C-terminal.	
		Combined mutants: AML with shorter latency than either mutant alone.	
	Mouse (Lin- BM) Retroviral transduction N-terminal mutant	Altered kinetics but no differentiation block *in vitro*.	[205]
	Human (CD34+ CB) Retroviral transduction N-terminal mutant	Block in differentiation at abnormal promyelocytic stage *in vitro*.	[205]
FLT3-ITD	**Mouse** Knock-in	Fatal myeloproliferative disorder. Median latency 10 months.	[82]
	Mouse (BM) Retroviral transduction	Lethal myeloproliferative disorder. Latency 40 – 60 days.	[81]
	Human (CD34⁺ CB) Retroviral transduction	Enhanced proliferation and self-renewal *in vitro*.	[83]
Flt3-TKD	**Mouse** (BM) Retroviral transduction	Lymphoid disease with long latency. T cell lymphoma or B-ALL.	[88]
cKit^V814	**Mouse** Transgenic – H-2L^d	ALL or lymphoma in 4/15 mice.	[89]
	Mouse (BM) Retroviral transduction.	Factor-independent growth *in vitro*. Lymphoid leukemia *in vivo*. Latency 6-19 weeks.	[89]
NPMc⁺	**Mouse** Transgenic – hMRP8	Non-fatal myeloproliferative disease from 6 months of age.	[93]
KRas^G12D	**Mouse** Conditional Knock-in	Fatal myeloproliferative disorder with complete penetrance.	[99]
	Mouse – Conditional knock-in. BM chimeras.	T cell malignancies and JMML depending on cell dosage used.	[103]
KRas^G12D	**Mouse** (BM) Retroviral transduction	CMML. Median latency 64 days.	[97]
NRas^G12D	**Mouse** (BM) Retroviral transduction	AML (latency 49.5 days) or CMML (latency 62.5 days).	[97]
NRAS^G13C	**Human** (CD34⁺ CB) Retroviral transduction	Enhanced myeloid proliferation and monocytic differentiation *in vitro* and *in vivo*.	[98]

Transgenic mice in which PML-RARα expression was driven from promoters expressed during the myeloid- promyelocytic stages of differentiation (*Cathepsin G* and *MRP8*), developed APL after long latency and low penetrance [25-27]. In contrast, mice in which PML-RARα expression was directed from a promoter expressed at a later stage of myeloid differentiation (*CD11b*), did not develop leukemia [28]. These studies highlight the importance of proper targeting of PML-RARα expression. The hMRP8-PML-RARα transgenic mice displayed a pre-leukemic phase which was associated with impaired neutrophil differentiation [25]. Impaired differentiation was also observed upon retroviral delivery of PML-RARα expression to both murine and human hematopoietic stem and progenitor cells (HSPCs) [29,30]. In contrast to the transgenic mice, the murine transduction/transplantation model gave rise to short latency APL with high penetrance. It is possible that retroviral insertional mutagenesis rapidly met the requirement for co-operating mutations in this model. Alternatively, the targeting of PML-RARα expression to more primitive hematopoietic progenitor cells rather than committed myeloid cells may explain the difference in penetrance and latencies.

The mechanism underlying the differentiation block induced by PML-RARα has been the subject of intense investigations. Both wild-type retinoic acid receptor (RARα) and PML-RARα mediate the transcriptional repression of retinoic acid (RA) target genes by binding the nuclear co-repressors NCOR and SMRT which recruit histone deacetylases (HDACs) – these are described in more detail in part II. During normal myeloid differentiation, physiological concentrations of retinoic acid (RA) induce the dissociation of the co-repressors and associated HDACs from RARα allowing the recruitment of transcriptional activators and normal myeloid differentiation. However, physiological concentrations of RA do not permit the dissociation of co-repressors and HDACs from the PML-RARα complex thus resulting in a block in differentiation [31]. This block is alleviated by higher concentrations of RA which is used in the clinic in combination with chemotherapy to achieve remission in the majority of patients.

Many AML cells exhibit enhanced survival upon genotoxic stress yet do not carry mutations of the *p53* tumour suppressor gene. In many cases the leukemic cells have acquired more subtle ways to inhibit p53 function. For example, the PML-RARα fusion protein retains the ability to interact with the product of the remaining wild-type *PML* allele which normally associates with p53. Recruitment of p53 to the PML-RARα/HDAC complex results in the inhibition of p53 acetylation and subsequent inactivation [32]. An alternative mechanism is proposed for AMLs with the t(8;21) translocation in which AML1-ETO has been shown to directly repress transcription of the p53 checkpoint mediator *p14ARF* [33].

NUP98 Fusion Genes

The *NUP98* gene undergoes reciprocal chromosomal translocations with many other partner genes and is hence one of the most promiscuous fusion partner genes in leukemia. *NUP98*-fusion genes are found in patients with AML, myelodysplastic syndrome, or blast crisis CML [34]. The *NUP98* nucleoporin gene encodes an important component of the nuclear pore complex. To date 21 fusion partners of NUP98 have been described of which the most common and extensively studied is NUP98-Hoxa9. Retroviral transduction of murine HSPCs with NUP98-HOXA9 enhanced the proliferation of myeloid progenitors *in vitro* and induced a myeloproliferative disorder *in vivo* which eventually progressed to AML. The latency of AML progression was markedly decreased upon co-expression of MEIS1 which also co-operates with wild-type HOXA9 to induce AML [35]. Retroviral transduction of human CD34[+] cells with NUP98-HOXA9 enhanced HSC proliferation and expansion *in vitro* and *in vivo*. Impaired neutrophil differentiation in response to G-CSF was also observed [36]. Gene expression profiling revealed that the Hox genes *Hoxa7*, *Hoxa9* and their co-factor *Meis1*, well recognized for their ability to induce AML in animal models [37], were up-regulated upon NUP98-HOXA9 expression in both murine and human models [36,38]. Several genes including *CEBPα* were also down-regulated upon NUP98-HOXA9 expression in human CD34[+] cells. Interestingly, restoration of *CEBPα* expression impaired the proliferation of NUP98-HOXA9 transduced cells suggesting that down-modulation of *CEBPα* expression by this fusion protein contributes to enhanced HSC proliferation and impaired differentiation [36]. A recent study using a transgenic Notch reporter mouse very elegantly demonstrated that NUP98-HOXA9 enhanced HSC self-renewal by increasing the number of HSCs undergoing symmetrical cell divisions. In contrast, the *BCR-ABL* fusion gene promoted proliferation but did not alter the ratio of symmetric versus asymmetric cell division [39].

MLL Fusion Genes

Like many of the genes involved in chromosomal translocations in acute leukemia, MLL plays an important role in normal hematopoietic development and is essential for definitive hematopoiesis [40]. Over 50 fusion partner genes of *MLL* have been identified so far of which the most common are *AF9*, *ENL* and *AF4*. Immortalized myeloid cell lines were efficiently generated following retroviral transduction of murine HSPCs with either MLL-ENL or MLL-AF9. Retrovirally transduced cells were able to induce AML with short latency and high penetrance upon transfer into mice [41,42]. Both fusion proteins were also able to enhance the proliferation of human cord blood cells and induce ALL upon transplantation into NOD/SCID mice [43]. However, the skew towards ALL in this model did not faithfully recapitulate the disease in humans. In patients the *MLL-ENL* fusion gene is found in both acute myeloid and lymphoid leukemia, while *MLL-AF9* is primarily associated with myeloid leukemia. Another study using human cord blood cells demonstrated that MLL-AF9 was able to give rise to either AML or ALL and this depended on the recipient strain of mice. AML was observed if the cells were transplanted into NOD/SCID-SGM3 (which are engineered to produce human SCF, GM-SCF and IL3) and ALL was observed if the mice were transplanted into NOD/SCID/β2m$^{-/-}$ mice [44]. These results suggest that the microenvironment plays an important role in the lineage of the leukemia.

Retroviral delivery of MLL-ENL to purified populations of murine HSCs, committed myeloid progenitors (CMPs) or granulocyte-macrophage progenitors (GMPs) followed by transplantation into recipient mice resulted in AML from all three populations [45]. This study demonstrated that MLL-fusions are able to impose self-renewal activity on committed progenitors which normally lack this ability. Using an MLL-AF9 retroviral transduction/transplantation model LSCs were identified which shared the same phenotype as the GMP from which they arose and expressed a self-renewal signature normally only observed in HSCs [46]. However, a recent study using MLL-AF9 'knock-in' mice in which MLL-AF9 expression was directed from the endogenous *MLL* promoter revealed that physiological levels of MLL-AF9 expression were not sufficient to transform GMPs [47].

The inter-chromosomal recombination model is perhaps the most elegant model to study the role of chromosomal translocations in leukemia. Gene targeting in mice was used to engineer *loxP* sites into the murine *MLL* and *ENL* loci. When these mice were crossed with *Lmo2-Cre* mice, the *de novo* translocation of *MLL* and *ENL* loci occurred specifically in hematopoietic cells and resulted in the generation of both reciprocal translocation products. The resultant MLL-ENL translocator mice developed AML rapidly within 4 months of birth suggesting that secondary alterations are not required in this model [48].

The models described above indicate that MLL-fusions promote the proliferation and self-renewal of hematopoietic progenitor cells. The mechanisms by which MLL-fusion proteins transform cells remain elusive although *HOX* genes and their associated co-factors play an important role. Multiple *HOXA* genes, the HOX co-factors *MEIS1* and *PBX3* and

FLT3 are up-regulated in patients with MLL translocations [49]. Several studies have shown that both wild-type MLL and MLL-fusion proteins directly regulate the expression of a subset of 5'*HoxA* genes [50-52]. Recent studies have shown that both HOXA9 and MEIS1 are required for the maintenance of immortalisation by MLL-fusion proteins and loss of expression of either gene induces growth arrest, apoptosis or differentiation of leukemic or immortalised cells [53-55].

BCR-ABL

The p210 BCR-ABL fusion protein is expressed as a result of the t(9;22)(q34;q11) chromosomal translocation. This translocation is found in the vast majority of CML patients and results in the generation of a constitutively active tyrosine kinase. Many murine retroviral transduction/transplantation models have been described which model the human disease with variable efficiency. Most of the studies demonstrated that BCR-ABL expression was sufficient to induce CML with a very short latency in recipient mice [56,57]. However, these studies were not very efficient at modeling the progression to myeloid blast crisis, which is eventually observed in CML patients if left untreated. Retroviral transduction of human Lin$^-$ cord blood cells with BCR-ABL resulted in enhanced erythroid differentiation *in vitro* and a low incidence of myeloproliferative disease upon transplantation into NOD/SCID/β2m$^{-/-}$ mice [58]. Targeting of BCR-ABL expression to the HSC compartment using the Sca1 promoter resulted in the most faithful model of CML so far although in this model BCR-ABL expression was limited to HSCs and was not expressed in more mature cells [59]. These mice developed CML with relatively long latency which progressed to either myeloid or lymphoid blast crisis. The CML cells from these mice displayed genomic instability as previously reported in CML patient samples [60]. Interestingly, the CML was reversible upon elimination of LSCs thus providing proof that elimination of LSCs is of therapeutic benefit [59].

It is assumed that transition to blast crisis is associated with the acquisition of secondary events. In support of this, activation of the Wnt signaling pathway through increased nuclear localization of β-catenin was observed in patients with accelerated phase and blast crisis CML. Furthermore, activation of the Wnt pathway endowed granulocyte-macrophage progenitors (GMPs) isolated from CML patients with self-renewal activity [61]. Although there are multiple lines of evidence to suggest that CML arises as a result of BCR-ABL expression in an HSC [62,63], this data suggests that during disease progression to blast crisis the LSC may evolve from an HSC to a GMP as a result of secondary genetic or epigenetic events. The study outlined previously by Wu et al showed that BCR-ABL acts to enhance proliferation rather than self-renewal of HSCs. Several studies showed that the Stat5 transcription factor is an important mediator of this effect [64-67]. In addition to STAT5, BCR-ABL is known to regulate several other signaling networks including RAS, ERK and CRKL [68]. In addition, RAC and Hedgehog signaling play an important part in leukemogenesis mediated by BCR-ABL. BCR-ABL hyper-activates RAC1 and RAC2 and both genes are required for BCR-ABL induced CML in mouse models [69]. Loss of Smoothened, an important component of the Hedgehog pathway also impairs CML induction by BCR-ABL [70].

Point Mutations/Insertions

CEBPα

AML patients without detectable chromosomal aberrations often harbor point mutations or insertions/deletions involving *CEBPα, FLT3, cKIT* or *NPM*. CEBPα is a transcription factor required for the CMP-GMP transition in normal hematopoiesis [71]. It is translated into two major polypeptides of 42 kDa (p42) and 30 kDa (p30) due to alternative translation initiation. Two major groups of *CEBPα* mutations are observed in AML; N-terminal and C-terminal mutations. Leukemic cells often possess mutations in both alleles of *CEBPα*; 1 allele harbors an N-terminal mutation and the other a C-terminal mutation [72]. Homozygous N- or C- terminal mutations are almost never observed in AML suggesting that there is selection for both types of mutation during leukemic progression. N-terminal mutations cause a frame shift leading to loss of the p42 isoform whereas C-terminal mutations involve insertions/deletions within the DNA binding domain of CEBPα [73]. The N-terminal mutation was very elegantly modeled by engineering the mouse *Cebp* locus to only express the p30 isoform. These mice uniformly developed AML within 1 year of birth. Interestingly, committed myeloid cells were capable of transferring disease to secondary recipients in this model implying that the CEBPα mutant confers self-renewal to this population [74]. The *Cebp* locus was also modified such that only the C-terminal CEBPα mutation was expressed. Since *CEBPα* mutations often result in embryonic lethality the combined effects of both N- and C-terminal mutations were studied in chimeric mice. Mice engrafted with fetal liver cells expressing only the C-terminal CEBPα mutation displayed an expansion of pre-malignant HSCs and developed leukemia which had an immature erythroid phenotype and a longer latency than chimeric mice expressing only the N-terminal mutation. Chimeric mice engrafted with cells expressing both N- and C-terminal mutations developed AML more rapidly than mice expressing either mutation alone suggesting that these mutations co-operate in AML progression [75]. Other mutations also result in the de-regulation of CEBPα function. The NUP98-HOXA9 and AML1-ETO fusion proteins down-regulate its expression [36,76]. Also PML-RARα can bind to CEBPα and prevent it from binding to its target gene promoters [77]. Therefore, alterations in CEBPα function may be a very common event in leukemogenesis and are thought to contribute to the differentiation block observed in AML.

FLT3 and cKIT

Mutations resulting in constitutive activation of receptor tyrosine kinases are frequently observed in AML. The FLT3 and cKIT receptors are normally activated by the ligands FLT3L and SCF respectively and are required for the survival, proliferation and normal differentiation of HSPCs [78,79]. *FLT3*-internal tandem duplications (ITDs) are frequently found in AML patients and are associated with a particularly poor prognosis. Point mutations in the tyrosine kinase domain (TKD) of *FLT3* are less common in AML. They are often observed in pediatric ALL patients with *MLL*-rearrangements and T-ALL [80]. Several models have provided insight into the role of these activated kinases in leukemia. Over-expression of FLT3-ITD in murine HSPCs resulted in a lethal myeloproliferative disorder when transplanted into mice [81]. The same outcome was observed when FLT3-ITD expression was directed from the endogenous *Flt3* promoter using a knock-in approach [82]. Retroviral delivery of FLT3-ITD to human CD34[+] cord blood cells resulted in enhanced progenitor self-renewal, proliferation and erythroid differentiation [83]. These effects were not observed upon over-expression of wild-type FLT3 in these models. This may be because FLT3-ITD, but not wild-type FLT3, is able to activate STAT5 [84] and several studies have demonstrated that this transcription factor is a critical mediator of FLT3-ITD activity. Co-expression of a dominant-negative STAT5 mutant in human cord blood cells abrogated FLT3-ITD-induced progenitor proliferation [83]. Furthermore, mice which expressed a mutated FLT3-ITD incapable of activating Stat5 failed to develop myeloproliferative disease (MPD) [85]. FLT3-ITD not only enhances proliferation but also survival of leukemic cells by up-regulating the expression of MCL1 and SURVIVIN [86,87].

Interestingly, FLT3-TKD mutants are much less effective at activating STAT5 and also display a distinct biology to FLT3-ITD mutants. Whereas mice expressing FLT3-ITD developed MPD, mice expressing FLT3-TKD developed lymphoid disorders (T cell lymphoma or B-ALL) instead [88]. A similar phenotype was observed upon over-expression of the cKIT^{V814} mutant in murine HSPCs. This mutant conferred growth factor independence to these cells and induced lymphoid leukemia with incomplete penetrance when transplanted into mice [89]. The lack of AML in these models suggests that by themselves these mutations are not sufficient to transform the myeloid lineage and require co-operating mutations to do so. This is consistent with the finding that *cKIT* mutations are frequently observed in AML patients expressing the *AML1-ETO* or *CBFβ-MYH11* fusion genes [90].

NPM

Mutations of the *Nucleophosmin1* gene (*NPM1*) occur in approximately 60% of AML cases with normal karyotype. NPM normally shuttles between the nucleus and the cytoplasm to fulfill its role in centrosome duplication and ribosome biogenesis. All NPM1 mutations lead to common alterations of the C-terminus, which result in exclusive cytoplasmic localization of the mutant (NPMc$^+$) protein [91]. Transformation assays have demonstrated that NPMc$^+$ behaves as an oncogene and antagonizes the tumor suppressor function of ARF [92]. Recently a transgenic mouse model was reported in which expression of NPMc$^+$ was directed from the human *MRP8* promoter. Although these mice developed a myeloproliferative disorder, they did not progress to AML [93].

RAS

Oncogenic *NRAS* and *KRAS* point mutations have been identified in myeloid and T cell disorders. Aberrant RAS signaling is particularly prevalent in juvenile myelomonocytic leukemia (JMML) [94]. RAS proteins are small GTPases which normally cycle between an active GTP-bound state and an inactive GDP-bound state. Activating *RAS* mutations prevent the hydrolysis of RAS-GTP and result in constitutive activation of the protein [95]. RAS proteins play a role in regulating multiple processes including proliferation, differentiation and survival [96]. Various models have successfully recapitulated the disorders associated with these mutations in humans. Murine HSPCs over-expressing KRAS^{G12D} or NRAS^{G12D} gave rise to CMML or AML upon transplantation into mice [97]. NRAS^{G12D} over-expression in human CD34$^+$ cord blood cells enhanced proliferation and monocytic differentiation but did not induce disease in NOD/SCID mice [98]. Conditional expression of the KRAS^{G12D} mutant from the endogenous *Ras* promoter resulted in a lethal myeloproliferative disease with complete penetrance [99,100]. The disease was found to originate from the HSC compartment in which elevated levels of pSTAT5, pERK and pS6 were induced by KRAS^{G12D} [101]. Due to possible non cell-autonomous effects in this model, bone marrow cells conditionally expressing KRAS^{G12D} from the endogenous promoter were used in competitive transplantation assays. Recipient mice developed T-cell leukemia, T cell lymphoma or a disease resembling JMML. Limiting dilution experiments revealed that the *Kras* mutation was insufficient for frank malignancy and co-operating events were acquired during the course of the experiment [102,103]. In addition to direct mutation of the *RAS* genes, the RAS signaling pathway is activated by a variety of other mechanisms including mutation of the *NF1* or *PTPN11* genes which regulate RAS-GTP levels but also by the BCR-ABL fusion protein [104] and mutant FLT3 [105].

II. EPIGENETIC ALTERATIONS IN LSCs THAT AFFECT SELF-RENEWAL AND/OR DIFFERENTIATION

Apart from genetic alterations acting as one of the steps in development of leukemia, epigenetic events have gained much interest for their role in leukemogenesis. The term epigenetics was coined by Sir Conrad Hall Waddington in 1942 but its definition in biology has been revisited and was recently described as: "an epigenetic trait is a stably heritable phenotype resulting from changes in a chromosome without alteration in the DNA sequence" [106,107]. This means that the phenotypical outcome of a genotype is not static, but can be modified by epigenetic processes. Epigenetic regulation of gene expression is regulated at the chromatin level. Microscopically, in interphase cell nuclei two types of chromatin can be observed: condensed chromatin (heterochromatin) and open chromatin (euchromatin). Heterochromatin is associated with silent genes whereas euchromatin contains mainly actively transcribed genes. The regulation of the chromatin structure is orchestrated at the level of the nucleosome, the structural unit of chromatin. A nucleosome is comprised of 146 bp DNA wrapped around a histone octamer, containing four different histones (H2A, H2B, H3 and H4) all present in duplicate. The amino-termini of the histones are unstructured and protrude from the nucleosomal core structure. These can be chemically altered by specific histone-modifying enzymes at various residues in several ways (acetylation, methylation, phosphorylation, ubiquitination etc.) [108]. Different modifications are involved in inducing either open or condensed chromatin. For example, acetylated histones are found in active chromatin and acetyl groups can be added to histones by histone acetyl transferases (HATs) and removed by histone deacetylases (HDACs). Histone methylation is present in both active and repressed chromatin, depending on the residue that is modified in the histone tail. DNA methylation is another well-known epigenetic modification which directly targets the genomic DNA. In mammals, cytosine residues in the context of CpG dinucleotides can be methylated by DNA methyltransferases (DNMTs). Methylation of CpG-dense regions (CpG islands, CGIs) in the promoters of genes causes repression of the transcriptional activity. Mechanistically, DNA methylation can act in two different ways. First, CpG methylation can interfere with the binding of activating transcription factors to CpG-containing sequences. Secondly, methylated CpGs can be targeted by methyl-CpG-binding proteins (i.e. MBDs), which can recruit HDACs resulting in deacetylation of genes that are targeted by DNA methylases [109,110]. In normal cells only a small fraction of the CGIs are methylated and the majority (~85%) are hypomethylated. In contrast, outside promoter regions and CGIs the genomic DNA is globally hypermethylated [111,112]. Data from multiple model organisms suggest a role for intra- and intergenic DNA methylation in maintenance of genome integrity, silencing of transposons and inhibition of cryptic transcription initiation.

Aberrant Epigenetic Regulation in AML

Given the fact that epigenetic regulation can induce a stable heritable gene expression profile in cells, a role for epigenetic events in generation and clonal expansion of cancer cells is very likely. Increasing knowledge about aberrant epigenetic activation of oncogenes and/or silencing of tumor suppressor genes underlines the importance of epigenetic events in tumor formation. Here we will discuss the role of abnormal epigenetic regulation in the process of leukemogenesis and more specifically in acute myeloid leukemia (AML). We will discuss important epigenetic pathways affected in AML and how this might contribute to development and progression of the disease.

DNA Methylation

DNA methylation was the first epigenetic modification found to be dramatically changed in cancer cells. Despite a reduction in global methylation levels in cancer cells, promoter-specific hypermethylation is observed. Together, this leads to unwanted transcription of repeats, activation of genes and abnormal silencing of tumor suppressor genes [113]. Inactivation of tumor suppressors is known to provide a major contribution to cancerous growth of cells and is suggested to take place in the initial steps of cancer development [114]. These tumor-suppressor genes are referred to as "epigenetic gatekeepers" and a classical example, which is commonly hypermethylated in various types of solid tumors, is the *p16INK4A* gene. Down-regulation of the p16INK4A transcript is known to result in increased self-renewal of stem cells and progenitors allowing more time for cells to develop secondary genetic abnormalities like mutations or translocations. In AML, *p16INK4A* hypermethylation is observed less frequently. In contrast, AML and myelodysplastic syndrome (MDS) patients often display hypermethylation of *p15INK4B*, a gene located directly upstream of *p16INK4A* in the genome [115-118]. p15INK4B is highly homologous to p16INK4A and most likely plays an important role in hematopoietic cell lineages. AML patients in clinical remission with a methylated *p15INK4B* show an increased risk of relapse and a significant reduction in survival [119]. Although *p15Ink4B$^{-/-}$* mouse models do not spontaneously develop myeloid leukemias, they do display extramedullary hematopoiesis and lymphoid hyperplasia in the spleen and reactive lymph nodes [120]. Furthermore, heterozygous deletion of *p15Ink4B* increases the frequency of retrovirus-induced myeloid leukemia in mice [121]. Apart from *p15INK4B* other frequently hypermethylated genes in AML include, among others, *CALCITONIN*, *E-CADHERIN*, *ER* and *MDR1*. Genome-wide analyses of DNA hypermethylation in AML patients at diagnosis and relapse showed an increase in DNA methylation at relapse, indicating that in myeloid malignancies DNA hypermethylation is not only involved in the initiation of disease but also during disease progression [122]. Very recently, genome-wide DNA methylation profiles of 344 AML patients were generated [123]. Clustering analysis identified 16 groups with distinct methylation profiles. Some of these groups correlated with known mutations (*CEBPα*) or translocations (*e.g. AML-ETO* and *PML-RARα*). Interestingly, 5 groups did not correlate with a specific genetic abnormality but did predict clinical outcome, underlining the biological and clinical relevance of these DNA methylation profiles in AML. Clinical intervention in aberrant DNA hypermethylation became possible with the approval of 5-azacytidine and 5-aza-2'-deoxycytidine (decitabine), which induce global hypomethylation. Decatibine treatment of MDS patients induces re-expression of the p15INK4B transcript and critically improved the survival of MDS patients [124,125].

Histone Acetylation

Histone acetylation is a chromatin mark associated with actively transcribed genes. Several lysine residues on the tails of histone H3 and H4 can be acetylated by histone acetyl transferases (HATs). The identified HATs can be categorized in three different families: GCN5/PCAF, MYST and p300/CBP. Within the MYST family, two members have been reported to be translocated in AML: MOZ (MYST3) and MORF (MYST4). Many different translocations producing *MOZ* fusions have been identified, including t(8;16)(p11;p13) [126] resulting in *MOZ-CBP* and t(8;22)(p11;q13) [127,128], inv(8)(p11;q13) [129,130] and t(8; 20)(p11;q13) [131] generating *MOZ-p300*, *MOZ-TIF2* and *MOZ-NcoA3* respectively. For the *MORF* gene only the t(10;16)(q22;p13) translocation has been identified which generates a *MORF-p300* fusion [132,133]. It is proposed that expression of these fusions leads to aberrant histone acetylation, thereby inducing leukemogenesis. Interestingly, HAT activity was dispensable for leukemic transformation by MOZ-TIF2 in mouse bone marrow transplants [134]. However, it was shown that MOZ-TIF2 expression leads to aberrant recruitment of CBP and p300 to target genes of nuclear receptors and p53 [135,136]. Gene targeting studies in mice revealed that MOZ is very important for maintenance of the HSC pool during early hematopoiesis and important for proper reconstitution of recipient mice in transplantation experiments [128,137]. Mice carrying a single point mutation in the HAT catalytic domain also display reduced numbers of HSCs and progenitors underlining the importance of HAT activity in normal hematopoiesis [138]. Gene expression analysis of AML patients with the *MOZ-CBP* t(8;16)(p11;p13) translocation showed increased expression of *HOXA9*, *HOXA10* and *MEIS1* [139]. Over-expression of these genes has been associated with leukemogenesis [37]. Up-regulation of *HOX* genes by MOZ-CBP does not reflect aberrant targeting of the fusion product since the wild-type MOZ protein is known to regulate *HOX* gene expression during development, but rather is a result of deregulation of HAT activity of the fusion protein [140-142].

Histone Methylation

Histone methylation is a chromatin modification that is found on both active and silent genes. Depending on the specific residue being methylated the mark poises activation or repression of a gene. A large group of highly conserved methyltransferases has been identified that target lysine or arginine residues on amino-termini of histone H3 and H4 [108]. The specificity of methyltransferases is much higher than that of histone acetyl transferases and in general they are specific for a single residue. In addition, residues can be either mono-, di- or tri-methylated, which cause different outcomes in terms of gene regulatory activity. In this chapter we will focus on two specific types of histone methylation, which are both involved in tumor formation and progression, despite their opposing activities in modulating gene activity.

H3K4 Methylation

A classical histone methyltransferase gene affected in leukemia is *Mixed Lineage Leukemia (MLL)*. A number of translocations generating *MLL* fusions have been introduced in this chapter already. The *MLL* gene was initially identified as a member of the Trithorax family of transcriptional activators in *Drosophila* [143]. The Su(var)3-9, Enhancer-of-zeste, Trithorax (SET) domain at the C-terminus of MLL possesses methyltransferase activity specific for lysine 4 on histone H3 (H3K4), a modification associated with transcriptional activation. Wild-type MLL resides in a multi-protein complex which regulates the maintenance, but not the initiation of *HOX* gene expression during early development [51,144]. Since *Mll* knockout mice are embryonic lethal, much attention has been directed to the role of *Mll* in fetal hematopoiesis. *Mll*$^{-/-}$ mice display defects in HSC maintenance and progenitor differentiation, which is at least in part dependent on correct expression of *Hox* genes, since re-expression of some *HOX* genes (*HOXA9*, *HOXA10* and *HOXB4*) can revert the progenitor phenotype [40,145,146]. Conditional *Mll*-null models revealed that MLL plays an important role in adult hematopoiesis since it is required to maintain the quiescence of the HSC pool [147,148].

Interestingly, MLL fusion proteins all lack a functional SET domain, since the part of the *MLL* gene encoding the SET domain is lost in the fusion gene [149]. However, they are still targeted to genes regulated by wild-type MLL and induce their aberrant activation. [50-52]. This activation is likely due to the fact that at least a set of MLL fusion proteins (*i.e.* MLL-ENL, MLL-AF4 and MLL-AF10) are capable of recruiting the non-SET domain containing histone methyltranferase DOT1L, which can methylate histone H3 at lysine 79 (H3K79), a modification associated with active transcription [150,151]. In addition, genome-wide analysis of MLL-AF4 induced histone modification patterns in a cell line model showed a dramatically changed chromatin interaction profile at target genes compared to wild-type MLL, which also likely contributes to aberrant gene expression [152]. The interaction between MLL fusions and DOT1L takes place via the ENL, AF4 or AF10 moiety of the fusion. This may imply that H3K79 methylation renders MLL target genes active (*e.g. HOX* genes), even in the absence of a functional MLL SET domain, thereby compensating for the loss of MLL H3K4 methyltransferase activity.

Although for a long time histone methylation was thought of as a stable epigenetic mark, the identification of a large family of histone demethylases showed that regulation of histone methylation is much more dynamic [153]. Recently, a translocation, t(11;21;12)(p15;p13;p13), was identified in AML patients generating a NUP98-JARID1A fusion, the latter being a H3K4 demethylase [154]. The fusion encodes the C-terminus of JARID1A, which contains a plant homeodomain (PHD) motif, which is known to 'read' the histone code and can bind di- and tri-methylated H3K4. Mice transplanted with retrovirally transduced lineage-negative bone marrow cells over-expressing the fusion protein quickly developed leukemia, which was dependent on the functionality of the PHD motif [155]. The authors show that NUP98-JARID1A prevents demethylation of H3K4 thereby interfering with down-regulation of transcription factors during lineage-commitment, including the *Hox* genes, *Meis1* and *Pbx1*. Taken together these data underline the importance of correct regulation of H3K4 methylation in prevention of leukemogenesis.

H3K27 Methylation

H3K4 methylation-dependent activation of transcription by the Trithorax family of transcriptional activators (including MLL) is counteracted by the Polycomb group family of transcriptional repressors, which were first identified in *Drosophila*, and are responsible for silencing the expression of many developmental genes [143,156]. The Polycomb group proteins are found in different multi-protein complexes, which together operate in initiating and maintaining silencing of their target genes. The complex believed to initiate Polycomb-mediated repression is the Polycomb repressive complex 2 (PRC2), consisting of the core components EZH2, EED, SUZ12 and RbAp46/48. EZH2 was found to be a SET-domain containing histone methyltransferase specific for lysine 27 on histone H3 (H3K27) [157]. Methylation of H3K27 is thought to be the initiating event in Polycomb silencing. PRC1, another Polycomb repressive complex consisting of RING1A/B, HPC, HPH, BMI1 and SCMH can recognize trimethylated H3K27 though the HPC protein [158]. PRC1 recruitment to promoters was shown to block chromatin remodeling and prevent initiation, but not binding, of RNA polymerase II [159,160]. The RING1 subunit of the PRC1 is capable of ubiquitinating lysine 119 at histone H2A (H2AK119) [161,162]. To what extent ubiquitination of H2AK119 is a key process in Polycomb-mediated silencing is not completely resolved. *Bmi1*$^{-/-}$ mice display loss of H2A ubiquitination at almost 700 gene promoters and leads to their increased expression (*i.e. Hox* genes), suggesting that H2A ubiquitination is important for Polycomb silencing [163,164]. Genome-wide localization analysis of PRC components have shown that not all Polycomb target genes are bound by both PRC1 and PRC2 complexes, indicating the existence of multiple modes of Polycomb-mediated repression [165-167].

Both the PRC1 and PRC2 complexes have been linked to tumor formation. A role for *EZH2* in cancer was suggested from work on both prostate and breast tumors showing over-expression of EZH2 correlates with a poor prognosis [168-170]. AML cell survival was shown to be significantly impaired when cells were treated with an EZH2 inhibitor, indicating that also in AML cells EZH2 plays an important role in disease progression. In addition, EZH2 over-expression prevents HSC exhaustion in a murine transplantation models, indicating that the protein is involved in dealing with replicative stress in HSPCs [171]. In the specific case of *PML-RARα* translocations, it was shown that EZH2 can be recruited by the fusion protein and represses its target genes, thereby contributing to the leukemogenic phenotype [172]

Another Polycomb group protein whose high expression correlates with poor prognosis in AML and other hematological diseases is BMI1 [173-175]. BMI1 was initially observed to be oncogenic in a retroviral integration site screen where it was identified as a collaborating hit in MMLV-induced B-cell lymphomas in Eµ-*myc* transgenic mice [176,177]. Knocking out the *Bmi1* gene results in reduced numbers of hematopoietic progenitors and more differentiated cells, eventually leading to hematopoietic failure [178]. More detailed analysis showed that BMI1 has a central regulatory role in self-renewal of HSCs by inducing symmetrical cell division both in mouse and human model systems [179-182]. Accordingly, *Bmi1*$^{-/-}$ mice display dramatically reduced HSC frequencies. BMI1 is also required for self-renewal of LSCs [181]. Over-expression of HOXA9 and MEIS1 in *Bmi1*$^{-/-}$ fetal liver cells and subsequent transplantation to irradiated recipients led to the development of AML. However, the leukemic cells could not repopulate secondary recipients suggesting that in the absence of Bmi1 the LSCs became exhausted. RNAi-mediated knockdown of BMI1 in both human cord blood and primary AML cells resulted in decreased self-renewal and led to induction of apoptosis [183]. Mechanistically, the role of BMI1 in regulating HSC self-renewal is partially explained by its ability to repress the *INK4A/ARF* locus [179,184]. Expression of p16INK4A and p19ARF in HSCs induces cell cycle arrest and p53-mediated cell death. Loss of BMI1 expression most likely results in a decreased H2AK119 ubiquitinating activity of the PRC1 complex at the *INK4A/ARF* locus, inducing expression of p16INK4A and p19ARF expression. Importantly, the hematopoietic phenotype of *Bmi1*$^{-/-}$ mice is not only dependent on the induction of *INK4A/ARF*. *Bmi1*$^{-/-}$ *Ink4A/Arf*$^{-/-}$ double knockout mice showed a partial recovery of hematopoietic cell counts but did not show a complete reversal of the Bmi1 null phenotype, suggesting that other pathways are also involved [185]. A candidate *INK4A/ARF*-independent pathway for BMI1 in controlling HSC and LSC self-renewal is regulation of reactive oxygen species (ROS) in the cell. Recently, it was shown that *Bmi1*$^{-/-}$ mice display impaired mitochondrial function due to increased expression of Polycomb target genes involved in ROS metabolism [186]. Long-term HSCs from *Bmi1*$^{-/-}$ mice showed increased levels of ROS and treatment of mice with the antioxidant N-acetylcysteine (NAC) resulted in a rescue of thymocyte cell numbers compared to non-treated *Bmi1*$^{-/-}$ mice. Furthermore, de-regulated ROS metabolism induced activation of the DNA damage response pathway. Knockout of *Chk2*, a component of the DNA damage response pathway, in a *Bmi*$^{-/-}$ background resulted in partial reversal of the thymocyte phenotype observed in *Bmi1*$^{-/-}$ mice. In addition, knockdown of BMI1 in human cord blood also induces increased ROS levels and apoptosis [183]. These data clearly show that apart from the well known role of BMI1 in regulating cell cycle and senescence through the *INK4A/ARF* locus, BMI1 is also implicated in other pathways regulating oxygen metabolism. It is clear that up-regulation of BMI1 in leukemic cells undoubtedly will give an advantage for these cells to cope with high oxygen levels. This is certainly advantageous for LSCs which are most likely not located in the oxygen-poor HSC niche and suffer from increased oxygen stress compared to normal HSCs.

III. MULTIPLE (EPI) GENETIC DEFECTS ARE REQUIRED FOR LEUKEMIC TRANSFORMATION

It is clear from the models summarized in part I that many if not all of the genetic events described are not sufficient to induce AML by themselves but require co-operating events to do so. The original two-step model of leukemogenesis was first proposed by Dash and Gilliland who postulated that two types of mutations (class I and class II) are required for the development of AML. Class I mutations are thought to confer a proliferative or survival advantage to the cell and class II mutations impair differentiation and enhance self-renewal. It has been generally considered that *FLT3*, *cKIT*, and *N-RAS* mutations are class I mutations and balanced translocations including *AML1/ETO*, *CBFB/MYH11*, *PML/RARA*, and *MLL* abnormalities are class II mutations [187]. This hypothesis has gained support from the findings that co-expression of various class I and class II mutations do indeed co-operate to induce leukemia in animal models. For example, the incidence of mice developing APL upon expression of PML-RARα was dramatically increased and the latency shortened following co-expression of FLT3-ITD or KRAS [188,189]. Furthermore, co-expression of FLT3-ITD and AML1-ETO, which individually are insufficient to cause disease, resulted in fatal acute leukemia [190]. These models are clinically relevant since the FLT3-ITD mutation is frequently found in patients harboring the t(8;21) or t(15;17) translocations. Activating cKIT mutations are frequently observed in patients with the t(8;21) or inv(16) translocations [90]. Consistent with this activated c-KIT co-operates with AML1-ETO to induce leukemia in a murine transduction/transplantation model [191]. The frequent co-existence of NPM1 and FLT3-ITD mutations in AML patients [192] suggests (according to the classical two-hit model) that NPM1 mutations block differentiation or enhance self-renewal.

However, as yet there is no evidence to support the idea that genetic mutations exclusively affect either the proliferation/survival (class I) or differentiation (class II). In fact, various genetic mutations often affect both of these pathways. Furthermore, many other cell biological properties of leukemic cells are frequently altered, including interactions with the bone marrow microenvironment, regulation of oxidative stress and DNA repair, and the process of self-renewal whereby the symmetry of stem cell divisions might be affected. Also, we hypothesize that leukemogenesis does not necessarily result as a consequence of two or more genetic events but may be mediated by a combination of genetic and epigenetic events.

Clearly, in some instances epigenetic changes can occur as a consequence of genetic abnormalities. Some epigenetic modifiers are directly targeted by a translocation (e.g. MLL, MOZ, JARID1A), which leads to aberrant epigenetic signaling. This could be due to either mis-targeting of a functional epigenetic modifier (including an active catalytic domain) or correct targeting of an inactive form which blocks other chromatin modifying enzymes or sequesters other epigenetic modifiers. A classical example of the latter situation is the MLL-AF9 translocation which leads to deregulated HOX gene expression due to aberrant targeting of DOT1L to its target genes [150,151]. Another example of translocations affecting the epigenetic state of genes are the PML-RARα and PLZF-RARα fusions, which are capable of recruiting the PRC2 and PRC1 complex respectively, leading to Polycomb-mediated silencing of their target genes [172,193].

On the other hand, epigenetic changes might be viewed as autonomous processes independent of genetic instability. Aging has dominant affects on the epigenetic landscape of hematopoietic stem cells, and myeloid leukemias arise particularly in elderly patients. Thus, it seems plausible that changes in epigenetic landscapes, for instance associated with aging, might contribute to the leukemic transformation process as well. The possibility to perform genome-wide analyses of epigenetic landscapes has set the stage for in depth analysis of epigenetic profiles in AML patients with known translocations or normal karyotypes. The recent publication by Figuero and colleagues is an example of how genome-wide analysis of DNA methylation levels in AML patients provides valuable information on the relation between DNA methylation and AML disease progression and how methylation profiles correlate with genetic hits [123]. Genome-wide DNA methylation analysis of 344 patients showed the existence of 16 distinct methylation profiles. A number of these profiles correlated with the presence of known translocations like CBFB-MYH11, AML1-ETO, PML-RARα or mutations in NPM1 or CEPBα. Surprisingly, 5 clusters were identified in a group of AMLs that did not share a common translocation or mutation. Most likely, AMLs clustered within these groups share unidentified mutations or deregulated expression of wild type epigenetic modifiers causing deregulated cell cycle control or a block in differentiation. A striking difference in clinical outcome was observed between these different groups, underlining the role of epigenetic regulation in disease progression and the importance of epigenetic analysis as a prognostic tool. The role of epigenetic analysis in survival prediction in AML was emphasized with the identification of a 15 gene methylation classifier which was predictive for clinical outcome in an independent patient cohort.

Most likely, in the near future more genome-wide epigenetic profiling studies on AML samples will be performed, leading to a better understanding of the contributing role of epigenetic hits in AML. As an example, genome-wide occupation analysis of over-expressed epigenetic modifiers like EZH2 and BMI1 and their associated epigenetic modification will be highly informative in elucidating the molecular mechanisms underlying the poor prognosis upon their over-expression. Identification of AML-specific target genes compared to normal hematopoietic cells will inevitably increase our knowledge of the role of epigenetic hits in the process of leukemogenesis, at what stage during disease progression they act and how they collaborate with genetic hits.

CONCLUSIONS

The generation of various genetic models using mouse or human cells has helped tremendously in gaining further insight into the process of leukemic transformation. From these models we have learned how genetic mutations might contribute to the development of hematological malignancies, but also that a single genetic alteration is most often not sufficient to induce overt leukemia. Besides genetic changes, epigenetic alterations, for instance as the consequence of aging, are likely to contribute as well. The challenge in the near future lies in establishing models in which these multiple hits are integrated in order to faithfully recapitulate leukemic development. These models will then provide excellent platforms to study molecular mechanisms involved in leukemic transformation and in which new drug entities can be tested.

REFERENCES

[1]   Passegue E, Jamieson CH, Ailles LE, Weissman IL. Normal and leukemic hematopoiesis: are leukemias a stem cell disorder or a reacquisition of stem cell characteristics? *Proc Natl Acad Sci U S A*. 2003;100 Suppl 111842-11849.

[2]   Bonnet D and Dick JE. Human acute myeloid leukemia is organized as a hierarchy that originates from a primitive hematopoietic cell. *Nat Med*. 1997;3(7):730-737.

[3]   Hope KJ, Jin L, Dick JE. Acute myeloid leukemia originates from a hierarchy of leukemic stem cell classes that differ in self-renewal capacity. *Nat Immunol*. 2004;5(7):738-743.

[4]   Lapidot T, Sirard C, Vormoor J, et al. A cell initiating human acute myeloid leukaemia after transplantation into SCID mice. *Nature*. 1994;367(6464):645-648.

[5]   Bhatia M, Wang JC, Kapp U, Bonnet D, Dick JE. Purification of primitive human hematopoietic cells capable of repopulating immune-deficient mice. *Proc Natl Acad Sci U S A*. 1997;94(10):5320-5325.

[6]   Taussig DC, Miraki-Moud F, Anjos-Afonso F, et al. Anti-CD38 antibody-mediated clearance of human repopulating cells masks the heterogeneity of leukemia-initiating cells. *Blood*. 2008;112(3):568-575.

[7]   Kelly LM and Gilliland DG. Genetics of myeloid leukemias. *Annu Rev Genomics Hum Genet*. 2002;3179-198.

[8]   Warner JK, Wang JC, Hope KJ, Jin L, Dick JE. Concepts of human leukemic development. *Oncogene*. 2004;23(43):7164-7177.

[9]   Jordan CT and Guzman ML. Mechanisms controlling pathogenesis and survival of leukemic stem cells. *Oncogene*. 2004;23(43):7178-7187.

[10]   Link KA, Chou FS, Mulloy JC. Core binding factor at the crossroads: determining the fate of the HSC. *J Cell Physiol*. 2010;222(1):50-56.

[11]   Fenske TS, Pengue G, Mathews V, et al. Stem cell expression of the AML1/ETO fusion protein induces a myeloproliferative disorder in mice. *Proc Natl Acad Sci U S A*. 2004;101(42):15184-15189.

[12]   Downing JR, Higuchi M, Lenny N, Yeoh AE. Alterations of the AML1 transcription factor in human leukemia. *Semin Cell Dev Biol*. 2000;11(5):347-360.

[13]   Higuchi M, O'Brien D, Kumaravelu P, Lenny N, Yeoh EJ, Downing JR. Expression of a conditional AML1-ETO oncogene bypasses embryonic lethality and establishes a murine model of human t(8;21) acute myeloid leukemia. *Cancer Cell*. 2002;1(1):63-74.

[14]   de Guzman CG, Warren AJ, Zhang Z, et al. Hematopoietic stem cell expansion and distinct myeloid developmental abnormalities in a murine model of the AML1-ETO translocation. *Mol Cell Biol*. 2002;22(15):5506-5517.

[15]   Basecke J, Schwieger M, Griesinger F, et al. AML1/ETO promotes the maintenance of early hematopoietic progenitors in NOD/SCID mice but does not abrogate their lineage specific differentiation. *Leuk Lymphoma*. 2005;46(2):265-272.

[16]   Mulloy JC, Cammenga J, MacKenzie KL, Berguido FJ, Moore MA, Nimer SD. The AML1-ETO fusion protein promotes the expansion of human hematopoietic stem cells. *Blood*. 2002;99(1):15-23.

[17]   Mulloy JC, Cammenga J, Berguido FJ, et al. Maintaining the self-renewal and differentiation potential of human CD34+ hematopoietic cells using a single genetic element. *Blood*. 2003;102(13):4369-4376.

[18]   Balkhi MY, Christopeit M, Chen Y, Geletu M, Behre G. AML1/ETO-induced survivin expression inhibits transcriptional regulation of myeloid differentiation. *Exp Hematol*. 2008;36(11):1449-1460.

[19]   Mori H, Colman SM, Xiao Z, et al. Chromosome translocations and covert leukemic clones are generated during normal fetal development. *Proc Natl Acad Sci U S A*. 2002;99(12):8242-8247.

[20]   Krejci O, Wunderlich M, Geiger H, et al. p53 signaling in response to increased DNA damage sensitizes AML1-ETO cells to stress-induced death. *Blood*. 2008;111(4):2190-2199.

[21]   Kuo YH, Landrette SF, Heilman SA, et al. Cbf beta-SMMHC induces distinct abnormal myeloid progenitors able to develop acute myeloid leukemia. *Cancer Cell*. 2006;9(1):57-68.

[22]   Landrette SF, Kuo YH, Hensen K, et al. Plag1 and Plagl2 are oncogenes that induce acute myeloid leukemia in cooperation with Cbfb-MYH11. *Blood*. 2005;105(7):2900-2907.

[23] Wunderlich M, Krejci O, Wei J, Mulloy JC. Human CD34+ cells expressing the inv(16) fusion protein exhibit a myelomonocytic phenotype with greatly enhanced proliferative ability. *Blood*. 2006;108(5):1690-1697.

[24] Turhan AG, Lemoine FM, Debert C, et al. Highly purified primitive hematopoietic stem cells are PML-RARA negative and generate nonclonal progenitors in acute promyelocytic leukemia. *Blood*. 1995;85(8):2154-2161.

[25] Brown D, Kogan S, Lagasse E, et al. A PMLRARalpha transgene initiates murine acute promyelocytic leukemia. *Proc Natl Acad Sci U S A*. 1997;94(6):2551-2556.

[26] Grisolano JL, Wesselschmidt RL, Pelicci PG, Ley TJ. Altered myeloid development and acute leukemia in transgenic mice expressing PML-RAR alpha under control of cathepsin G regulatory sequences. *Blood*. 1997;89(2):376-387.

[27] He LZ, Triboli C, Rivi R, et al. Acute leukemia with promyelocytic features in PML/RARalpha transgenic mice. *Proc Natl Acad Sci U S A*. 1997;94(10):5302-5307.

[28] Early E, Moore MA, Kakizuka A, et al. Transgenic expression of PML/RARalpha impairs myelopoiesis. *Proc Natl Acad Sci U S A*. 1996;93(15):7900-7904.

[29] Grignani F, Valtieri M, Gabbianelli M, et al. PML/RAR alpha fusion protein expression in normal human hematopoietic progenitors dictates myeloid commitment and the promyelocytic phenotype. *Blood*. 2000;96(4):1531-1537.

[30] Minucci S, Monestiroli S, Giavara S, et al. PML-RAR induces promyelocytic leukemias with high efficiency following retroviral gene transfer into purified murine hematopoietic progenitors. *Blood*. 2002;100(8):2989-2995.

[31] Minucci S, Nervi C, Lo Coco F, Pelicci PG. Histone deacetylases: a common molecular target for differentiation treatment of acute myeloid leukemias? *Oncogene*. 2001;20(24):3110-3115.

[32] Insinga A, Monestiroli S, Ronzoni S, et al. Impairment of p53 acetylation, stability and function by an oncogenic transcription factor. *EMBO J*. 2004;23(5):1144-1154.

[33] Linggi B, Muller-Tidow C, van de Locht L, et al. The t(8;21) fusion protein, AML1 ETO, specifically represses the transcription of the p14(ARF) tumor suppressor in acute myeloid leukemia. *Nat Med*. 2002;8(7):743-750.

[34] Moore MA, Chung KY, Plasilova M, et al. NUP98 dysregulation in myeloid leukemogenesis. *Ann N Y Acad Sci*. 2007;1106114-142.

[35] Kroon E, Thorsteinsdottir U, Mayotte N, Nakamura T, Sauvageau G. NUP98-HOXA9 expression in hemopoietic stem cells induces chronic and acute myeloid leukemias in mice. *EMBO J*. 2001;20(3):350-361.

[36] Chung KY, Morrone G, Schuringa JJ, et al. Enforced expression of NUP98-HOXA9 in human CD34(+) cells enhances stem cell proliferation. *Cancer Res*. 2006;66(24):11781-11791.

[37] Argiropoulos B and Humphries RK. Hox genes in hematopoiesis and leukemogenesis. *Oncogene*. 2007;26(47):6766-6776.

[38] Calvo KR, Sykes DB, Pasillas MP, Kamps MP. Nup98-HoxA9 immortalizes myeloid progenitors, enforces expression of Hoxa9, Hoxa7 and Meis1, and alters cytokine-specific responses in a manner similar to that induced by retroviral co-expression of Hoxa9 and Meis1. *Oncogene*. 2002;21(27):4247-4256.

[39] Wu M, Kwon HY, Rattis F, et al. Imaging hematopoietic precursor division in real time. *Cell Stem Cell*. 2007;1(5):541-554.

[40] Ernst P, Mabon M, Davidson AJ, Zon LI, Korsmeyer SJ. An Mll-dependent Hox program drives hematopoietic progenitor expansion. *Curr Biol.* 2004;14(22):2063-2069.

[41] Lavau C, Szilvassy SJ, Slany R, Cleary ML. Immortalization and leukemic transformation of a myelomonocytic precursor by retrovirally transduced HRX-ENL. *EMBO J.* 1997;16(14):4226-4237.

[42] Somervaille TC and Cleary ML. Identification and characterization of leukemia stem cells in murine MLL-AF9 acute myeloid leukemia. *Cancer Cell.* 2006;10(4):257-268.

[43] Barabe F, Kennedy JA, Hope KJ, Dick JE. Modeling the initiation and progression of human acute leukemia in mice. *Science.* 2007;316(5824):600-604.

[44] Wei J, Wunderlich M, Fox C, et al. Microenvironment determines lineage fate in a human model of MLL-AF9 leukemia. *Cancer Cell.* 2008;13(6):483-495.

[45] Cozzio A, Passegue E, Ayton PM, Karsunky H, Cleary ML, Weissman IL. Similar MLL-associated leukemias arising from self-renewing stem cells and short-lived myeloid progenitors. *Genes Dev.* 2003;17(24):3029-3035.

[46] Krivtsov AV, Twomey D, Feng Z, et al. Transformation from committed progenitor to leukaemia stem cell initiated by MLL-AF9. *Nature.* 2006;442(7104):818-822.

[47] Chen W, Kumar AR, Hudson WA, et al. Malignant transformation initiated by Mll-AF9: gene dosage and critical target cells. *Cancer Cell.* 2008;13(5):432-440.

[48] Forster A, Pannell R, Drynan LF, et al. Engineering de novo reciprocal chromosomal translocations associated with Mll to replicate primary events of human cancer. *Cancer Cell.* 2003;3(5):449-458.

[49] Kohlmann A, Schoch C, Dugas M, et al. New insights into MLL gene rearranged acute leukemias using gene expression profiling: shared pathways, lineage commitment, and partner genes. *Leukemia.* 2005;19(6):953-964.

[50] Horton SJ, Grier DG, McGonigle GJ, et al. Continuous MLL-ENL expression is necessary to establish a "Hox Code" and maintain immortalization of hematopoietic progenitor cells. *Cancer Res.* 2005;65(20):9245-9252.

[51] Milne TA, Briggs SD, Brock HW, et al. MLL targets SET domain methyltransferase activity to Hox gene promoters. *Mol Cell.* 2002;10(5):1107-1117.

[52] Milne TA, Martin ME, Brock HW, Slany RK, Hess JL. Leukemogenic MLL fusion proteins bind across a broad region of the Hox a9 locus, promoting transcription and multiple histone modifications. *Cancer Res.* 2005;65(24):11367-11374.

[53] Faber J, Krivtsov AV, Stubbs MC, et al. HOXA9 is required for survival in human MLL-rearranged acute leukemias. *Blood.* 2009;113(11):2375-2385.

[54] Kumar AR, Li Q, Hudson WA, et al. A role for MEIS1 in MLL-fusion gene leukemia. *Blood.* 2009;113(8):1756-1758.

[55] Wong P, Iwasaki M, Somervaille TC, So CW, Cleary ML. Meis1 is an essential and rate-limiting regulator of MLL leukemia stem cell potential. *Genes Dev.* 2007;21(21):2762-2774.

[56] Gishizky ML, Johnson-White J, Witte ON. Efficient transplantation of BCR-ABL-induced chronic myelogenous leukemia-like syndrome in mice. *Proc Natl Acad Sci U S A.* 1993;90(8):3755-3759.

[57] Pear WS, Miller JP, Xu L, et al. Efficient and rapid induction of a chronic myelogenous leukemia-like myeloproliferative disease in mice receiving P210 bcr/abl-transduced bone marrow. *Blood.* 1998;92(10):3780-3792.

[58] Chalandon Y, Jiang X, Christ O, et al. BCR-ABL-transduced human cord blood cells produce abnormal populations in immunodeficient mice. *Leukemia.* 2005;19(3):442-448.

[59] Perez-Caro M, Cobaleda C, Gonzalez-Herrero I, et al. Cancer induction by restriction of oncogene expression to the stem cell compartment. *EMBO J.* 2009;28(1):8-20.

[60] Melo JV and Barnes DJ. Chronic myeloid leukaemia as a model of disease evolution in human cancer. *Nat Rev Cancer.* 2007;7(6):441-453.

[61] Jamieson CH, Ailles LE, Dylla SJ, et al. Granulocyte-macrophage progenitors as candidate leukemic stem cells in blast-crisis CML. *N Engl J Med.* 2004;351(7):657-667.

[62] Fialkow PJ, Singer JW, Raskind WH, et al. Clonal development, stem-cell differentiation, and clinical remissions in acute nonlymphocytic leukemia. *N Engl J Med.* 1987;317(8):468-473.

[63] Takahashi N, Miura I, Saitoh K, Miura AB. Lineage involvement of stem cells bearing the philadelphia chromosome in chronic myeloid leukemia in the chronic phase as shown by a combination of fluorescence-activated cell sorting and fluorescence in situ hybridization. *Blood.* 1998;92(12):4758-4763.

[64] de Groot RP, Raaijmakers JA, Lammers JW, Jove R, Koenderman L. STAT5 activation by BCR-Abl contributes to transformation of K562 leukemia cells. *Blood.* 1999;94(3):1108-1112.

[65] Scherr M, Chaturvedi A, Battmer K, et al. Enhanced sensitivity to inhibition of SHP2, STAT5, and Gab2 expression in chronic myeloid leukemia (CML). *Blood.* 2006;107(8):3279-3287.

[66] Sillaber C, Gesbert F, Frank DA, Sattler M, Griffin JD. STAT5 activation contributes to growth and viability in Bcr/Abl-transformed cells. *Blood.* 2000;95(6):2118-2125.

[67] Ye D, Wolff N, Li L, Zhang S, Ilaria RL, Jr. STAT5 signaling is required for the efficient induction and maintenance of CML in mice. *Blood.* 2006;107(12):4917-4925.

[68] Ren R. Mechanisms of BCR-ABL in the pathogenesis of chronic myelogenous leukaemia. *Nat Rev Cancer.* 2005;5(3):172-183.

[69] Thomas EK, Cancelas JA, Chae HD, et al. Rac guanosine triphosphatases represent integrating molecular therapeutic targets for BCR-ABL-induced myeloproliferative disease. *Cancer Cell.* 2007;12(5):467-478.

[70] Zhao C, Chen A, Jamieson CH, et al. Hedgehog signalling is essential for maintenance of cancer stem cells in myeloid leukaemia. *Nature.* 2009;458(7239):776-779.

[71] Zhang P, Iwasaki-Arai J, Iwasaki H, et al. Enhancement of hematopoietic stem cell repopulating capacity and self-renewal in the absence of the transcription factor C/EBP alpha. *Immunity.* 2004;21(6):853-863.

[72] Barjesteh van Waalwijk van Doorn-Khosrovani, Erpelinck C, Meijer J, et al. Biallelic mutations in the CEBPA gene and low CEBPA expression levels as prognostic markers in intermediate-risk AML. *Hematol J.* 2003;4(1):31-40.

[73] Leroy H, Roumier C, Huyghe P, Biggio V, Fenaux P, Preudhomme C. CEBPA point mutations in hematological malignancies. *Leukemia.* 2005;19(3):329-334.

[74] Kirstetter P, Schuster MB, Bereshchenko O, et al. Modeling of C/EBPalpha mutant acute myeloid leukemia reveals a common expression signature of committed myeloid leukemia-initiating cells. *Cancer Cell.* 2008;13(4):299-310.

[75] Bereshchenko O, Mancini E, Moore S, et al. Hematopoietic stem cell expansion precedes the generation of committed myeloid leukemia-initiating cells in C/EBPalpha mutant AML. *Cancer Cell.* 2009;16(5):390-400.

[76] Pabst T, Mueller BU, Harakawa N, et al. AML1-ETO downregulates the granulocytic differentiation factor C/EBPalpha in t(8;21) myeloid leukemia. *Nat Med.* 2001;7(4):444-451.

[77] Tenen DG. Abnormalities of the CEBP alpha transcription factor: a major target in acute myeloid leukemia. *Leukemia.* 2001;15(4):688-689.

[78] Lennartsson J, Jelacic T, Linnekin D, Shivakrupa R. Normal and oncogenic forms of the receptor tyrosine kinase kit. *Stem Cells.* 2005;23(1):16-43.

[79] Mackarehtschian K, Hardin JD, Moore KA, Boast S, Goff SP, Lemischka IR. Targeted disruption of the flk2/flt3 gene leads to deficiencies in primitive hematopoietic progenitors. *Immunity.* 1995;3(1):147-161.

[80] Stirewalt DL and Radich JP. The role of FLT3 in haematopoietic malignancies. *Nat Rev Cancer.* 2003;3(9):650-665.

[81] Kelly LM, Liu Q, Kutok JL, Williams IR, Boulton CL, Gilliland DG. FLT3 internal tandem duplication mutations associated with human acute myeloid leukemias induce myeloproliferative disease in a murine bone marrow transplant model. *Blood.* 2002;99(1):310-318.

[82] Li L, Piloto O, Nguyen HB, et al. Knock-in of an internal tandem duplication mutation into murine FLT3 confers myeloproliferative disease in a mouse model. *Blood.* 2008;111(7):3849-3858.

[83] Chung KY, Morrone G, Schuringa JJ, Wong B, Dorn DC, Moore MA. Enforced expression of an Flt3 internal tandem duplication in human CD34+ cells confers properties of self-renewal and enhanced erythropoiesis. *Blood.* 2005;105(1):77-84.

[84] Mizuki M, Fenski R, Halfter H, et al. Flt3 mutations from patients with acute myeloid leukemia induce transformation of 32D cells mediated by the Ras and STAT5 pathways. *Blood.* 2000;96(12):3907-3914.

[85] Rocnik JL, Okabe R, Yu JC, et al. Roles of tyrosine 589 and 591 in STAT5 activation and transformation mediated by FLT3-ITD. *Blood.* 2006;108(4):1339-1345.

[86] Fukuda S, Singh P, Moh A, et al. Survivin mediates aberrant hematopoietic progenitor cell proliferation and acute leukemia in mice induced by internal tandem duplication of Flt3. *Blood.* 2009;114(2):394-403.

[87] Yoshimoto G, Miyamoto T, Jabbarzadeh-Tabrizi S, et al. FLT3-ITD up-regulates MCL-1 to promote survival of stem cells in acute myeloid leukemia via FLT3-ITD-specific STAT5 activation. *Blood.* 2009;114(24):5034-5043.

[88] Grundler R, Miething C, Thiede C, Peschel C, Duyster J. FLT3-ITD and tyrosine kinase domain mutants induce 2 distinct phenotypes in a murine bone marrow transplantation model. *Blood.* 2005;105(12):4792-4799.

[89] Kitayama H, Tsujimura T, Matsumura I, et al. Neoplastic transformation of normal hematopoietic cells by constitutively activating mutations of c-kit receptor tyrosine kinase. *Blood.* 1996;88(3):995-1004.

[90] Frohling S, Scholl C, Gilliland DG, Levine RL. Genetics of myeloid malignancies: pathogenetic and clinical implications. *J Clin Oncol.* 2005;23(26):6285-6295.

[91] Falini B, Nicoletti I, Bolli N, et al. Translocations and mutations involving the nucleophosmin (NPM1) gene in lymphomas and leukemias. *Haematologica.* 2007;92(4):519-532.

[92] Cheng K, Grisendi S, Clohessy JG, et al. The leukemia-associated cytoplasmic nucleophosmin mutant is an oncogene with paradoxical functions: Arf inactivation and induction of cellular senescence. *Oncogene.* 2007;26(53):7391-7400.

[93] Cheng K, Sportoletti P, Ito K, et al. The cytoplasmic NPM mutant induces myeloproliferation in a transgenic mouse model. *Blood.* 2009.

[94] Tartaglia M, Niemeyer CM, Fragale A, et al. Somatic mutations in PTPN11 in juvenile myelomonocytic leukemia, myelodysplastic syndromes and acute myeloid leukemia. *Nat Genet.* 2003;34(2):148-150.

[95] Bos JL, Rehmann H, Wittinghofer A. GEFs and GAPs: critical elements in the control of small G proteins. *Cell.* 2007;129(5):865-877.

[96] Boguski MS and McCormick F. Proteins regulating Ras and its relatives. *Nature.* 1993;366(6456):643-654.

[97] Parikh C, Subrahmanyam R, Ren R. Oncogenic NRAS, KRAS, and HRAS exhibit different leukemogenic potentials in mice. *Cancer Res.* 2007;67(15):7139-7146.

[98] Shen SW, Dolnikov A, Passioura T, et al. Mutant N-ras preferentially drives human CD34+ hematopoietic progenitor cells into myeloid differentiation and proliferation both in vitro and in the NOD/SCID mouse. *Exp Hematol.* 2004;32(9):852-860.

[99] Braun BS, Tuveson DA, Kong N, et al. Somatic activation of oncogenic Kras in hematopoietic cells initiates a rapidly fatal myeloproliferative disorder. *Proc Natl Acad Sci U S A.* 2004;101(2):597-602.

[100] Chan IT, Kutok JL, Williams IR, et al. Conditional expression of oncogenic K-ras from its endogenous promoter induces a myeloproliferative disease. *J Clin Invest.* 2004;113(4):528-538.

[101] Van Meter ME, Diaz-Flores E, Archard JA, et al. K-RasG12D expression induces hyperproliferation and aberrant signaling in primary hematopoietic stem/progenitor cells. *Blood.* 2007;109(9):3945-3952.

[102] Sabnis AJ, Cheung LS, Dail M, et al. Oncogenic Kras initiates leukemia in hematopoietic stem cells. *PLoS Biol.* 2009;7(3):e59.

[103] Zhang J, Wang J, Liu Y, et al. Oncogenic Kras-induced leukemogeneis: hematopoietic stem cells as the initial target and lineage-specific progenitors as the potential targets for final leukemic transformation. *Blood.* 2009;113(6):1304-1314.

[104] Alvarado Y and Giles FJ. Ras as a therapeutic target in hematologic malignancies. *Expert Opin Emerg Drugs.* 2007;12(2):271-284.

[105] Scholl C, Gilliland DG, Frohling S. Deregulation of signaling pathways in acute myeloid leukemia. *Semin Oncol.* 2008;35(4):336-345.

[106] Goldberg AD, Allis CD, Bernstein E. Epigenetics: a landscape takes shape. *Cell.* 2007;128(4):635-638.

[107] Berger SL, Kouzarides T, Shiekhattar R, Shilatifard A. An operational definition of epigenetics. *Genes Dev.* 2009;23(7):781-783.

[108] Kouzarides T. Chromatin modifications and their function. *Cell.* 2007;128(4):693-705.

[109] Bird A. DNA methylation patterns and epigenetic memory. *Genes Dev.* 2002;16(1):6-21.

[110] Jones PL, Veenstra GJ, Wade PA, et al. Methylated DNA and MeCP2 recruit histone deacetylase to repress transcription. *Nat Genet.* 1998;19(2):187-191.

[111] Suzuki MM and Bird A. DNA methylation landscapes: provocative insights from epigenomics. *Nat Rev Genet.* 2008;9(6):465-476.

[112] Weber M and Schubeler D. Genomic patterns of DNA methylation: targets and function of an epigenetic mark. *Curr Opin Cell Biol.* 2007;19(3):273-280.

[113] Ting AH, McGarvey KM, Baylin SB. The cancer epigenome--components and functional correlates. *Genes Dev.* 2006;20(23):3215-3231.

[114] Jones PA and Baylin SB. The epigenomics of cancer. *Cell.* 2007;128(4):683-692.

[115] Claus R and Lubbert M. Epigenetic targets in hematopoietic malignancies. *Oncogene.* 2003;22(42):6489-6496.

[116] Herman JG, Civin CI, Issa JP, Collector MI, Sharkis SJ, Baylin SB. Distinct patterns of inactivation of p15INK4B and p16INK4A characterize the major types of hematological malignancies. *Cancer Res.* 1997;57(5):837-841.

[117] Kim WY and Sharpless NE. The regulation of INK4/ARF in cancer and aging. *Cell.* 2006;127(2):265-275.

[118] Uchida T, Kinoshita T, Nagai H, et al. Hypermethylation of the p15INK4B gene in myelodysplastic syndromes. *Blood.* 1997;90(4):1403-1409.

[119] Agrawal S, Unterberg M, Koschmieder S, et al. DNA methylation of tumor suppressor genes in clinical remission predicts the relapse risk in acute myeloid leukemia. *Cancer Res.* 2007;67(3):1370-1377.

[120] Latres E, Malumbres M, Sotillo R, et al. Limited overlapping roles of P15(INK4b) and P18(INK4c) cell cycle inhibitors in proliferation and tumorigenesis. *EMBO J.* 2000;19(13):3496-3506.

[121] Wolff L, Garin MT, Koller R, et al. Hypermethylation of the Ink4b locus in murine myeloid leukemia and increased susceptibility to leukemia in p15(Ink4b)-deficient mice. *Oncogene.* 2003;22(58):9265-9274.

[122] Kroeger H, Jelinek J, Estecio MR, et al. Aberrant CpG island methylation in acute myeloid leukemia is accentuated at relapse. *Blood.* 2008;112(4):1366-1373.

[123] Figueroa ME, Lugthart S, Li Y, et al. DNA Methylation Signatures Identify Biologically Distinct Subtypes in Acute Myeloid Leukemia. *Cancer Cell.* 2010.

[124] Daskalakis M, Nguyen TT, Nguyen C, et al. Demethylation of a hypermethylated P15/INK4B gene in patients with myelodysplastic syndrome by 5-Aza-2'-deoxycytidine (decitabine) treatment. *Blood.* 2002;100(8):2957-2964.

[125] Garcia-Manero G. Demethylating agents in myeloid malignancies. *Curr Opin Oncol.* 2008;20(6):705-710.

[126] Borrow J, Stanton VP, Jr., Andresen JM, et al. The translocation t(8;16)(p11;p13) of acute myeloid leukaemia fuses a putative acetyltransferase to the CREB-binding protein. *Nat Genet.* 1996;14(1):33-41.

[127] Chaffanet M, Gressin L, Preudhomme C, Soenen-Cornu V, Birnbaum D, Pebusque MJ. MOZ is fused to p300 in an acute monocytic leukemia with t(8;22). *Genes Chromosomes Cancer.* 2000;28(2):138-144.

[128] Kitabayashi I, Aikawa Y, Yokoyama A, et al. Fusion of MOZ and p300 histone acetyltransferases in acute monocytic leukemia with a t(8;22)(p11;q13) chromosome translocation. *Leukemia.* 2001;15(1):89-94.

[129] Carapeti M, Aguiar RC, Goldman JM, Cross NC. A novel fusion between MOZ and the nuclear receptor coactivator TIF2 in acute myeloid leukemia. *Blood.* 1998;91(9):3127-3133.

[130] Liang J, Prouty L, Williams BJ, Dayton MA, Blanchard KL. Acute mixed lineage leukemia with an inv(8)(p11q13) resulting in fusion of the genes for MOZ and TIF2. *Blood.* 1998;92(6):2118-2122.

[131] Esteyries S, Perot C, Adelaide J, et al. NCOA3, a new fusion partner for MOZ/MYST3 in M5 acute myeloid leukemia. *Leukemia.* 2008;22(3):663-665.

[132] Kojima K, Kaneda K, Yoshida C, et al. A novel fusion variant of the MORF and CBP genes detected in therapy-related myelodysplastic syndrome with t(10;16)(q22;p13). *Br J Haematol.* 2003;120(2):271-273.

[133] Panagopoulos I, Fioretos T, Isaksson M, et al. Fusion of the MORF and CBP genes in acute myeloid leukemia with the t(10;16)(q22;p13). *Hum Mol Genet.* 2001;10(4):395-404.

[134] Deguchi K, Ayton PM, Carapeti M, et al. MOZ-TIF2-induced acute myeloid leukemia requires the MOZ nucleosome binding motif and TIF2-mediated recruitment of CBP. *Cancer Cell.* 2003;3(3):259-271.

[135] Collins HM, Kindle KB, Matsuda S, et al. MOZ-TIF2 alters cofactor recruitment and histone modification at the RARbeta2 promoter: differential effects of MOZ fusion proteins on CBP- and MOZ-dependent activators. *J Biol Chem.* 2006;281(25):17124-17133.

[136] Kindle KB, Troke PJ, Collins HM, et al. MOZ-TIF2 inhibits transcription by nuclear receptors and p53 by impairment of CBP function. *Mol Cell Biol.* 2005;25(3):988-1002.

[137] Thomas T, Corcoran LM, Gugasyan R, et al. Monocytic leukemia zinc finger protein is essential for the development of long-term reconstituting hematopoietic stem cells. *Genes Dev.* 2006;20(9):1175-1186.

[138] Perez-Campo FM, Borrow J, Kouskoff V, Lacaud G. The histone acetyl transferase activity of monocytic leukemia zinc finger is critical for the proliferation of hematopoietic precursors. *Blood.* 2009;113(20):4866-4874.

[139] Camos M, Esteve J, Jares P, et al. Gene expression profiling of acute myeloid leukemia with translocation t(8;16)(p11;p13) and MYST3-CREBBP rearrangement reveals a distinctive signature with a specific pattern of HOX gene expression. *Cancer Res.* 2006;66(14):6947-6954.

[140] Crump JG, Swartz ME, Eberhart JK, Kimmel CB. Moz-dependent Hox expression controls segment-specific fate maps of skeletal precursors in the face. *Development.* 2006;133(14):2661-2669.

[141] Miller CT, Maves L, Kimmel CB. moz regulates Hox expression and pharyngeal segmental identity in zebrafish. *Development.* 2004;131(10):2443-2461.

[142] Voss AK, Collin C, Dixon MP, Thomas T. Moz and retinoic acid coordinately regulate H3K9 acetylation, Hox gene expression, and segment identity. *Dev Cell.* 2009;17(5):674-686.

[143] Schuettengruber B, Chourrout D, Vervoort M, Leblanc B, Cavalli G. Genome regulation by polycomb and trithorax proteins. *Cell.* 2007;128(4):735-745.

[144] Nakamura T, Mori T, Tada S, et al. ALL-1 is a histone methyltransferase that assembles a supercomplex of proteins involved in transcriptional regulation. *Mol Cell.* 2002;10(5):1119-1128.

[145] Hess JL, Yu BD, Li B, Hanson R, Korsmeyer SJ. Defects in yolk sac hematopoiesis in Mll-null embryos. *Blood*. 1997;90(5):1799-1806.

[146] Ernst P, Fisher JK, Avery W, Wade S, Foy D, Korsmeyer SJ. Definitive hematopoiesis requires the mixed-lineage leukemia gene. *Dev Cell*. 2004;6(3):437-443.

[147] Jude CD, Climer L, Xu D, Artinger E, Fisher JK, Ernst P. Unique and independent roles for MLL in adult hematopoietic stem cells and progenitors. *Cell Stem Cell*. 2007;1(3):324-337.

[148] McMahon KA, Hiew SY, Hadjur S, et al. Mll has a critical role in fetal and adult hematopoietic stem cell self-renewal. *Cell Stem Cell*. 2007;1(3):338-345.

[149] Krivtsov AV and Armstrong SA. MLL translocations, histone modifications and leukaemia stem-cell development. *Nat Rev Cancer*. 2007;7(11):823-833.

[150] Krivtsov AV, Feng Z, Lemieux ME, et al. H3K79 methylation profiles define murine and human MLL-AF4 leukemias. *Cancer Cell*. 2008;14(5):355-368.

[151] Okada Y, Feng Q, Lin Y, et al. hDOT1L links histone methylation to leukemogenesis. *Cell*. 2005;121(2):167-178.

[152] Guenther MG, Lawton LN, Rozovskaia T, et al. Aberrant chromatin at genes encoding stem cell regulators in human mixed-lineage leukemia. *Genes Dev*. 2008;22(24):3403-3408.

[153] Shi Y and Whetstine JR. Dynamic regulation of histone lysine methylation by demethylases. *Mol Cell*. 2007;25(1):1-14.

[154] van Zutven LJ, Onen E, Velthuizen SC, et al. Identification of NUP98 abnormalities in acute leukemia: JARID1A (12p13) as a new partner gene. *Genes Chromosomes Cancer*. 2006;45(5):437-446.

[155] Wang GG, Song J, Wang Z, et al. Haematopoietic malignancies caused by dysregulation of a chromatin-binding PHD finger. *Nature*. 2009;459(7248):847-851.

[156] Schwartz YB and Pirrotta V. Polycomb silencing mechanisms and the management of genomic programmes. *Nat Rev Genet*. 2007;8(1):9-22.

[157] Cao R, Wang L, Wang H, et al. Role of histone H3 lysine 27 methylation in Polycomb-group silencing. *Science*. 2002;298(5595):1039-1043.

[158] Cao R and Zhang Y. The functions of E(Z)/EZH2-mediated methylation of lysine 27 in histone H3. *Curr Opin Genet Dev*. 2004;14(2):155-164.

[159] Dellino GI, Schwartz YB, Farkas G, McCabe D, Elgin SC, Pirrotta V. Polycomb silencing blocks transcription initiation. *Mol Cell*. 2004;13(6):887-893.

[160] Shao Z, Raible F, Mollaaghababa R, et al. Stabilization of chromatin structure by PRC1, a Polycomb complex. *Cell*. 1999;98(1):37-46.

[161] Wang H, Wang L, Erdjument-Bromage H, et al. Role of histone H2A ubiquitination in Polycomb silencing. *Nature*. 2004;431(7010):873-878.

[162] de NM, Mermoud JE, Wakao R, et al. Polycomb group proteins Ring1A/B link ubiquitylation of histone H2A to heritable gene silencing and X inactivation. *Dev Cell*. 2004;7(5):663-676.

[163] Cao R, Tsukada Y, Zhang Y. Role of Bmi-1 and Ring1A in H2A ubiquitylation and Hox gene silencing. *Mol Cell*. 2005;20(6):845-854.

[164] Kallin EM, Cao R, Jothi R, et al. Genome-wide uH2A localization analysis highlights Bmi1-dependent deposition of the mark at repressed genes. *PLoS Genet*. 2009;5(6):e1000506.

[165] Boyer LA, Plath K, Zeitlinger J, et al. Polycomb complexes repress developmental regulators in murine embryonic stem cells. *Nature*. 2006;441(7091):349-353.

[166] Lee TI, Jenner RG, Boyer LA, et al. Control of developmental regulators by Polycomb in human embryonic stem cells. *Cell*. 2006;125(2):301-313.

[167] Bracken AP, Dietrich N, Pasini D, Hansen KH, Helin K. Genome-wide mapping of Polycomb target genes unravels their roles in cell fate transitions. *Genes Dev*. 2006;20(9):1123-1136.

[168] Varambally S, Dhanasekaran SM, Zhou M, et al. The polycomb group protein EZH2 is involved in progression of prostate cancer. *Nature*. 2002;419(6907):624-629.

[169] Kleer CG, Cao Q, Varambally S, et al. EZH2 is a marker of aggressive breast cancer and promotes neoplastic transformation of breast epithelial cells. *Proc Natl Acad Sci U S A*. 2003;100(20):11606-11611.

[170] Bracken AP, Pasini D, Capra M, Prosperini E, Colli E, Helin K. EZH2 is downstream of the pRB-E2F pathway, essential for proliferation and amplified in cancer. *EMBO J*. 2003;22(20):5323-5335.

[171] Kamminga LM, Bystrykh LV, de BA, et al. The Polycomb group gene Ezh2 prevents hematopoietic stem cell exhaustion. *Blood*. 2006;107(5):2170-2179.

[172] Villa R, Pasini D, Gutierrez A, et al. Role of the polycomb repressive complex 2 in acute promyelocytic leukemia. *Cancer Cell*. 2007;11(6):513-525.

[173] Sawa M, Yamamoto K, Yokozawa T, et al. BMI-1 is highly expressed in M0-subtype acute myeloid leukemia. *Int J Hematol*. 2005;82(1):42-47.

[174] Bea S, Tort F, Pinyol M, et al. BMI-1 gene amplification and overexpression in hematological malignancies occur mainly in mantle cell lymphomas. *Cancer Res*. 2001;61(6):2409-2412.

[175] Chowdhury M, Mihara K, Yasunaga S, Ohtaki M, Takihara Y, Kimura A. Expression of Polycomb-group (PcG) protein BMI-1 predicts prognosis in patients with acute myeloid leukemia. *Leukemia*. 2007;21(5):1116-1122.

[176] Haupt Y, Alexander WS, Barri G, Klinken SP, Adams JM. Novel zinc finger gene implicated as myc collaborator by retrovirally accelerated lymphomagenesis in E mu-myc transgenic mice. *Cell*. 1991;65(5):753-763.

[177] van LM, Verbeek S, Scheijen B, Wientjens E, van der GH, Berns A. Identification of cooperating oncogenes in E mu-myc transgenic mice by provirus tagging. *Cell*. 1991;65(5):737-752.

[178] van der Lugt NM, Domen J, Linders K, et al. Posterior transformation, neurological abnormalities, and severe hematopoietic defects in mice with a targeted deletion of the bmi-1 proto-oncogene. *Genes Dev*. 1994;8(7):757-769.

[179] Park IK, Qian D, Kiel M, et al. Bmi-1 is required for maintenance of adult self-renewing haematopoietic stem cells. *Nature*. 2003;423(6937):302-305.

[180] Iwama A, Oguro H, Negishi M, et al. Enhanced self-renewal of hematopoietic stem cells mediated by the polycomb gene product Bmi-1. *Immunity*. 2004;21(6):843-851.

[181] Lessard J and Sauvageau G. Bmi-1 determines the proliferative capacity of normal and leukaemic stem cells. *Nature*. 2003;423(6937):255-260.

[182] Rizo A, Dontje B, Vellenga E, de HG, Schuringa JJ. Long-term maintenance of human hematopoietic stem/progenitor cells by expression of BMI1. *Blood*. 2008;111(5):2621-2630.

[183] Rizo A, Olthof S, Han L, Vellenga E, de HG, Schuringa JJ. Repression of BMI1 in normal and leukemic human CD34(+) cells impairs self-renewal and induces apoptosis. *Blood*. 2009;114(8):1498-1505.

[184] Jacobs JJ, Kieboom K, Marino S, DePinho RA, van LM. The oncogene and Polycomb-group gene bmi-1 regulates cell proliferation and senescence through the ink4a locus. *Nature*. 1999;397(6715):164-168.

[185] Bruggeman SW, Valk-Lingbeek ME, van der Stoop PP, et al. Ink4a and Arf differentially affect cell proliferation and neural stem cell self-renewal in Bmi1-deficient mice. *Genes Dev*. 2005;19(12):1438-1443.

[186] Liu J, Cao L, Chen J, et al. Bmi1 regulates mitochondrial function and the DNA damage response pathway. *Nature*. 2009;459(7245):387-392.

[187] Dash A and Gilliland DG. Molecular genetics of acute myeloid leukaemia. *Best Pract Res Clin Haematol*. 2001;14(1):49-64.

[188] Chan IT, Kutok JL, Williams IR, et al. Oncogenic K-ras cooperates with PML-RAR alpha to induce an acute promyelocytic leukemia-like disease. *Blood*. 2006;108(5):1708-1715.

[189] Kelly LM, Kutok JL, Williams IR, et al. PML/RARalpha and FLT3-ITD induce an APL-like disease in a mouse model. *Proc Natl Acad Sci U S A*. 2002;99(12):8283-8288.

[190] Schessl C, Rawat VP, Cusan M, et al. The AML1-ETO fusion gene and the FLT3 length mutation collaborate in inducing acute leukemia in mice. *J Clin Invest*. 2005;115(8):2159-2168.

[191] Zheng X, Oancea C, Henschler R, Ruthardt M. Cooperation between constitutively activated c-Kit signaling and leukemogenic transcription factors in the determination of the leukemic phenotype in murine hematopoietic stem cells. *Int J Oncol*. 2009;34(6):1521-1531.

[192] Suzuki T, Kiyoi H, Ozeki K, et al. Clinical characteristics and prognostic implications of NPM1 mutations in acute myeloid leukemia. *Blood*. 2005;106(8):2854-2861.

[193] Boukarabila H, Saurin AJ, Batsche E, et al. The PRC1 Polycomb group complex interacts with PLZF/RARA to mediate leukemic transformation. *Genes Dev*. 2009;23(10):1195-1206.

[194] Yergeau DA, Hetherington CJ, Wang Q, et al. Embryonic lethality and impairment of haematopoiesis in mice heterozygous for an AML1-ETO fusion gene. *Nat Genet*. 1997;15(3):303-306.

[195] Castilla LH, Wijmenga C, Wang Q, et al. Failure of embryonic hematopoiesis and lethal hemorrhages in mouse embryos heterozygous for a knocked-in leukemia gene CBFB-MYH11. *Cell*. 1996;87(4):687-696.

[196] Castilla LH, Garrett L, Adya N, et al. The fusion gene Cbfb-MYH11 blocks myeloid differentiation and predisposes mice to acute myelomonocytic leukaemia. *Nat Genet*. 1999;23(2):144-146.

[197] Iwasaki M, Kuwata T, Yamazaki Y, et al. Identification of cooperative genes for NUP98-HOXA9 in myeloid leukemogenesis using a mouse model. *Blood*. 2005;105(2):784-793.

[198] Corral J, Lavenir I, Impey H, et al. An Mll-AF9 fusion gene made by homologous recombination causes acute leukemia in chimeric mice: a method to create fusion oncogenes. *Cell*. 1996;85(6):853-861.

[199] Dobson CL, Warren AJ, Pannell R, et al. The mll-AF9 gene fusion in mice controls myeloproliferation and specifies acute myeloid leukaemogenesis. *EMBO J.* 1999;18(13):3564-3574.

[200] Honda H, Fujii T, Takatoku M, et al. Expression of p210bcr/abl by metallothionein promoter induced T-cell leukemia in transgenic mice. *Blood.* 1995;85(10):2853-2861.

[201] Voncken JW, Kaartinen V, Pattengale PK, Germeraad WT, Groffen J, Heisterkamp N. BCR/ABL P210 and P190 cause distinct leukemia in transgenic mice. *Blood.* 1995;86(12):4603-4611.

[202] Honda H, Oda H, Suzuki T, et al. Development of acute lymphoblastic leukemia and myeloproliferative disorder in transgenic mice expressing p210bcr/abl: a novel transgenic model for human Ph1-positive leukemias. *Blood.* 1998;91(6):2067-2075.

[203] Huettner CS, Zhang P, Van Etten RA, Tenen DG. Reversibility of acute B-cell leukaemia induced by BCR-ABL1. *Nat Genet.* 2000;24(1):57-60.

[204] Chalandon Y, Jiang X, Hazlewood G, et al. Modulation of p210(BCR-ABL) activity in transduced primary human hematopoietic cells controls lineage programming. *Blood.* 2002;99(9):3197-3204.

[205] Schwieger M, Lohler J, Fischer M, Herwig U, Tenen DG, Stocking C. A dominant-negative mutant of C/EBPalpha, associated with acute myeloid leukemias, inhibits differentiation of myeloid and erythroid progenitors of man but not mouse. *Blood.* 2004;103(7):2744-2752.

In: Cancer Stem Cells
Editor: Melissa E. Jordan, pp. 31-61

ISBN: 978-1-61668-971-1
© 2010 Nova Science Publishers, Inc.

Chapter II

CANCER STEM CELLS IN LUNG CANCER: DISTINCT DIFFERENCES BETWEEN SMALL CELL LUNG CARCINOMA AND NON-SMALL CELL LUNG CARCINOMA

Koji Okudela[1], Noriyuki Nagahara[2], Akira Katayama[2] and Hitoshi Kitamura[1,*]

[1]Graduate School of Medicine, Yokohama City University, Yokohama, Japan[
[2]Graduate School of Medicine, Nippon Medical School, Tokyo, Japan.

ABSTRACT

Of the many markers for cancer stem cells (CSCs) in lung cancer reported to date, the cell surface antigen CD133, nuclear β-catenin accumulation, the side population phenotype, and high aldehyde dehydrogenase (ALDH) activity seem to be most reliable. In this chapter, we review the results of studies on lung CSCs and discuss the significance of these markers from a biological, pathological, and clinical viewpoint. In addition, we present our own data, focusing primarily upon ALDH1A1. Twenty-seven lung cancer cell lines (nine small cell lung carcinoma (SCLC) cell lines and eighteen non-small cell lung carcinoma (NSCLC) cell lines) were examined for mRNA and protein expression and fractions of cells with activity. ALDH1A1 mRNA was strongly expressed in five cell lines, of which three were SCLC cell lines and two were NSCLC cell lines. Two of the SCLC cell lines consistently expressed the protein and had a large fraction of cells with ALDH activity, but the third did not. Both the NSCLC cell lines expressed the protein, but only one had a large fraction of cells with strong ALDH activity. In brief, the level of ALDH1A1 mRNA did not always parallel that of the protein in SCLC cell lines, while the level of ALDH1A1 protein did not necessarily parallel that of ALDH activity in

---

* Correspondence concerning this article should be addressed to: Dr. Hitoshi Kitamura, M.D., Ph.D. Department of Pathology, Graduate School of Medicine, Yokohama City University, 3-9 Fukuura, Kanazawa-ku, Yokohama 236-0004, Japan. (Tel: +81-45-787-2583; Fax: +81-45-789-0588; E-mail address: pathola@med.yokohama-cu.ac.jp)

NSCLC cell lines. The ALDH1A1 protein level or ALDH activity level was well associated with the mRNA level of CD133, which is the most commonly used marker for CSCs, in SCLC cell lines, but not in NSCLC cell lines, suggesting an abundance of CSC populations in SCLC compared to in NSCLC. From the current findings, the mechanism and pathway that regulate the expression of ALDH1A1 mRNA and its protein, and its enzymatic activity as well differ greatly between SCLC and NSCLC cells. We speculate that ALDH (its expression and activity) is only one of the factors determining the stemness of CSCs in lung cancers. In conclusion, the CSCs in SCLC and NSCLC differ distinctly in terms not only of their abundance but also of the regulatory mechanism of ALDH1A1 expression and activity, as well as its role in the maintenance/activation of stemness. Exploring the mechanism of ALDH's activation and its role in the maintenance of the stemness not only of CSCs but also of normal stem cells would provide a novel paradigm for stem cell biology.

Keywords: Cancer stem cell; Small cell lung carcinoma; Non-small cell lung carcinoma; Aldehyde dehydrogenase.

ABBREVIATIONS

SCLC: small cell lung carcinoma;
NSCLC: non-small cell lung carcinoma;
SQC: squamous cell carcinoma;
DC: adenocarcinoma;
LCC: large cell carcinoma;
RB: retinoblastoma;
TP53: tumor protein 53;
EGFR: epidermal growth factor receptor;
ASCL1: achaete-scute complex homolog 1;
TTF-1: thyroid transcription factor-1;
ALDH: aldehyde dehydrogenase;
CSC: cancer stem cell;
ABCG2, ATP binding cassette transporter superfamily member G2;
CIC: cancer initiating cell;
SP: side population;
FACS: fluorescence activating cell sorting;
UV: ultraviolet;
uPAR: urokinase plasminogen activator receptor;
uPA: urokinase plasminogen activator;
Shh: Sonic hedgehog;
BMP: bone morphogenetic protein;
Bmi1: B cell-specific Mo-MuLV integration site 1;
PODXL-1: podocalyxin-like protein 1;
RT-PCR: reverse transcription polymerase chain reaction;
mRNA, messenger ribonucleic acid: cDNA;
complementary deoxyribonucleic acid;
siRNA: small interfering RNA;
PI: propidium iodide.

INTRODUCTION

Lung cancer is one of the most common malignancies worldwide and a leading cause of cancer-related deaths. It is increasing year by year in almost all areas of the world, except for a slight decrease in certain countries [1]. Lung cancer consists of heterogeneous groups in terms of pathological features and is commonly classified into the following two major types, small cell lung carcinoma (SCLC) and non-small cell lung carcinoma (NSCLC). NSCLC also is a group of heterogeneous histological types, the majority of which are squamous cell carcinoma (SQC) and adenocarcinoma (ADC) with roughly similar frequencies (30-40% each), and large cell carcinoma (LCC) with a lower frequency (< 10%). SCLC comprises nearly 20% of lung cancer. ADC and LCC are further sub-classified into several categories, respectively. The classification of lung cancer is not only of academic interest but also of practical necessity, because the biological aggressiveness, responsiveness to therapeutic intervention and patients' prognosis are greatly different among the respective types [2].

Lung cancer originates from the airway epithelia of larger and smaller bronchi as well as of alveoli. While it is generally accepted that cancer cells are derived from progenitor or tissue stem cells, relatively little has been elucidated with regard to the identification of airway stem cells and the molecular mechanisms underlying their self-renewal and differentiation abilities [3-5], in contrast to other epithelial tissues such as the intestine, mammary gland, and skin [6].

The heterogeneity of lung cancer likely reflects differences in the site of origin (proximal versus peripheral), and, more importantly, in the type of cell of origin, i.e., progenitor (tissue stem) cells. The diversity of etiologic factors and target genes, the types of genetic insults, and the ensuing effects, activation or inactivation, on the genes involved, would also be responsible for the heterogeneity of lung cancer. In fact, tobacco smoke, containing more than 60 carcinogens, is generally accepted as the most important cause of almost all types of lung cancer, among which the genetic and molecular mechanisms of carcinogenesis differ considerably. The ensuing genetic alteration and epigenetic changes as well, could lead to dysfunction of molecular signal transduction pathways, which relate directly or indirectly to proliferation, differentiation, and death of the cell.

In our recent review article, we underscored that silencing alterations of both the *RB* and *TP53* genes are most likely to be important and early events in the development of SCLC, whereas alterations of the epidermal growth factor receptor (EGFR) signaling pathway play significant and important roles in NSCLC carcinogenesis [7]. We also emphasized that alterations of both the *RB* and *TP53* genes are central to the carcinogenesis of SCLC, while many other factors including achaete-scute complex homolog 1 (ASCL1) and thyroid transcription factor-1 (TTF-1) contribute to the development and biological behavior of SCLC [8].

The cancer stem cell (CSC) theory has proposed that a tumor cell subpopulation possessing self-renewal capacity which forms only a small fraction of tumor tissue is central in sustaining neoplastic lesions and is a potentially crucial target of cancer therapy [9-23]. The CSCs are possibly produced by either transformation of normal stem cells or multistep dedifferentiation of specialized progenitor cells through a progressive accumulation of genetic aberrations. Rapp, *et al.* [12] proposed a model of oncogene-induced plasticity for CSC origin by demonstrating reprogramming events triggered by a specific combination of oncogenes.

Li, *et al.* [16] suggested that genomic instability is a driving force for transforming normal stem cells into CSCs and, in CSCs, a potential mechanism for cancer cell heterogeneity. The origin of CSCs and this mechanism are discussed in more detail in other chapters [The publisher may modify this part].

The CSCs of lung cancers can be considered to originate from either airway stem cells, which have not been identified yet, or respective committed progenitor cells, such as bronchioloalveolar progenitor cells, basal/mucous secretory bronchial progenitor cells, and neuroendocrine progenitor cells (see the section Origin of CSCs in lung cancer).

The CSC theory is tremendously attractive to both researchers and physicians, because the CSC is central to cancer cell biology and cancer therapy. The discovery of specific markers of CSCs in the respective types of cancers is particularly important. Furthermore, it is necessary to clarify the function of these molecules, as the disruption of the signaling pathways and gene transcriptions that control the activity of CSCs is the final goal of CSC-targeting therapy. We emphasized that a knowledge of CSC signaling pathways may lead to new treatment that kill or induce differentiation of CSCs and could better contribute to cures [24]. These treatments could be designed to target CSCs in order to induce the differentiation of CSCs, or eliminate CSCs by inhibiting the maintenance of the stem-cell state. For instance, side population (SP) cells that are considered to represent CSCs (see below), of a human lung cancer cell line (A549) totally disappeared after treatment with the selective ATP-binding cassette transporter G2 (ABCG2) inhibitor fumitremorgin C [25]. As another example, a Hedgehog signaling inhibitor cyclopamine strikingly reduced the *in vitro* invasive capacity of pancreatic cancer cell lines and also profoundly inhibited metastatic spread in an orthotopic xenograft model [26].

In regard to lung cancer, we also stressed the extreme importance of identifying specific CSC markers for the respective subtypes of lung cancer, for instance SCLC and NSCLC (ADC, SQC, LCC, and others), since they are quite different not only in phenotype but also in pathogenesis and biological behavior. In particular, SCLC is highly metastatic, drug-resistant, and rapidly fatal. The aggressiveness of SCLC may be attributable to an abundance of CSCs, as CSCs are drug-resistant and play a crucial role in cancer recurrence and metastasis. Alternatively, it is also possible that the CSCs of SCLC are endowed with specific biological properties, for instance niche-independency or strong drug-resistance, or both. If SCLC-specific CSC markers were discovered, they would be extremely useful as targets of chemotherapy, for the establishment of therapeutic regimens, and for predictions of the prognosis (outcome) of patients.

In this chapter, we discuss the characteristics of normal airway stem/progenitor cells and CSCs in lung cancer by reviewing hitherto described study results. In addition, we demonstrate the potentially distinct differences in the mechanism of maintenance of CSCs between SCLC and NSCLC, primarily focusing upon aldehyde dehydrogenase (ALDH) based on our own experiments currently underway.

Stem Cells in Healthy and Injured Lungs

Although the airway stem cell in a strict sense has not been identified yet, several lines of evidence support the existence of regional progenitors cells, such as bronchioloalveolar progenitor cells, basal/mucous secretory bronchial progenitor cells, and neuroendocrine progenitor cells, which maintain normal homeostasis as well as play roles in repair [3-5]. These progenitor cells expand their populations in response to various insults including toxic substances, but do not become tumorigenic unless at least one genetic or epigenetic event occurs, for instance by tobacco smoke carcinogens [4,27].

Table 1. Cancer stem cell markers in small cell lung carcinoma and non-small cell lung carcinoma

Category	Molecule	SCLC	NSCLC
Cell surface marker	CD133	1. Eramo A, *et al.* [42] Cancer cells isolated from surgical specimens 2. Jiang T, *et al.* [52] H1688 cell line 3. Meng X, *et al.* [48] *H446 cell line	1. Eramo A, *et al.* [42] Cancer cells isolated from surgical specimens 2. Jiang T, *et al.* [52] H460, H125, H322, and H358 cell lines 3. Levina V, *et al.* [50] H460 cell line 4. Chen YC, *et al.* [51] Cancer cells isolated from surgical specimens 5. Meng X, *et al.* [48] *A549 cell line
	PODXL-1	Koch LK, *et al.* [69] Immunohistochemical analysis in surgical specimen tissue sections	
	uPAR	Gutova M, *et al.* [54] H1417, H69AR, H211, H1688, H1882, and H250 cell lines	
Transporter	SP	1. Meng X, *et al.* [48] *H446 cell line	1. Ho MM, *et al.* [48] A549, H23, H460, HTB-58, H2170, and H441 cell lines 2. Meng X, *et al.* [48] *A549 cell line
	ABCG2		Sung JM, *et al.* [25] A549 cell line
Enzymatic activity	ALDH	Jiang T, *et al.* [52] Aldefluor assay in H1618 cell line Moreb JS, *et al.* [93] RT-PCR, Western blotting, spectrophotometrical analysis and Aldefluor assay in SW210.5, H82, and SCLC-16HC cell lines	Ucar D, *et al.* [95] Spectrophotometrical analysis and Aldefluor assay in H522 cell line Patel M, *et al.* [96]. Immunohistochemical analysis in surgical specimen tissue sections Jiang F, *et al.* [49] Aldefluor assay in H460, H125, H322, and H358 cell lines Moreb JS, *et al.* [93] RT-PCR, Western blotting, spectrophotometrical analysis and Aldefluor assay in A549, H522, H322, H157, H125, H460, H1299, LCLC-103H and ADLC-5M2H lung cancer cell lines, as well as Beas-2B non-cancerous airway cell line

Table 1. (Continued)

Category	Molecule	SCLC	NSCLC
Signaling pathway	Shh	Watkins DN, *et al.* [77] NCI-H1618, NCI-H60, NCI-H146, NCI-H209, NCI-H249, NCI-H82, and NCI-H417 cell lines Yagui-Beltrán A, *et al.* [78] Review Peacock CD, *et al.* [79] Review	Yagui-Beltrán A, *et al.* [78] Review Peacock CD, *et al.* [79] Review
	Wnt/β-catenin	Yagui-Beltrán A, *et al.* [78] Review Peacock CD, *et al.* [79] Review	Yagui-Beltrán A, *et al.* [78] Review Peacock CD, *et al.* [79] Review 3. Levina V, *et al.* [50] H460 cell line
Transcription factor	Bmi1	Koch LK, *et al.* [69] Immunohistochemical analysis in surgical specimen tissue sections	Dovey JS, *et al.* [85] Bronchioloalveolar carcinoma (mouse)
	Oct-4		1. Levina V, *et al.* [50] H460 cell line 2. Chen YC, *et al.* [51] Cancer cells isolated from surgical specimens

SCLC: small cell lung carcinoma; NSCLC: non-small cell lung carcinoma; PODXL-1: podocalyxin-like protein 1; uPAR: urokinase plasminogen activator receptor;

SP: side population; ABCG2: ATP binding cassette transporter superfamily member G2; ALDH: aldehyde dehydrogenase; Shh: Sonic hedgehog; Bmi1: B cell-specific Mo-MuLV integration site 1.

*These authors reported that both of CD133+ and CD133- cells and of SP cells and non-SP cells exhibited the cancer initiating activity.

The methods for analysis of ALDH activity and protein expression are specifically described, because the procedures employed may potentially lead to the differences in results.

Origin of CSCs in Lung Cancers

As in hematological malignancies and other solid cancers, the presence of subpopulations of cells endowed with CSC properties has been recognized in lung cancers. Like CSCs in other tissues, the CSCs of lung cancers can be considered to originate from either airway stem cells, which have not been identified yet, or respective committed progenitor cells, such as bronchioloalveolar progenitor cells, basal/mucous secretory bronchial progenitor cells, and neuroendocrine progenitor cells [3-5], resulting in the initiation of region-specific lung cancers [4].

Cell markers for CSCs in Lung Cancers

CSC markers for lung cancer are a matter of some controversy, probably reflecting the tremendous heterogeneity of lung cancers in terms of cell of origin, etiology, pathology, biology, and molecular/genetic pathogenesis [2,7]. We herein briefly discuss these markers, paying special attention to the differences between SCLC and NSCLC; representative lung CSC markers reported to date are listed in Table 1.

CD133

CD133 was first reported as a novel marker for human hematopoietic stem and progenitor cells [28], and later found in some types of leukemic cells [29]. Prominin-1, which was identified on neuroepithelial stem cells in mice in 1997, is a mouse homolog of the human CD133 antigen [30]. The expression of CD133 has been detected in human central nervous system stem cells [31], human trophoblasts [32], human lymphatic/vascular endothelial precursor cells [33], and human prostatic epithelial stem cells [34]. The CD133 antigen is a 120kDa five-transmembrane domain glycoprotein, and its chromosomal location (4p16.2-p12) and amino acid sequence have been clarified [35]. Although its function is still unknown, CD133 may have a role in stem cell activation/maintenance, as shown by its coexpression with β1-integrin in the epidermal basal cells [36], release of CD133-carrying membrane particles into the extracellular space from neural progenitors and some epithelial cells [37], and potential regulatory activity of cell-cell contacts [38].

Recent studies have demonstrated that CD133 is a specific marker of CSCs in a wide spectrum of malignant tumors including brain tumors, colorectal cancers, pancreatic cancers, breast cancers, prostate cancers, ovarian cancers [39-41], and some lung cancers [42]. In contrast to the general consensus that CD133 is a ubiquitous CSC marker, several studies demonstrated that CD133-negative cells in certain human tumors also possess tumorigenic activity upon xenotransplantation into immunocompromised rodents [43-45]. These results imply that the CD133-negative subpopulation also contains cells with cancer initiating cell (CIC) activity. Mizrak, *et al.* [46] pointed out that CD133 is actually detected by its glycosylated epitope, AC133, and it is likely that AC133, but not CD133, is a more reliable CSC marker. Bidlingmaier, *et al.* [47] also suggested that the use of CD133 expression as a marker for CSC should be critically evaluated. These reports may explain the discrepancy observed in the results from different studies.

In regard to lung cancers, Eramo, *et al.* [42] reported that CD133 is a useful CSC marker in both SCLC and NSCLC. In contrast, Meng, *et al.* [48] reported more than 45% of A549 (NSCLC) and H446 (SCLC) cells to be CICs regardless of CD133 expression based on the results of cloning and tumorigenic analyses. Jiang, *et al.* [49] reported that, in NSCLC, cancer cells with strong ALDH activity (see below), showed CSC features and CD133 expression. Levina, *et al.* [50] demonstrated that NSCLC cells (H460) propagated a CD133-positive CSC-like cell population, in association with the expression of Oct-4 and high nuclear β-catenin (see below), after an *in vitro* treatment with anti-cancer drugs. Chen, *et al.* [51] reported that CD133-positive NSCLC cell lines display self-renewal and chemo-radio-resistant properties. Intriguingly, in SCLC, Jiang, *et al.* [52] demonstrated that achaete-scute complex homolog 1 (ASCL1) directly regulates ALDH1A1 and CD133 and that the CD133^{high}-ALDH1A1^{high}-ASCL1^{high} subpopulation exhibits the features of CSCs both *in vitro* and *in vivo*. ASCL1 is a specific marker of SCLC and thought to play important roles in its phenotypic expression and biological aggressiveness [8,53].

Side Population

Hoechst 33342 dye-efflux side population (SP) bone marrow cells were first discovered as hematopoietic stem cells in mice [54]. Since then, SP cells with stem-cell-like capabilities have been found in a variety of human hematologic and solid malignancies. These cells show the features of CSCs characterized by self-renewal activity, differentiated progeny production, tumorigenicity, as well as the expression of CSC markers and stem cell genes [55]. Thus, SP cells can be assumed to be CSCs. Importantly, SP cells are highly resistant to chemotherapeutic agents and crucial in therapy resistance and tumor recurrence [55-57]. Zhou, *et al.* [58] showed that expression of the *ATP binding cassette transporter superfamily member G2 (ABCG2)* gene is an important determinant of the SP phenotype, and that it might serve as a marker for stem cells from various sources. SP cells are usually isolated and purified by fluorescence activating cell sorting (FACS) using an ultraviolet (UV) laser. Recently, a new technique using a Violet-excited cell-permeable DNA-binding dye has been reported [59]. This method is inexpensive and yields the same results as UV-excited FACS [59]. In contrast, Wu, *et al.* [55] pointed out the following problems in using the SP phenotype as a CSC marker: 1) cells resistant to the Hoechst dye's toxicity do not consist only of stem-like cells, 2) variables in staining times, dye concentrations, and cellular concentrations can greatly affect the SP phenotype, and 3) cytometric gating strategies used to isolate SP cells lack the consistency of gating strategies used when staining with markers. These problems potentially lead to cross contamination of the SP and the non-SP fractions ultimately resulting in the production of confounding data. They emphasized that more stringent gating strategies are necessary and that a combination of isolation methods are required to enhance the purity of CSCs.

In lung cancers, Ho, *et al.* [60] reported that the SP cells in NSCLC cell lines were an enriched source of tumor-initiating cells with stem cell properties. Sung, *et al.* [25] suggested that ABCG2 played an important role in the multidrug resistance phenotype of SP cells in a NSCLC cell line, A549. In contrast, Meng, *et al.* [48] reported more than 45% of A549 (NSCLC) and H446 (SCLC) cells to be CICs regardless of SP features based on the results of cloning and tumorigenic analyses.

Aldehyde Dehydrogenase

The ALDH superfamily represents a divergently related group of enzymes that metabolize a wide variety of endogenous and exogenous aldehydes. In the human genome, at least 19 functional genes and 3 pseudogenes have been identified [61]. ALDH also contributes to the oxidation of retinol to retinoic acid, a modulator of cell proliferation, which may also modulate stem cell proliferation [62]. Murine and human hematopoietic stem cells [63-64], murine neural stem cells [65], normal and malignant human mammary stem cells [66], and normal and malignant human colorectal stem cells [62,67] exhibit ALDH activity and express this enzyme, strongly suggesting that strong ALDH activity and/or antigen expression can be used as a marker for stem cells in a variety of cancers. ALDH activity has been measured as substrate-oxidizing activity in whole cell lysate, and the expression of the enzyme has been detected by immunoreactions with specific antibodies, such as Western blot and immunohistochemical analyses. Since the development of a new method using an

ALDH-activated fluorescent substrate as a marker for the isolation of human hematopoietic stem cells [68], the so-called Aldefluor assay has been widely applied to the measurement and isolation of normal and malignant stem-cell-like cells in a variety of tissues [49,64-67]. This method is useful for isolating and purifying viable cells with high levels of ALDH activity for assays of the CSC properties of these cell populations.

Other Lung CSC Markers

Koch, *et al.* [69] demonstrated that a majority of SCLC were immunohistochemically positive for the antibody against podocalyxin-like protein 1 (PODXL-1) and hypothesized that PODXL-1 is a potential CSC marker of SCLC. PODXL-1, belonging to a large family of cell surface sialomucins and being most closely related to CD34 and endoglycan [33,70,71], is expressed in primitive hematopoietic progenitors and thought to be a marker of embryonic and hematopoietic stem cells [72].

Gutova, *et al.* [73] found that SCLC cells positive for urokinase plasminogen activator receptor (uPAR) were resistant to traditional chemotherapies and speculated that they contain a putative CSC population. Urokinase plasminogen activator (uPA) and its receptor uPAR are instrumental in controlling membrane-associated extracellular proteolysis and transmembranous signaling, thus affecting cell migration and invasion [74]. uPAR is up-regulated by several oncogenic pathways including mutations of multiple oncogenes. Alfano, *et al.* [74] underlined the importance of uPAR signaling in the prevention of apoptosis.

Signaling Pathways in CSCs of Lung Cancers

Sonic Hedgehog

Sonic hedgehog (Shh) is expressed by the epithelial cells, and binds and signals to Patched1/2 receptors in the underlying mesenchyme [6,75,76].

Watkins, *et al.* [77] reported the significance of Hedgehog signaling in a subset of SCLCs. Yagui-Beltrán, *et al.* [78] and Peacock, *et al.* [79] reviewed the results of studies on CSC markers and signaling pathways in pulmonary carcinogenesis with special attention to the differences between SCLC and NSCLC. Both papers emphasized the potential importance of the Hedgehog and Wnt signaling pathways in SCLC and NSCLC (see below). Interestingly, human primary or immortalized bronchial epithelial cells exposed to cigarette smoke for only eight days in culture became tumorigenic in nude mice, in association with the activation of the Hedgehog and Wnt signaling pathways [80].

Wnt Signaling Pathway and nuclear β-Catenin

For the maintenance and activation of normal stem cells, the Wnt/β-catenin signaling pathway is crucial, as distinctly demonstrated in the intestinal mucosa epithelia, epidermis, mammary gland [6], and other tissue [81]. The importance of Wnt signaling in cancer cells has been emphasized [82], and the Wnt/β-catenin signaling cascade is a critical regulator not only of normal stem cells but also of CSCs [83]. Disruption of this signaling pathway at any step potentially causes disorders of stem cell activity and plays a crucial role in the development of cancer. For instance, sustained Wnt signaling mediated by the membrane receptor Frizzled stimulates the release of β-catenin from a cytoplasmic degradation complex composed of APC, Axin, GSK3-β and Dsh, resulting in its movement into the nucleus and activation of Lef/Tcf transcription factors for c-Myc and cyclin D1 [82]. As another example, inactivation of APC due to a gene mutation also results in the release of β-catenin from the degradation complex, leading to the neoplastic transformation of colonic epithelial stem cells [11]. Thus, nuclear β-catenin is a hallmark for active Wnt signaling [75].

As described above, Yagui-Beltrán, *et al.* [87] and Peacock, *et al.* [79] emphasized the potential importance of the Wnt signaling pathway in SCLC and NSCLC in addition to the Hedgehog signaling pathway. Also as described above, human primary or immortalized bronchial epithelial cells exposed to cigarette smoke became tumorigenic in nude mice, being associated with the activation of not only the Hedgehog signaling pathway but also the Wnt signaling pathway [80].

Other Signaling Pathways and Transcription Factors in Lung CSCs

While the Wnt/β-catenin signaling pathway has been extensively investigated in many tissues including the lung, other signaling pathways are also important for controlling stem cell activity, including transmembranous Notch signaling and bone morphogenetic protein (BMP) signaling mediated by the cell membrane receptor Bmpr1a [8,75]. However, we are only beginning to understand the roles these pathways play in CSC populations of lung cancers.

B cell-specific Mo-MuLV integration site 1 (Bmi1) is a member of the Polycomb group family of proteins and a downstream effector of the extracellular signaling molecule Shh. Bmi1 is implicated in the self-renewal of multiple stem cells including hematopoietic and neural stem cells [84]. Dovey, *et al.* [85] suggested that Bmi1 is critical for both normal and tumor bronchioloalveolar stem cell expansion in mice. Koch, *et al.* [69] demonstrated that a majority of SCLCs were immunohistochemically positive for antibodies against Bmi1. From these results, they hypothesized that Bmi1 is a potential CSC marker of SCLC.

A couple of studies suggest that Oct-4 is a potential CSC marker for lung cancers. Levina, *et al.* [50] demonstrated that a human large cell cancer cell line (H460) propagated a CSC-like cell population that showed CD133, Oct-4, and high nuclear β-catenin expression after an *in vitro* treatment with anti-cancer drugs. Chen, *et al.* [51] reported that Oct-4 expression plays a crucial role in maintaining the self-renewing, CSC-like, and chemo-radio-resistant properties of CD133-positive NSCLC cell lines. Oct-4 is a member of the POU transcription factor family known to be expressed in pluripotent stem cells and to function as a transcriptional regulator of multiple genes related to stemness [86].

In Vitro Assay

Several *in vitro* assays have been used to identify CSCs, including sphere-formation assays, serial colony-forming unit assays (re-plating assays), and label-retention assays

[10,14]. Among them, sphere-formation assays are utilized in a wide range of tissue systems including lung cancers [42,87]. However, each of these methods has potential pitfalls that complicate interpretation of the results. For instance, difficulty in confirming clonality (single cell origin) has been pointed out [10]. In addition, the culture conditions used for these assays potentially exert selection pressures upon the cultured cells, resulting in the selection of only cell populations that are able to survive and proliferate under such specific conditions. The limitations of these *in vitro* assays should be kept in mind, and a combination of methods including *in vivo* assays is necessary for the identification and isolation of CSCs.

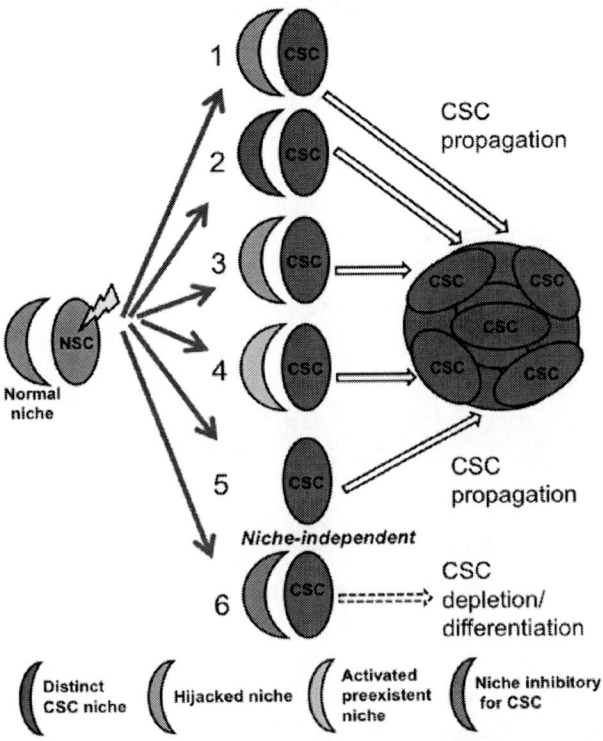

Figure 1. Hypothesis for the relationship between cancer stem cells (CSCs) and their niche. At least one genetic or epigenetic event (yellow arrow) is required to occur in a normal stem cell (NSC; or progenitor cell, not shown here) for a CSC initiation to develop (closed arrows). The CSCs may utilize the normal niche (1), require the distinct CSC niche (2), instruct an otherwise quiescent niche to become activated by providing signals ("hijacking the niche") (3), amplify an already existent activated niche (4), or become niche-independent (5). Furthermore, there may be a discrete niche that is inhibitory for CSC maintenance (6). (Modified from [24]).

CSC Niche

The microenvironment surrounding normal and cancer stem cells, which provides the stem cell niche, plays multiple roles including as a mechanical anchorage for the stem cells and in cross-talk communication mediated by direct contact and/or indirect extracellular factors. For instance, Wnt ligands are produced and released from both stem cells and niche cells, BMP and Shh are released from niche cells and epithelial cells respectively, and Notch signaling is transmembranously transmitted between neighboring cells. The micro environment may also provide signaling via the cell receptor integrin as suggested by its expression in prostatic CSCs [88] and its co-expression with AC133 (CD133) in the epidermal basal cells [36], as well as through metalloprotease-mediated lysophopholipid signaling [89].

The concept of a CSC niche is a matter of debate [90]. Two fundamental questions need to be answered: 1) Does a specific CSC niche exist? 2) If it does, what are the differences between the normal stem cell niche and CSC niche? Sneddon, *et al.* [23] removed some of the confusion regarding the CSC niche by proposing several possible models (Figure 1): 1) CSCs are capable of surviving in the normal stem cell niche, 2) a distinct CSC niche is necessary for activation, 3) CSCs may be capable of providing signals that instruct an otherwise quiescent niche to become activated ("hijacking the niche"), 4) CSCs could amplify an already existent activated niche, 5) CSCs may be niche-independent, that is, they themselves acquire the ability to maintain activity, and 6) there may be a discrete niche that is inhibitory for CSC maintenance. Accumulating evidence suggests that no single model fits all the diverse types of cancer. Further study is required to establish a universally acceptable CSC niche theory.

While the niche may also play an important role in the maintenance of CSCs from lung cancers, little has been elucidated yet. Hilbe, *et al.* [91] demonstrated by immunohisto chemistry a significant increase in CD133-positive vascular endothelial cells in patients with NSCLC and suggested an involvement of endothelial progenitor cells in the tumor vasculature and tumor growth, as well as possibly the maintenance and activation of CSCs. More studies of the lung CSC niche are required not only to understand the biological relationship between lung CSCs and their niche but also for the development of therapeutic strategies for lung cancers.

Brief Summary of Lung CSC Markers and Potential Problems

While investigations into the CSC markers of lung cancer are insufficient at this time, as discussed above and summarized in Table 1, we tentatively summarize the findings to date as follows: 1) CD133 expression and the SP phenotype are common CSC markers for SCLC and NSCLC. 2) The Wnt/β-catenin signaling pathway is also important in the maintenance and activation of CSCs in SCLC and NSCLC. 3) PODXL-1 and uPAR are potential CSC markers for SCLC, but their expression has not been well examined in NSCLC. 4) In regard to ALDH, results reported to date appear to be complicated. Its enzymatic activity has been demonstrated in SCLC and NSCLC cells by the Aldefluor assay, as well as by a spectrophotometrical assay [92-97]. On the other hand, an immunohistochemical analysis using antibodies against ALDH1A1 and ALDH3A1 in tissue sections of surgical specimens of lung cancer demonstrated the expression of these ALDH isozymes in NSCLC cases, but not in SCLC cases, suggesting that the ALDH protein expression was limited to CSCs in NSCLC [96]. In contrast, Moreb, *et al.* [93] reported that in their studies using several SCLC and NSCLC cell lines there were good correlations between the results of a Western blot analysis, a spectrophotometrical analysis, and the Aldefluor assay, in spite of a few exceptions (see below). The discrepancy among these results may be attributable to the difference in the antibodies used, and the difference between the *in vitro* and *in vivo* conditions as well.

Though evidence is still poor, it is supposed that distinct differences in the mechanism of ALDH expression and activity, as well as the role of ALDH in the maintenance/activation of CSCs, exist between SCLC and NSCLC. Furthermore, the exact mechanism and role of ALDH in the maintenance of the stemness of normal stem cells and CSCs are still unknown. To try to resolve these issues, we have carried out investigations, which are described in the following section.

Recent Findings in ALDH and CSC of the Lung

As described above, ALDH activity and its protein expression have been reported to be useful normal stem cell and CSC markers in a wide range of tissues [66,92,96-98]. These ALDHs play pluripotent roles in endobiotic and xenobiotic metabolism through specific metabolic pathways. One important issue to be addressed is which ALDH isozymes are responsible for the ALDH activity used to identify stem cell progenitors. Several studies have demonstrated that ALDH activity is needed for the differentiation of primitive progenitors into mature cells, thus fulfilling one of the defining characteristics of multipotent stem cells, and some lines of evidence suggest that ALDH1A1 is an important marker of hematopoietic stem cell progenitors [92]. In fact, ALDH1A1 is one of the enzymes involved in the production of retinoic acid from retinol, and retinoic acid is considered significantly important in maintaining a balance between hematopoietic stem cell self-renewal and differentiation [92].

Moreb, *et al.* [93] systemically evaluated ALDH expression in several lung cancer cells lines (SCLC and NSCLC cell lines) utilizing the Aldefluor assay, a Western blotting, and a spectrophotometry and found a very good correlation between the results of all three. They concluded that the Aldefluor assay can be adapted successfully to measure ALDH activity in lung cancer cells, providing real time changes in ALDH activity in viable cells treated with chemotherapy or siRNA. They emphasized the importance of the use of mixed populations of cells with high ALDH levels and cells lacking ALDH activity when ALDH activity is measured by the Aldefluor assay in cells known to have high ALDH levels. Importantly, they carried out double Aldefluor and propidium iodide (PI) staining to delineate dead cells. According to their results, while ALDH expression levels were heterogeneous among the cell lines examined, overall findings revealed low levels of ALDH activity in SCLC cell lines, while higher levels were detected in some, but not all, NSCLC cell lines. The results correlated very well with protein and enzymatic activity as measured by the Western blot analysis and the spectrophotometrical assay, respectively. Intriguingly, there was one exception: The SW210.5 (SCLC) cell line registered only a small amount of ALDH activity in the spectrophotometrical assay and expressed only small amounts of ALDH1A1 and ALDH3A1 proteins in the Western blot analysis, whereas the Aldefluor assay showed high levels of ALDH activity (50% of the cells). This SCLC cell line (SW210.5) was shown to express mRNA for ALDH1A1 and ALDH2, but not ALDH3A1, by the semi-quantitative reverse transcription polymerase chain reaction (RT-PCR) assay.

Our preliminary experiments revealed very high levels of ALDH1A1 mRNA expression in some SCLC and NSCLC cell lines. We also observed considerable discrepancies between mRNA levels detected by the quantitative RT-PCR assay, protein levels analyzed by Western blotting, and the proportion of cells with enzymatic activity measured by the Aldefluor assay in several SCLC and NSCLC cell lines.

Aiming to elucidate the mechanism underlying the discrepancies observed in preliminary experiments and the previous study, we carried out the following experiments.

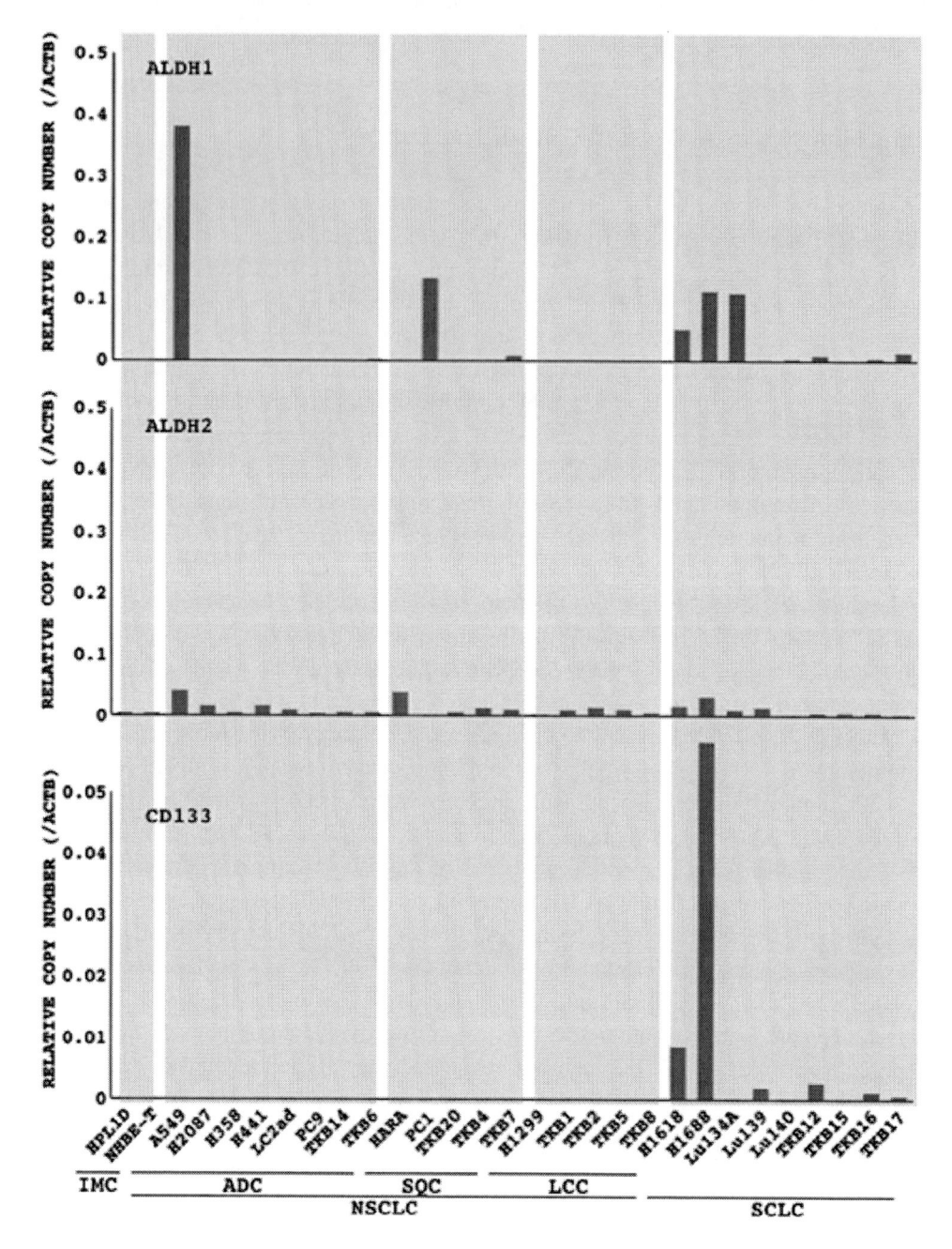

Figure 2. Expression of ALDH1, ALDH2 and CD133 mRNA in immortalized human airway cell and lung cancer cell lines. Levels of mRNA of ALDH1, ALDH2 and CD133 and β-actin (ACTB) were measured by quantitative RT-PCR. The mRNA levels of ALDH1 (upper panel), ALDH2 (second panel) and CD133 (lower panel) relative to that of ACTB in immortalized human airway cells and lung cancer

cells are presented. IMC, immortalized human airway cell lines; ADC, adenocarcinoma cell lines; SQC, squamous cell carcinoma cell lines; LCC, large cell carcinoma cell lines; NSCLC, non-small cell lung carcinoma cell lines; SCLC, small cell lung carcinoma cell lines. The experimental materials and methods are as follows. An immortalized human airway epithelial cell line (16HBE14o, Simian virus 40 (SV40)-transformed human bronchial epithelial cells) described by Cozens AL, *et al.* [102] was kindly provided by Gruenert DC (California Pacific Medical Center Research Institute, CA) via Kaneko T (Division of Respiratory Disease Center, Yokohama City Medical Center Hospital, Yokohama, Japan). A sub-clone of 16HBE14o cells, described as NHBE-T in this chapter, was used. An immortalized airway epithelial cell line (HPL1D, SV40-transformed human small airway epithelial cells) established by Masuda A, *et al.* [103], was provided by Takahashi T (Division of Molecular Carcinogenesis, Center for Neurological Disease and Cancer, Nagoya University Graduate School of Medicine, Nagoya, Japan). Human lung cancer cell lines (A549, H358, H2087, H1618, H1688 and H1299) were purchased from American Type Culture Collection (ATCC, Manassas, VA). Human lung cancer cell lines, LC2/ad, Lu134A and Lu140 were obtained form Riken Cell Bank (Tsukuba, Japan), and PC9, PC1 and HARA from Immuno-Biological Laboratories Co. (Gunma, Japan). Human lung cancer cell lines, TKB1, TKB2, TKB4, TKB5, TKB6, TKB7, TKB8, TKB12, TKB15, TKB16, TKB17 and TKB20, were kindly provided by Kamma H (Department of Pathology, Kyorin University School of Medicine, Tokyo, Japan) via Yazawa T (Department of Pathology, Yokohama City University School of Medicine, Yokohama Japan). The cells were cultured and grown in DEMEM (Sigma Aldrich, St. Louis, MO) (NHBE-T, HPL1D, A549, H358, H2087, PC9, PC1, HARA, LC2/ad, TKB1, TKB2, TKB4, TKB5, TKB6, TKB7, TKB8, TKB20 and H1299) or RPMI1640 medium (Sigma) (H1618, H1688, Lu130, Lu134A, Lu140, TKB12, TKB15, TKB16 and TKB17) supplemented with 10% heat-inactivated fetal bovine serum (FBS) (Sigma), 100 units/ml of penicillin (Sigma), and 100 μg/ml of streptomycin (Sigma). Total RNA was extracted from the cells with Isogen reagents (NIPPON GENE, Tokyo, Japan). First-strand cDNA was synthesized from total RNA using the SuperScript First-Strand Synthesis System according to the protocols of the manufacturer (Invitrogen, Carlsbad, CA). The cDNA generated was used as a template in real-time PCR with SYBR Premix EXTaq (Takara, Kyoto, Japan). The primer set used for ALDH1A1 was forward (F), 5'- agtgcccctttggtggattc; reverse (R), 5'- aagagcttctctccactcttg. That for ALDH2 was, F, 5'- ctacacacgccatgaacctg; R, 5'- caaccacgtttccagttg. That for CD133 was, F, 5'- ttgtggcaaatcaccaggta; R, 5'- gatgttgggtctcagtcggt. That for ACTB was, F, 5'-tggcacccagcacaatgaa; R, 5'- ctaagtcatagtccgcctagaagca. The mean of the copy number of ALDH1A1, ALDH2 or CD133 normalized to the value for ACTB mRNA was obtained from triplicate reactions.

ALDH mRNA Expression - its Correlation with the most Common CSC Marker CD133 -

The quantitative RT-PCR assay revealed that ALDH1A1 mRNA was expressed at detectable levels in seven out of nine SCLC cell lines (77.8%), three of which expressed it at unequivocally high levels (33.3%), while it was expressed in four of the 18 NSCLC cell lines, two of which expressed it at high levels (11.1%) (Figure 2). On the other hand, ALDH2 was expressed in eight of the nine SCLC cell lines and 17 of the 18 NSCLC cell lines. The levels were lower on the whole than those of ALDH1A1 and did not remarkably differ among the cell lines. mRNA of CD133, most commonly used CSC marker, was expressed only in SCLC cell lines (66.7%, six out of nine cell lines), and its level in SCLC cell lines tended to be associated with the level of ALDH1A1, but not ALDH2. The findings suggested ALDH1A1 to have an important significance in the maintenance of stemness in lung cancer cells, and might account for the highly malignant activity of SCLCs.

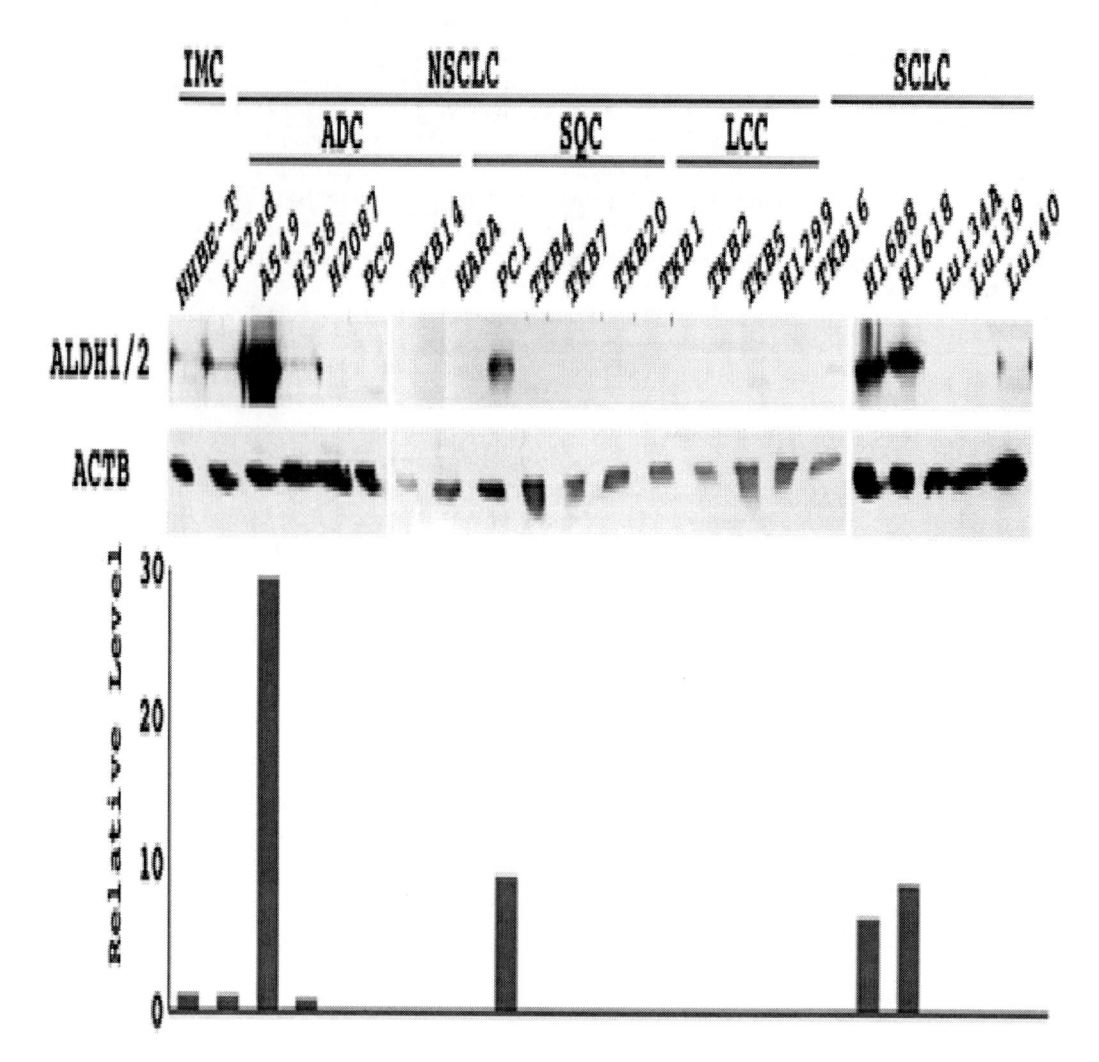

Figure 3. Expression of ALDH1A1/ALDH2 (ALDH1/2) protein in lung cancer cell lines. ALDH1/2 (top panel) and β-actin (ACTB) (second panel) protein expressions were analyzed by Western blotting. Levels of ALDH1/2 and ACTB protein were semi-quantified with a densitometer (NIH Image; National Institute of Mental Health at Bethesda, MD). The level of ALDH1/2 normalized to that of ACTB is presented in a graph (third panel). IMC, immortalized human airway epithelial cell lines; ADC, adenocarcinoma cell lines; SQC, squamous cell carcinoma cell lines; LCC, large cell carcinoma cell lines; NSCLC, non-small cell lung carcinoma cell lines; SCLC, small cell lung carcinoma cell lines. The experimental materials and methods are as follows. The cell lines (the details of the experimental materials are described in the legend for Figure 2) grown to sub-confluence were solved with extraction buffer, as described elsewhere [104]. After centrifugation, supernatants were recovered as protein extracts. The extracts were mixed with equal volumes of 2×sample buffer [104], and then boiled. The samples were subjected to sodium dodecyl sulfate-polyacrylamide gel electrophoresis, and transferred onto PVDF membranes (Amersham, Arlington Heights, IL). The membranes were incubated with nonfat dry milk in 0.01 M Tris-buffered saline containing 0.1% Tween-20 (TBS-T) to block non-immunospecific protein binding, and then with 0.1 μg/ml of a primary antibody which non-selectively binds to both ALDH1A1 and ALDH2 (clone 44, BD Transduction, San Jones, CA) or a primary antibody against ACTB (Sigma). After washing with TBS-T, the membranes were incubated with animal-matched horseradish peroxidase-conjugated secondary antibodies (Amersham). Immunoreactivity was visualized with the enhanced chemiluminescence system (ECL, Amersham).

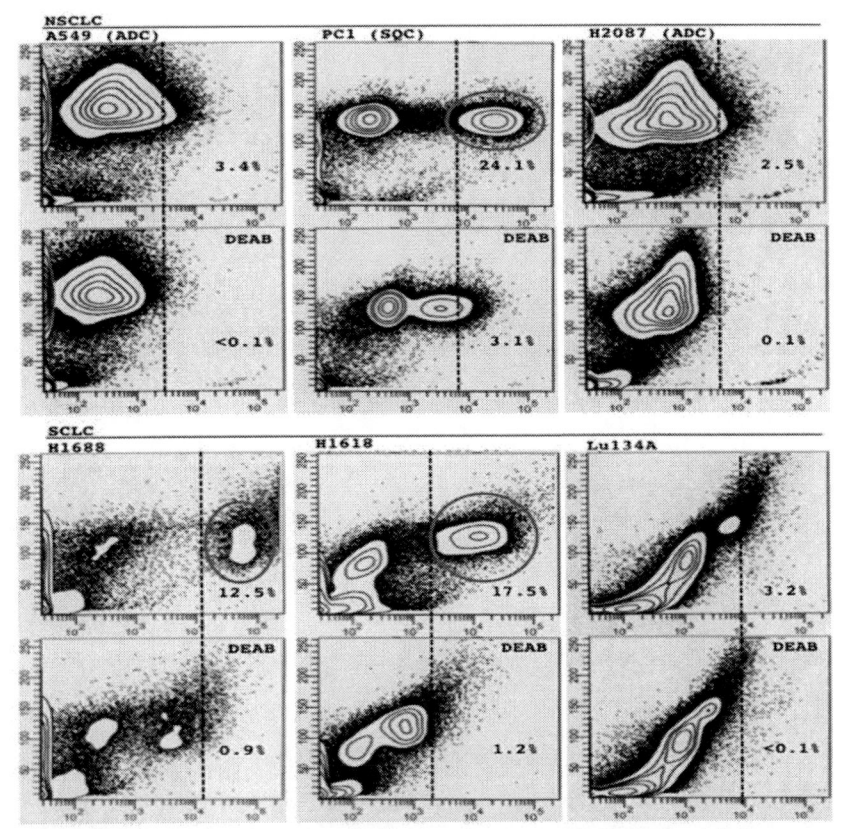

Figure 4. Measurement of fraction of cells with ALDH activity (Aldefluor assay) in lung cancer cell lines. Cells were labeled with Aldefluor (BODIPY-aminoacetaldehyde [BAAA]) (Stem cell technology Inc., Vancouver, Canada) with or without the ALDH inhibitor diethylaminobenzaldehyde (DEAB) (Stem cell technology). The proportion of fraction of cells with ALDH activity was measured by flow cytometer. The X-axis is fluorescence intensity (log scale), and the Y-axis is forward scatter level (linear scale). The fraction of cells with strong ALDH activity is shown (red circle). NSCLC, non-small cell lung carcinoma cell lines; ADC, adenocarcinoma cell lines; SQC, squamous cell carcinoma cell lines; SCLC, small cell lung carcinoma cell lines. The experimental materials and methods are as follows. The details of the cell lines examined are described in the legend for Figure 1. Cells with ALDH activity was labeled using Aldefluor assay kit (Stem cell technology) according to the manufacturer's instructions. Briefly, 1.0×10^6 cells in 1 ml of Aldefluor assay buffer with BAAA at a concentration of 1.5 mM were incubated for 45 min at 37C. In each experiment, a sample of cells was treated under identical conditions with 50 mM of a specific ALDH inhibitor (DEAB) to serve as a negative control. The fraction of cells with ALDH activity labeled by Aldefluor was measured with a flow cytometer (BD Science, San Jose, CA) (excitation wave length 488 nm and emission wave length 525 nm (green fluorescence)). Data for 1.0×10^5 cells were collected.

ALDH Protein Expression in Lung Cancer Cell Lines

ALDH protein was detected by Western blotting using a non-selective antibody, which binds both ALDH1A1 and ALDH2 proteins (clone 44, BD transduction, Palo Alto, CA). The protein was expressed at high levels in two of the nine SCLC cell lines (22.2%), and two of the 18 NSCLC cell lines (11.1%) (Figure 3). The level of protein paralleled well the level of ALDH1A1 mRNA, but not ALDH2 mRNA, in NSCLC cell lines, suggesting that the protein detected by the Western blot analysis was ALDH1A1 rather than ALDH2 (Figure 2 and

Figure 3). Thus, we describe the protein detected here by the Western blot analysis as ALDH1A1. Interestingly, one SCLC cell line (Lu134) with a high level of ALDH1A1 mRNA did not express ALDH1A1 (either ALDH1A1 or ALDH2) (Figure 2). This result is similar to a previous observation that a SCLC cell line, SW210.5, expressed ALDH1 mRNA, but only a very small amount of protein [93]. These findings suggest a potential post-translational mechanism to be involved in ALDH1A1 protein expression in some SCLC cells.

A

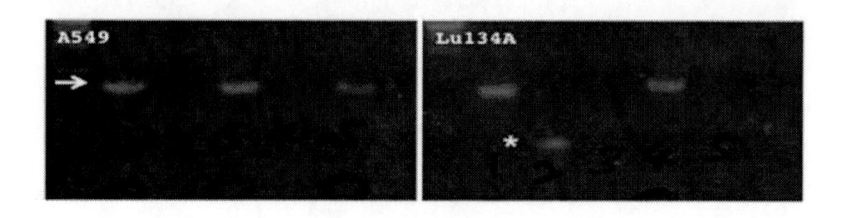

B

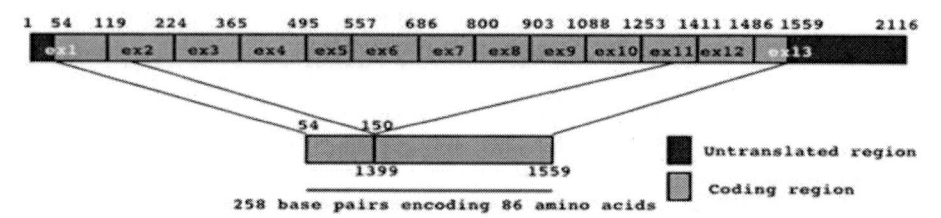

Figure 5. Analysis of primary structure of mRNA of ALDH1A1. The protein-coding sequence in ALDH1A1 mRNA was amplified by RT-PCR using primers, forward, 5'-aggagccgaatcagaaatgtc; reverse, 5'-aagagcttctctccactcttg, according to the method descried in the legend for Figure 2. The PCR product was sub-cloned into the plasmid vector pT7Blue (Novagen, Darmstadt, Germany), and then its size was checked by PCR using universal primers (T7 promoter primer and M13M4 primer (Novagen)). (A) A representative result from A549 (ADC) and Lu134A (SCLC) cells is shown. Shorter PCR products (faster migrating band (asterisk)) were found in some sub-clones from Lu134A. Bands of expected size with a full-length coding region of ALDH1A1 (NCBI accession # NM_000689) are indicated with an arrow. (B) Schema of the primary structure of the consensus mRNA and the shorter variant with their mRNA spliced sites in the *ALDH1A1* gene, is shown. The shorter novel variant consists of parts of exon 1, exon2, exon 11, exon 12, and exon 13. "ex" in figure means exon.

ALDH Activity in Lung Cancer Cell Lines

The fraction of cells with ALDH activity was measured with the Aldefluor assay. The two SCLC cell lines with high ALDH1A1 protein levels (H1688 and H1618) had fractions of cells with strong ALDH activity (Figure 4). All of the SCLC cell lines with very weak ALDH protein expression (the faint bands detected by Western blotting in these cell lines were presumably ALDH2, because these cell lines expressed only ALDH2, not ALDH1A1, mRNA) had only a small fraction (less than 10%) of cells with ALDH activity. On the other hand, among NSCLC cell lines examined (A549, PC1, H441, H2087 and H1299) (not all data shown), only one (PC1) had fraction of cells with strong ALDH activity (Figure 4). One cell line with high ALDH1A1 protein levels (A549) unexpectedly had only a very small fraction of cells with strong ALDH activity. Summarizing the findings, ALDH1A1 protein expression was closely associated with ALDH activity in SCLC cells, but not necessarily in NSCLC cells, suggesting the potential post-translational mechanism to be involved in activation of ALDH1A1 protein in NSCLCs.

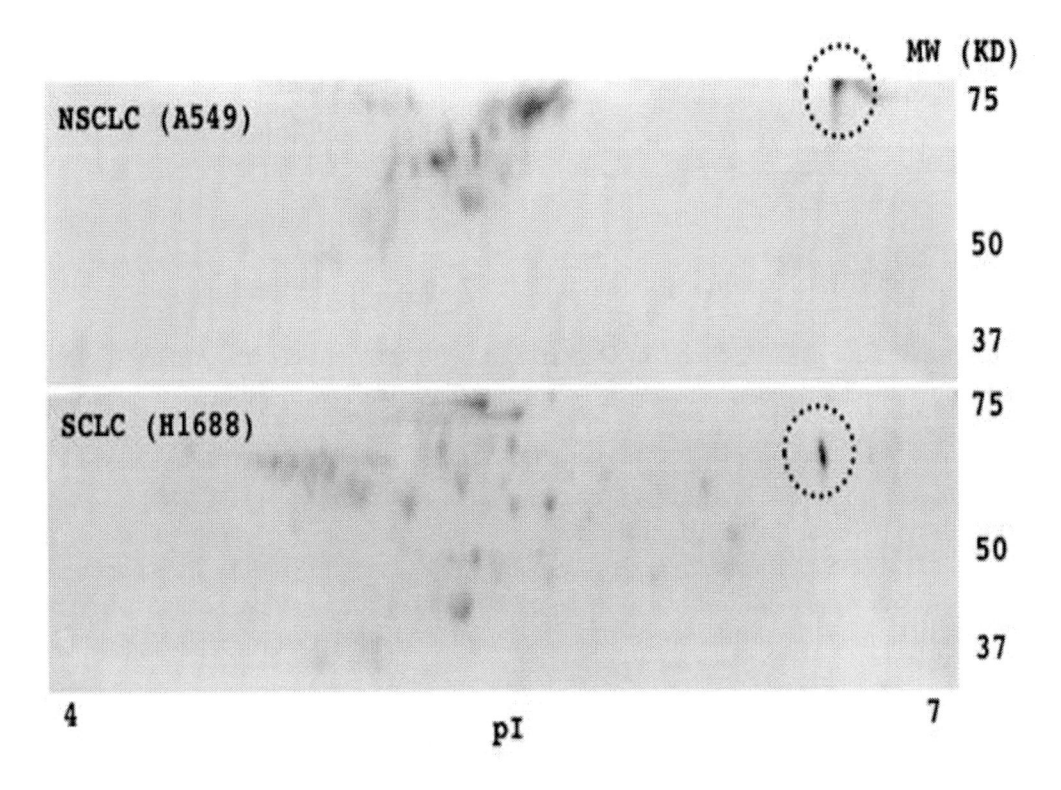

Figure 6. Two-dimensional Western blotting analysis of ALDH1A1/ALDH2 (ALDH1/2) protein in a NSCLC cell line (top panel; A549) and SCLC cell line (Bottom panel; H1688). Spots of ALDH1/2 protein were circulated with dashed lines. MW, molecular weight; KD, kilo-dalton; pI, isoelectric point plugin. The experimental materials and methods are as follows. Two-dimensional electrophoresis (2-DE) was carried out using a horizontal electrophoresis system (Maltiphor II; Amersham) according to the manufacture's instruction. Briefly, equal amount of protein sample was subjected to the first-dimensional isoelectric focusing, and followed by the second dimensional sodium dodecyl sulfate-polyacrylamide gel electrophoresis. The details of method are described elsewhere [105,106]. The separated proteins on the 2-DE gels were transferred onto a polyvinylidene difluoride membrane (FluoroTrans® PVDF Membrane, Nippon Genetics, Tokyo, Japan). The membranes were incubated with nonfat dry milk in 0.01 M Tris-buffered saline containing 0.1% Tween-20 (TBS-T) to block non-immunospecific protein binding, and then with 0.1 µg/ml of a primary antibody, which non-selectively binds to both ALDH1A1 and ALDH2 (clone 44, BD Transduction). After washing with TBS-T, the membranes were incubated with animal-matched horseradish peroxidase-conjugated secondary antibodies (Amersham). Immunoreactivity was visualized with the enhanced chemiluminescence system (ECL, Amersham).

Primary Structure of ALDH1A1 mRNA

To elucidate the possible involvement of a mutation (or polymorphism) or splicing disorder in the difference among the levels of mRNA, protein and activity, which was observed in Lu134 SCLC and A549 NSCLC cells, the nucleotide sequence of open reading frames of cDNA were analyzed. No mutation (or polymorphism) causing an amino acid substitution was found in either cell line (data not shown). However, interestingly, short mRNA variant (258 base pairs in the open reading frame, encoding 86 amino acids: see Figure 5) was found in the Lu134A cell line. This variant was found in three of eight sub-clones (37.5%) in our sub-cloning experiment (part of the result is shown in Figure 5). The result suggested the possible involvement of such a variant in the post-transcriptional regulation of ALHD1A1 expression, and also implied a potential difference between SCLC and NSCLC, although further screening of a larger number of cell lines and primary lung cancers is required to test this idea.

Post-translational Modification of ALDH1A1 Protein

Since no mutation was found in the cell line with the lag between ALDH1/2 protein expression and ALDH activity (A549 cells), we next verified the possible involvement of a post-translational modification. To screen for such a modification, two-dimensional Western blot analysis was performed with A549 (NSCLC) and H1688 (SCLC) cells (Figure 6). While the results did not reveal unequivocal evidence of a modification, the ALDH1A1 protein migrated slightly faster in A549 cells (Figure 6). To elucidate the mechanism underlying the lag between ALDH1A1 protein expression and ALDH activity, further investigations of protein structure and modifications such as glycosylation, phosphorylation and acetylation status, are required.

ALDH Protein Expression in Primary Lung Cancers

ALDH protein expression in primary lung tumors was examined by immunohistochemistry using a non-selective antibody (clone 44, BD transduction, Palo Alto, CA), which binds both ALDH1A1 and ALHD2 proteins (ALDH1/2). The protein expression was detected in three of nine SCLCs (33.3%) and in 41 of 70 NSCLCs (58.6%) (Table 2). The levels tended to be higher in NSCLC, especially SQC, than in SCLC (Figure 5). The results were similar to those reported by Patel, *et al.* [96], who found in their immunohistochemical analysis that the ALDH isozymes 1A1 and 1A3 were expressed at significantly higher levels in NSCLC than in SCLC [96]. However, we have found that there is a discrepancy between the results of Western blotting for cancer cell lines and immunohistochemistry for primary lung cancers. The frequency of ALDH1/2 protein expression was considerably higher in primary cancers than in cell lines among NSCLCs, whereas it was similar between the two among SCLCs (Figure 3 and Table 2). Moreover, non-cancerous airway cells *in vivo*, i.e., both the bronchial, bronchiole and alveolar epithelial cells, exhibited high levels of immunohistochemical expression of ALHD1/2 protein compared to cancer cells in all cases examined (Figure 7 and Table 2). Interestingly, the two non-cancerous immortalized airway epithelial cell lines (NHBE-T and HPL1D) showed very weak expression of ALDH1/2 protein *in vitro*. The ALDH family is expressed in response to toxic stress [99-101]. The marked expression of ALDH1/2 protein in non-cancerous airway epithelial cells *in vivo* is supposed to be induced by external stimuli such as dust, cigarette smoke and so on. In NSCLCs, ALDH1/2 protein tended to be expressed more strongly among *in situ* parts than invasive parts (data not shown), in support of our supposition. Furthermore ALDH1/2 protein expression tended to decrease in parallel with the dedifferentiation process, as a large proportion of poorly differentiated NSCLCs expressed the protein only faintly (data not shown). In well-differentiated and *in situ* NSCLCs, ALDH1/2 expression may still be regulated by the physiological system (it may be lost during progression process to develop poorly differentiated ones). Although further investigation is required to elucidate the mechanism and significance of such a downregulation of ALDH1/2 protein expression in primary lung cancers, the results obtained here imply that ALDH1/2 protein plays diverse roles in different situations is not a universal stem cell marker. The mechanism to induce ALDH1/2 protein expression and its significance are likely to differ among the non-cancerous airway epithelia, NSCLCs and SCLCs.

Table 2. Positive rate of immunohistochemical ALDH1/2 expression among NSCLC and SCLC

		NSCLC		SCLC
No. of cases analyzed	ADC [49]	SQC [16]	LCC [5]	[9]
Positive rate % [No.]	51.0% [25]	87.5% [14]	40.0% [2]	33.3% [3]

NSCLC, non-small cell lung carcinoma; SCLC, small cell lung carcinoma; ADC, adenocarcinoma; SQC, squamous cell carcinoma; LCC, large cell carcinoma;
Chi-square test (among all, $P = 0.0254$; NSCLC versus SCLC, $P = 0.154$)
Immunohistochemical analysis was performed in formalin-fixed tumor sections using a primary antibody against
ALDH (BD transduction, Palo Alto, CA). Immunoreactivity was visualized with an Envision detection system (DAKO).
If 5% or more of neoplastic cells in a tumor showed immunohistochemical expression of ALDH, it was judged as positive.

CONCLUSION

As is widely accepted, among lung cancers, SCLC and NSCLC are distinctly different in terms of biological behavior and pathogenesis. We have hypothesized that the CSCs of these two major subtypes of lung cancer possess different biological properties and that the abundance of CSCs population differs between the two. We have here focused upon ALDH to confirm such a potential difference.

The proportion of cells with strong ALDH activity tended to be associated with the CD133 mRNA level especially in SCLC cell lines (Figure 2). Recently, Jiang, *et al.* [52] demonstrated, in SCLC cell lines, that the ALDH1A1[high]-CD133[high]-ASCL1[high] subpopulation

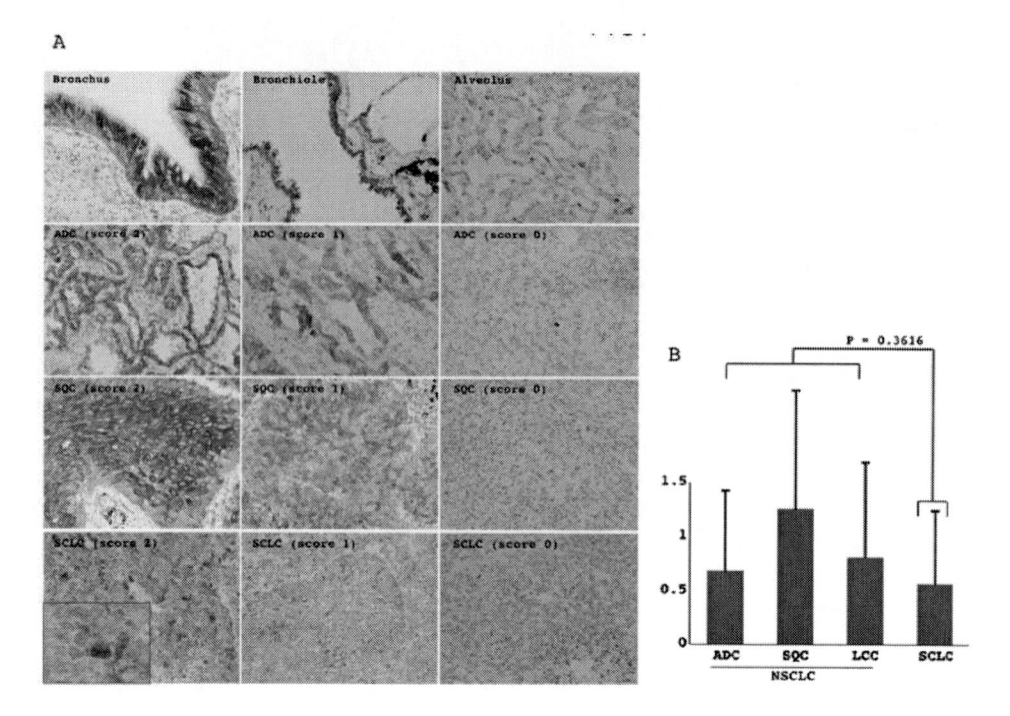

Figure 7. Expression of ALDH1A1/ALDH2 (ALDH1/2) protein in non-cancerous airway epithelia and primary lung cancers. (A) Representative photographs of immunohistochemistry of surgical specimens of non-cancerous airway epithelia (top panels) and lung cancers (the other panels) are shown. Magnifications are ×200 in, non-cancerous airway epithelia (bronchus, bronchiole and alveolus), adenocarcinoma (ADC), squamous cell carcinoma (SQC) and small cell lung carcinoma (SCLC), and ×400 in the inset of SCLC. Levels of ALDH1/2 expression were evaluated according to a scoring system; negative (score 0), unequivocally strong (score 2), and positive but weaker than a score of 2 (score 1). (B) Seventy-nine tumors (49 ADCs, 16 SQCs, 5 large cell carcinomas, and 9 SCLCs) were examined. The mean and standard deviation (error bar) among each histological type are shown in graph. Differences were analyzed with Student's t-test, and P value is indicated. The experimental materials and methods are as follows. All cases examined were of lung cancer patients who underwent surgical resection at the Kanagawa Prefectural Cardiovascular and Respiratory Disease Center Hospital (Yokohama, Japan) between 2001 and 2008. Informed consent for research use was obtained from all the subjects providing materials. Tissue sections (4 µm thick), cut from the formalin-fixed and paraffin-embedded tissue block with largest tumor dimension, were deparaffinized and rehydrated, and incubated with 3% hydrogen peroxide to block endogenous peroxidase activities. The sections were incubated with 5% goat serum to block non-immunospecific protein binding. After antigen retrieval treatment, boiling in citrated buffer (0.01 M, pH6.0) to restore the masked epitope, the sections were incubated with a primary antibody, which non-selectively binds to both ALDH1A1 and ALDH2 (clone 44, BD Transduction). Immunoreactivity was visualized with an Envision detection system (DAKOcytomation, Carpinteria, CA), and the nuclei were counterstained with hematoxylin.

exhibits the features of CSCs and that ASCL1 directly regulates ALDH1A1 and CD133 both *in vitro* and *in vivo*. Previous observations [60] are consistent with our results and also support the hypothesis that the size of the CSC fraction (population) could be one causes of highly malignant activity of SCLC. Importantly, however, not all SCLCs among cell lines and primary tumors were found to have either protein expression or a fraction of cells with high ALDH activity (Figure 4, Figure 7 and Table 2). We thus speculate that the ALDH activity is only one of the factors determining the stemness of CSCs in SCLCs. Alternatively, ALDH1A1 protein expression or ALDH activity is just part of the machinery to maintain stemness and might have significance only in some fractions of SCLCs. On the other hand, Ucar, *et al.* [95] proposed ALDH activity to be a CSC marker in a NSCLC cell line (NIH-H522 LCC cell line). Moreover, Jiang, *et al.* [49] reported that, in NSCLCs, cancer cells with strong ALDH1A1 activity, which were isolated using the Aldefluor assay followed by fluorescence-activated cell sorting, showed CSC features and CD133 expression. They proposed that ALDH1A1 is a lung cancer stem cell-associated marker, being a potential prognostic factor and therapeutic target for the treatment of patients with lung cancer. In our experiments, one NSCLC cell line (PC1 [SQC]) had a high ALDH1A1 protein level and a large fraction of cells with strong ALDH activity (Figure 3 and Figure 5), but did not express CD133 mRNA. Taken together, it is supposed that there is considerable heterogeneity in the mechanism maintaining the stemness of CSCs of SCLCs and NSCLCs.

Aside from the maintenance of stemness, another interesting finding of our experiments was that the level of ALDH1A1 mRNA did not always parallel the level of protein in SCLC cell lines, whereas, in NSCLC cell lines (Figure 3 and Figure 4), the level of protein was not always consistent with that of activity. Furthermore, the *in vivo* findings revealed that either non-cancerous airway epithelia or low-grade neoplasms such as well-differentiated or *in situ* NSCLCs showed stronger immunohistochemical expression of ALDH1A1 (possibly ALDH2 too) protein than less-differentiated cancer cells.

From the current findings, the mechanism and pathway which regulate the expression of ALDH1A1 mRNA and its protein as well as its enzymatic activity, and its role vary in different situations and among non-cancerous airway cells, NSCLCs and SCLCs, as well as among individual tumors. We speculate that ALDH1A1, its expression and/or activity, is only one of the factors determining the stemness in lung cancers.

In conclusion, the CSCs in SCLC and NSCLC differ distinctly from each other in terms not only of their abundance (suggested by CD133 mRNA levels) but also of the regulatory mechanism of ALDH1A1 expression and its activity, as well as its role in the maintenance/activation of stemness. The investigation of the mechanism of ALDH activation and its role in the maintenance of the stemness not only of CSCs but also of normal stem cells would provide a novel paradigm for stem cell biology and the development of a molecular targeting therapy for lung cancer.

ACKNOWLEDGMENTS

This work was supported by the Japanese Ministry of Education, Culture, Sports, and Science (Tokyo Japan), Smoking Research Foundation (Tokyo, Japan), and by a grant from Yokohama Medical Facility (Yokohama, Japan). We especially thank Hideaki Mitsui (Department of Pathology, Yokohama City University Graduate School of Medicine, Yokohama, Japan), Shigeko Iwanade (Division of Pathology, Kanagawa Prefectural Cardiovascular and Respiratory Center Hospital, Yokohama, Japan), and Tetsukan Woo (Department of General Thoracic Surgery, Kanagawa Prefectural Cardiovascular and Respiratory Center Hospital, Yokohama, Japan) for assistance.

REFERENCES

[1] Parkin, M., Tyczynski, JE., Boffetta, P., Samet, J., Shields, P., Caporaso, N. Lung cancer epidemiology and etiology. In: Travis, W.D., Brambilla, E., Muller-Hermelink, H.K., Harris, C.C. (eds). *Tumours of the lung. Tumours of the lung, pleura, thymus and heart. World Health Organization Classification of Tumours. Pathology & Genetics.* Lyon, IARC Press 2004; 12-15.

[2] Travis, W.D., Brambilla, E., Muller-Hermelink, H.K., Harris, C.C. (eds). IARC Press: Lyon, 2004; 9-124. Working group that convened for an editorial and consensus conference in Lyon, France, March 12-16, 2003. Tumours of the Lung. In: *World Health Organization Classification of Tumours. Pathology and Genetics of Tumours of the Lung, Pleura, Thymus and Heart.*

[3] Otto, W.R. (2002) Lung epithelial stem cells. *J Pathol, 197*, 527-535.

[4] Giangreco, A., Groot, K.R., Janes, S.M. (2007) Lung cancer and lung stem cells: strange bedfellows? *Am J Respir Crit Care Med, 175*, 547-553.

[5] Giangreco, A., Arwert, E.N., Rosewell, I.R., Snyder, J., Watt, F.M., Stripp, B.R. (2009) Stem cells are dispensable for lung homeostasis but restore airways after injury. *Proc Natl Acad Sci USA, 106*, 9286-9291.

[6] Blanpain, C., Horsley, V., Fuchs, E. Epithelial stem cells: turning over new leaves. (2007) *Cell, 128*, 445-458.

[7] Kitamura, H., Yazawa, T., Shimoyamada, H., Okudela, K., Sato, H. (2008) Molecular and genetic pathogenesis of lung cancer: differences between small-cell and non-small-cell carcinomas. *Open Pathol J, 2*, 106-114. Doi:10.2174/1874375700802010106

[8] Kitamura, H., Yazawa, T., Sato, H., Okudela, K., Shimoyamada, H. (2009) Small cell lung cancer: significance of RB alterations and TTF-1 expression in its carcinogenesis, phenotype, and biology. *Endcr Pathol, 20*, 101-107.

[9] Nuciforo, P., Fraggetta, F. (2004) Cancer stem cell theory: pathologists' considerations and ruminations about wasting time and wrong evaluations. *J Clin Pathol, 7*, 782-783.

[10] Clarke, M.F., Dick, J.E., Dirks, P.B., Eaves, C.J., Jamieson, C.H., Jones, D.L. (2006) Cancer stem cells--perspectives on current status and future directions: AACR Workshop on cancer stem cells. *Cancer Res, 66*, 9339-9344.

[11] Lobo, N.A., Shimono, Y., Qian, D., Clarke, M.F. (2007) The biology of cancer stem cells. *Annu Rev Cell Dev Biol, 23*, 675-699.

[12] Rapp, U.R., Ceteci, F., Schreck, R. (2008) Oncogene-induced plasticity and cancer stem cells. *Cell Cycle, 7*, 45-51.

[13] Kim, C.F., Dirks, P.B. (2008) Cancer and stem cell biology: how tightly intertwined? *Cell Stem Cell, 3*, 147-150.

[14] Yang, Y.M., Chang, J.W. (2008) Current status and issues in cancer stem cell study. *Cancer Invest, 26*, 741-755.

[15] Li, X., Lewis, M.T., Huang, J., Gutierrez, C., Osborne, C.K., Wu, M.F. (2008) Intrinsic resistance of tumorigenic breast cancer cells to chemotherapy. *J Natl Cancer Inst, 100*, 672-679.

[16] Li, L., Borodyansky, L., Yang, Y. (2009) Genomic instability en route to and from cancer stem cells. *Cell Cycle, 8*, 1000-1002.

[17] Hill, R.P. (2006) Identifying cancer stem cells in solid tumors: case not proven. *Cancer Res, 66,* 1883-1890.

[18] Kelly, P.N., Dakic, A., Adams, J.M., Nutt, S.L., Strasser, A. (2007) Tumor growth need not be driven by rare cancer stem cells. *Science, 317,* 337.

[19] Lewis, M.T. (2008) Faith, heresy and the cancer stem cell hypothesis. *Future Oncol, 4,* 585-589.

[20] Yoo, M.H., Hatfield, D.L. (2008) The cancer stem cell theory: is it correct? *Mol Cells, 26,* 514-516.

[21] Vezzoni, L., Parmiani, G. (2008) Limitations of the cancer stem cell theory. *Cytotechnology, 58,* 3-9.

[22] Rowan, K. (2009) Are cancer stem cells real? After four decades, debate still simmers. *J Natl Cancer Inst, 101,* 546-547.

[23] Sneddon, J.B., Werb, Z. (2007) Location, location, location: the cancer stem cell niche. *Cell Stem Cell, 1,* 607-611.

[24] Kitamura, H., Okudela, K., Yazawa, T., Sato, H., Shimoyamada, H. (2009) Cancer stem cell: implications in cancer biology and therapy with special reference to lung cancer. *Lung Cancer, 66,* 275-281.

[25] Sung, J.M., Cho, H.J., Yi, H., Lee, C.H., Kim, H.S., Kim, D.K. (2008) Characterization of a stem cell population in lung cancer A549 cells. *Biochem Biophys Res Commun, 371,* 163-167.

[26] Feldmann, G., Dhara, S., Fendrich, V., Bedja, D., Beaty, R., Mullendore, M., Karikari, C., Alvarez, H., Iacobuzio-Donahue, C., Jimeno, A., Gabrielson, K.L., Matsui, W., Maitra, A. (2007) Blockade of hedgehog signaling pancreatic cancer invasion and metastases: a new paradigm for combination therapy in solid cancers. *Cancer Res, 67,* 2187-96.

[27] Besson, A., Hwang, H.C., Cicero, S., Donovan, S.L., Gurian-West, M., Johnson, D. (2007) Discovery of an oncogenic activity in p27Kip1 that causes stem cell expansion and a multiple tumor phenotype. *Genes Dev, 21,* 1731-1746.

[28] Yin, A.H., Miraglia, S., Zanjani, E.D., Almeida-Porada, G., Ogawa, M., Leary, A.G., et al. (1997) AC133, a novel marker for human hematopoietic stem and progenitor cells. *Blood, 90,* 5002-5012.

[29] Wuchter, C., Ratei, R., Spahn, G., Schoch, C., Harbott, J., Schnittger, S., *et al.* (2001) Impact of CD133 (AC133) and CD90 expression analysis for acute leukemia immunophenotyping. *Haematologica, 86,* 154-161.

[30] Shmelkov, S.V., St. Clair, R., Lyden, D., Rafii, S. (2005) AC133/CD133/Prominin-1. *Int J Biochem Cell Biol, 37,* 715-719.

[31] Uchida, N., Buck, D.W., He, D., Reitsma, M.J., Masek, M., Phan, T.V., *et al.* (2000) Direct isolation of human central nervous system stem cells. *Proc Natl Acad Sci USA, 97,* 14720-14725.

[32] Pötgens, A.J., Bolte, M., Huppertz, B., Kaufmann, P., Frank, H.G. (2001) Human trophoblast contains an intracellular protein reactive with an antibody against CD133--a novel marker for trophoblast. *Placenta, 22,* 39-645.

[33] Salven, P., Mustjoki, S., Alitalo, R., Alitalo, K., Rafii, S. (2003) VEGFR-3 and CD133 identify a population of CD34+ lymphatic/vascular endothelial precursor cells. *Blood, 101,* 168-172.

[34] Richardson, G.D., Robson, C.N., Lang, S.H., Neal, D.E., Maitland, N.J., Collins, A.T. (2004) CD133, a novel marker for human prostatic epithelial stem cells. *Cell Science, 117 pt16,* 3539-3545.

[35] Piechaczek, C. (2001) CD133. *J Biol Regul Homeost Agents, 15,* 101-102.

[36] Yu, Y., Flint, A., Dvorin, E.L., Bischoff, J. (2002) AC133-2, a novel isoform of human AC133 stem cell antigen. *J Biol Chem, 277,* 20711-20716.

[37] Marzesco, A.M., Janich, P., Wilsch-Bräuninger, M., Dubreuil, V., Langenfeld, K., Corbeil, D., *et al.* Release of extracellular membrane particles carrying the stem cell marker prominin-1 (CD133) from neural progenitors and other epithelial cells *J Cell Science, 118 pt13,* 2849-2858.

[38] Taïeb, N., Maresca, M., Guo, X.J., Garmy, N., Fantini, J., Yahi, N. (2009) The first extracellular domain of the tumour stem cell marker CD133 contains an antigenic ganglioside-binding motif. *Cancer Lett, 278,* 164-173.

[39] Choi, D., Lee, H.W., Hur, K.Y., Kim, J.J., Park, G.S., Jang, S.H., et al. Cancer stem cell markers CD133 and CD24 correlate with invasiveness and differentiation in colorectal adenocarcinoma. *World J Gastroenterol, 15,* 2258-2264.

[40] Ahn, S.M., Goode, R.J., Simpson, R.J. (2008) Stem cell markers: insights from membrane proteomics? *Proteomics, 8,* 4946-4957.

[41] Klonisch, T., Wiechec, E., Hombach-Klonisch, S., Ande, S.R., Wesselborg, S., Schulze-Osthoff, K., *et al.* Cancer stem cell markers in common cancers - therapeutic implications. *Trends Mol Med, 14,* 450-460.

[42] Eramo, A., Lotti, F., Sette, G., Pilozzi, E., Biffoni, M., Di Virgilio. A., *et al.* (2008), Identification and expansion of the tumorigenic lung cancer stem cell population. *Cell Death Differ, 15,* 504-514.

[43] Wang, J., Sakariassen, P.Ø., Tsinkalovsky, O., Immervoll, H., Bøe, S.O., Svendsen, A., *et al.* (2008) CD133 negative glioma cells form tumors in nude rats and give rise to CD133 positive cells. *Int J Cancer, 122,* 761-768.

[44] Ogden, A.T., Waziri, A.E., Lochhead, R.A., Fusco, D., Lopez, K., Ellis, J.A., *et al.* (2008) Identification of A2B5+CD133- tumor-initiating cells in adult human gliomas. *Neurosurgery, 60,* 505-514.

[45] Shmelkov, S.V., Butler, J.M., Hooper, A.T., Hormigo, A., Kushner, J., Milde, T., *et al.* (2008) CD133 expression is not restricted to stem cells, and both CD133+ and CD133- metastatic colon cancer cells initiate tumors. *J Clin Invest, 188,* 2111-2120.

[46] Mizrak, D., Brittan, M., Alison, M.R. CD133: molecule of the moment. *J Pathol, 214,* 3-9.

[47] Bidlingmaier, S., Zhu, X., Liu, B. (2008) The utility and limitations of glycosylated human CD133 epitopes in defining cancer stem cells. *J Mol Med, 86,* 1025-1032.

[48] Meng, X., Wang, X., Wang, Y. (2009) More than 45% of A549 and H446 cells are cancer initiating cells: evidence from cloning and tumorigenic analyses. *Oncol Rep, 12,* 995-1000.

[49] Jiang, F., Qiu, Q., Khanna, A., Todd, N.W., Deepak, J., Xing, L, *et al.* (2009) Aldehyde dehydrogenase 1 is a tumor stem cell-associated marker in lung cancer. *Mol Cancer Res, 7,* 330-338

[50] Levina, V., Marrangoni, A.M., DeMarco, R., Gorelik, E., Lokshin, A.E. (2008) Drug-selected human lung cancer stem cells: cytokine network, tumorigenic and metastatic properties. *PLoS ONE, 2,* e3077.

[51] Chen, Y.C., Hsu, H.S., Chen, Y.W., Tsai, T.H., How, C.K., Wang, C.Y., *et al.* (2008) Oct-4 expression maintained cancer stem-like properties in lung cancer-derived CD133-positive cells. *PLoS ONE, 3,* e2637.

[52] Jiang, T., Collins, B.J., Jin, N., Watkins, D.N., Brock, M.V., Matsui, W., *et al.* (2009) Achaete-scute complex homologue 1 regulates tumor-initiating capacity in human small cell lung cancer. *Cancer Res, 69,* 845-854.

[53] Ito, T., Udaka, N., Okudela, K., Yazawa, T., Kitamura, H. (2003) Mechanisms of neuroendocrine differentiation in pulmonary neuroendocrine cells and small cell carcinoma. *Endocr Pathol, 14,* 133-139.

[54] Goodell, M.A., Brose, K., Paradis, G., Conner, A.S., Mulligan, R.C. (1996) Isolation and functional properties of murine hematopoietic stem cells that are replicating in vivo. *J Exp Med, 183,* 1797-1806.

[55] Wu, C., Alman, B.A. Side population cells in human cancers. *Cancer Lett, 268,* 1-9.

[56] Hirschmann-Jax, C., Foster, A.E., Wulf, G.G., Nuchtern, J.G., Jax, T.W., Gobel, U., *et al.* (2004) A distinct "side population" of cells with high drug efflux capacity in human tumor cells. *Proc Natl Acad Sci USA, 101,* 14228-14233.

[57] Hirschmann-Jax, C., Foster, A.E., Wulf, G.G., Goodell, M.A., Brenner, M.K. (2005) A distinct "side population" of cells in human tumor cells: implications for tumor biology and therapy. *Cell Cycle,* 4, 203-205

[58] Zhou, S., Schuetz, J.D., Bunting, K.D., Colapietro, A.M., Sampath, J., Morris, J.J., *et al.* (2001) The ATP binding cassette transporter Bcrp1/ABCG2 is expressed in a wide variety of stem cells and is a molecular determinant of the side-population phenotype. *Nat Med, 7,* 1028-1034.

[59] Telford, W.G., Bradford, J., Godfrey, W., Robey, R.W., Bates, S.E. (2007) Side population analysis using a violet-excited cell-permeable DNA dye. *Stem Cells, 25,* 1029-1036.

[60] Ho MM, Ng AV, Lam S, Hung JY. Side population in human lung cancer cell lines and tumors is enriched with stem-like cancer cells. *Cancer Res* 2007; 67:4827-4833.

[61] Sophos, N.A., Vasiliou, V. (2003) Aldehyde dehydrogenase gene superfamily: the 2009 update. *Chem Biol Interact, 143-144, 5-22.*

[62] Huang, E.H., Hynes, M.J., Zhang, T., Ginestier, C., Dontu, G., Appelman, H., *et al.* (2009) Aldehyde dehydrogenase 1 is a marker for normal and malignant human colonic stem cells (SC) and tracks SC overpopulation during colon tumorigenesis. *Cancer Res, 69,* 3382-3389.

[63] Jones, R.J., Barber, J.P., Vala, M.S., Collector, M.I., Kaufmann, S.H., Ludeman, S.M., *et al.* (1995) Assessment of aldehyde dehydrogenase in viable cells. *Blood, 85,* 2742-2746.

[64] Armstrong, L., Stojkovic, M., Dimmick, I., Ahmad, S., Stojkovic, P., Hole, N., *et al.* (2004) Phenotypic characterization of murine primitive hematopoietic progenitor cells isolated on basis of aldehyde dehydroganse activity. *Stem Cells, 22,* 1142-1151.

[65] Corti, S., Locatelli, F., Papadimitriou, D., Donadoni, C., Salani, S., Del Bo, R., *et al.* (2006) Identification of a primitive brain-derived neural stem cell population based on aldehyde dehydrogenase activity. *Stem Cells, 24,* 975-985.

[66] Ginestier, C., Hur, M.H., Charafe-Jauffret, E., Monville, F., Dutcher, J., Brown, M., et *al.* (2007) ALDH1 is a marker of normal and malignant human mammary stem cells and a predictor of poor clinical outcome. *Cell Stem Cell, 1,* 555-567.

[67] Dylla, S.J., Beviglia, L., Park, I.K., Chartier, C., Raval, J., Ngan, L., *et al.* (2008) Colorectal cancer stem cells are enriched in xenogeneic tumors following chemotherapy. *PLoS ONE, 3,* e2428.

[68] Storms, R.W., Trujillo, A.P., Springer, J.B., Shah, L., Colvin, O.M., Ludeman, S.M., *et al.* (1999) Isolation of primitive human hematopoietic progenitors on the basis of aldehyde dehydrogenase activity. *Proc Natl Acad Sci USA, 96,* 9118-9123.

[69] Koch, L.K., Zhou, H., Ellinger, J., Biermann, K., Höller, T., von Rücker, A., *et al.* (2008) Stem cell marker expression in small cell lung carcinoma and developing lung tissue. *Hum Pathol, 39,* 1597-1605.

[70] Lanza, F., Healy, L., Sutherland, D.R. Structural and functional features of the CD34 antigen: an update. *J Biol Regul Homeost Agents, 15,* 1-13.

[71] Nielsen, J.S., McNagny, K.M. (2008) Novel functions of the CD34 family. *J Cell Sci, 121pt22,* 3683-92.

[72] Doyonnas, R., Nielsen, J.S., Chelliah, S., Drew, E., Hara, T., Miyajima, A., McNagny, K.M. (2005) *Blood, 105,* 4170-4178.

[73] Gutova, M., Najbauer, J., Gevorgyan, A., Metz, M.Z., Weng, Y., Shih, C.C., *et al.* (2007) Identification of uPAR-positive chemoresistant cells in small cell lung cancer. *PLoS ONE, 2,* e243.

[74] Alfano, D., Franco, P., Vocca, I., Gambi, N., Pisa, V., Mancini, A., Caputi, M., Carriero, M.V., Iaccarino, I., Stoppelli, M.P. (2009) The urokinase plasminogen activator and its receptor: role in cell growth and apoptosis. *Thromb Haemost, 93,* 205-211.

[75] Van der Flier, L.G., Clevers, H. (2009) Stem cells, self-renewal, and differentiation in the intestinal epithelium. *Annu Rev Physiol, 71,* 5.1-5.20.

[76] Liao, X., Siu, M.K., Au, C.W., Chan, Q.K., Chan, H.Y., Wong, E.S., et al. (2009) Aberrant activation of hedgehog signaling pathway contributes to endometrial carcinogenesis through β-catenin. *Mod Pathol, 22,* 839-847.

[77] Watkins, D.N., Berman, D.M., Burkholder, S.G., Wang, B., Beachy, P.A., Baylin, S.B. (2003) Hedgehog signalling within airway epithelial progenitors and in small-cell lung cancer. *Nature, 422,* 313-317.

[78] Yagui-Beltrán, A., He, B., Jablons, D.M. (2008) The role of cancer stem cells in neoplasia of the lung: past, present and future. *Clin Transl Oncol, 10,* 719-725.

[79] Peacock, C.D., Watkins, D.N. (2008) Cancer stem cells and the ontogeny of lung cancer. *J Clin Oncol, 26,* 2883-2889.

[80] Lemjabbar-Alaoui, H., Dasari, V., Sidhu, S.S., Mengistab, A., Finkbeiner, W., Gallup, M., *et al.* (2006) Wnt and Hedgehog are critical mediators of cigarette smoke-induced lung cancer. *PLoS ONE, 1,* e93.

[81] Alison, M.R., Islam, S. (2009) Attributes of adult stem cells. *J Pathol, 217,* 144-160.

[82] Polakis, P. (2000) Wnt signaling and cancer. *Genes Dev, 14,* 1837-1851.

[83] Reya, T., Clevers, H. (2005) Wnt signalling in stem cells and cancer. *Nature, 434,* 843-850.

[84] Valk-Lingbeek, M.E., Bruggenman, S.W.M., van Lohuizen, M. (2004) Stem cell and cancer: poly-comb connection. *Cell, 118,* 409-418.

[85] Dovey, J.S., Zacharek, S.J., Kim, C.F., Lees, J.A. (2008) Bmi1 is critical for lung tumorigenesis and bronchioalveolar stem cell expansion. *Proc Natl Acad Sci USA. 105,* 11857-11862.

[86] Ovitt, C.E., Schöler, H.R. (1998) The molecular biology of Oct-4 in the early mouse embryo. *Mol Hum Reprod, 4,* 1021-1031.

[87] Basak, S.K., Veena, M.S., Oh, S., Huang, G., Srivatsan, E., Huang, M., Sharma, S., Batra, R.K. (2009) The malignant pleural effusion as a model to investigate intratumoral heterogeneity in lung cancer. *PLoS One, 4,* e5884.

[88] Collins, A.T., Berry, P.A., Hyde, C., Stower, M.J., Maitland, N.J. (2005) Prospective identification of tumorigenic prostate cancer stem cells. *Cancer Res, 65,* 10946-10951.

[89] Annabi, B., Lachambre, M.P., Plouffe, K., Sartelet, H., Béliveau, R. (2009) Modulation of invasive properties of CD133(+) glioblastoma stem cells: a role for MT1-MMP in bioactive lysophospholipid signaling. *Mol Carcinog, 48,* 910-919.

[90] Li, L., Neaves, W.B. (2006) Normal stem cells and cancer stem cells: the niche matters. *Cancer Res, 66,* 4553-4557.

[91] Hilbe, W., Dirnhofer, S., Oberwasserlechner, F., Schmid, T., Gunsilius, E., Hilbe, G., *et al.* (2004) CD133 positive endothelial progenitor cells contribute to the tumour vasculature in non-small cell lung cancer. *J Clin Pathol, 57,* 965-969.

[92] Moreb, J.S., Baker, H.V., Chang, L.J., Amaya, M., Lopez, M.C., Ostmark, B., Chou, W. (2008) ALDH isozymes downregulation affects cell growth, cell motility and gene expression in lung cancer cells. *Mol Cancer, 7,* 87.

[93] Moreb, J.S., Zucali, J.R., Ostmark, B., Benson, N.A. (2007) Heterogeneity of aldehyde dehydrogenase expression in lung cancer cell lines is revealed by Aldefluor flow cytometry-based assay. *Cytometry B Clin Cytom, 72,* 281-9.

[94] Moreb, J.S. (2008) Aldehyde dehydrogenase as a marker for stem cells. *Curr Stem Cell Res Ther, 3,* 237-46.

[95] Ucar, D., Cogle, C.R., Zucali, J.R., Ostmark, B., Scott, E.W., Zori, R., *et al.* (2009) Aldehyde dehydrogenase activity as a functional marker for lung cancer. *Chem Biol Interact, 178,* 48-55.

[96] Patel, M., Lu, L., Zander, D.S., Sreerama, L., Coco, D., Moreb, J.S. (2008) ALDH1A1 and ALDH3A1 expression in lung cancers: correlation with histologic type and potential precursors. *Lung Cancer, 59,* 340-349.

[97] Carpentino, J.E., Hynes, M.J., Appelman, H.D., Zheng, T., Steindler, D.A., Scott, E.W., Huang, E.H. (2008) Aldehyde dehydrogenase-expressing colon stem cells contribute to tumorigenesis in the transition from colitis to cancer. *Cancer Res, 69,* 8208-8215.

[98] Christ, O., Lucke, K., Imren, S., Leung, K., Hamilton, M., Eaves, A., Smith, C., Eaves, C. (2007) Improved purification of hematopoietic stem cells based on their elevated aldehyde dehydrogenase activity. *Haematologica, 92,* 1165-1172.

[99] Sisson, J.H. (2007) Alcohol and airways function in health and disease. *Alcohol, 41,* 293-307.

[100] Moriwaki, Y., Yamamoto, T., Higashino, K. (1997) Distribution and pathophysiologic role of molybdenum-containing enzymes. *Histol Histopathol, 12,* 513-524.

[101] Yin SJ. Alcohol dehydrogenase: enzymology and metabolism. Alcohol Alcohol Suppl. 1994;2:113-9.

[102] Cozens, A.L., Yezzi, M.J., Kunzelmann, K., Ohrui, T., Chin, L., Eng, K., Finkbeiner, W.E., Widdicombe, J.H., Gruenert, D.C. CFTR expression and chloride secretion in polarized immortal human bronchial epithelial cells. *Am J Respir Cell Mol Biol, 10,* 38-47.

[103] Masuda, A., Kondo, M., Saito, T., Yatabe, Y., Kobayashi, T., Okamoto, M., Suyama, M., Takahashi, T., Takahashi, T. (1997) Establishment of human peripheral lung epithelial cell lines (HPL1) retaining differentiated characteristics and responsiveness to epidermal growth factor, hepatocyte growth factor, and transforming growth factor β1. *Cancer Res, 57,* 4898-4904.

[104] Okudela, K., Hayashi, H., Ito, T., Yazawa, T., Suzuki, T., Nakane, Y., Sato, H., Ishi, H., KeQin, X., Masuda, A., Takahashi, T., Kitamura, H. (2004) K-ras gene mutation enhances motility of immortalized airway cells and lung adenocarcinoma cells via Akt activation: possible contribution to non-invasive expansion of lung adenocarcinoma. *Am J Pathol, 164,* 91-100.

[105] Deshusses JM, Burgess JA, Scherl A, Wenger Y, Walter N, Converset V, Paesano S, Corthals GL, Hochstrasser DF, Sanchez JC. (2003) Exploitation of specific properties of trifluoroethanol for extraction and separation of membrane proteins. *Proteomics, 3,* 1418-1424.

[106] Zhan X, Desiderio DM. (2003) Spot volume vs. amount of protein loaded onto a gel: a detailed, statistical comparison of two gel electrophoresis systems. *Electrophoresis, 24,* 1818-1833.

In: Cancer Stem Cells
Editor: Melissa E. Jordan, pp. 63-77

ISBN: 978-1-61668-971-1
© 2010 Nova Science Publishers, Inc.

Chapter III

MESENCHYMAL STEM CELLS AND THEIR ROLE IN TUMOR PROGRESSION

Jürgen Dittmer[*]

Clinic for Gynecology, University of Halle, Germany.

ABSTRACT

Mesenchymal stem cells (MSCs) are adult stem cells that derive from the bone marrow. A major feature of these cells is their ability to differentiate into adipocytes, chondrocytes or osteocytes. They are also defined by the expression of certain markers, such as CD105, CD73 and CD90, and the lack of others (CD45, CD34, CD14, CD79a and HLA-DR). This expression profile makes them distinct from other bone-derived cells. Several functions have been attributed to MSCs. E.g., MSCs modulate immune responses by suppressing the activities of a number of immune cells. This function is thought to be important to prevent excessive inflammation in the wound healing process. MSCs are chemoattracted to wounds. Probably mistaking tumors for wounds, MSCs also enter solid tumors, where they modulate the activities of tumor cells by exposing them to a plethora of cyto- and chemokines. Recently, MSC-secreted CCL5 has been shown to trigger breast cancer cells to metastasize to lung. Moreover, MSCs are able to differentiate into carcinoma-associated fibroblasts (CAF) which are known to have tumor-promoting activity. This review will summarize the current knowledge on the functions of MSCs in tumor progression.

---

[*] Correspondence concerning this article should be addressed to: Jürgen Dittmer, Clinic for Gynecology, University of Halle, Ernst-Grube-Str. 40, 06120 Halle, Germany. Tel: +49-345-557-1338; Fax: +49-345-557-5261; e.mail: juergen.dittmer@medizin.uni-halle.de.

1. DEFINING MESENCHYMAL STEM CELLS

Mesenchymal stem cells (MSCs) or also called multipotent mesenchymal stromal cells were discovered by Alexander Friedenstein. Friedenstein found a population of bone marrow stromal cells that are distinct from haematopoietic progenitor cells in that they were able to form osseous tissues instead of giving rise to haematopoietic cells [1]. These osteogenic cells are clonogenic cells with fibroblast-like appearance. Owing to their capability of self-maintenance they were classified as stem cells [2,3]. These stem cells are able to differentiate to a number of mesenchymal cells, such as adipocytes, chondroblasts and osteoblasts [4]. MSCs are rare in the bone marrow (1 MSC per 34000 nucleated cells) [5] and are a heterogenous population of cells that show varying developmental potentials (reviewed in [6]). When maintained in vitro, they may quickly lose their potential to differentiate to chondrocytes and adipocytes. Up to now, there are no specific markers defined that allow to clearly identify a cell as an MSC. Instead, a list of minimal criteria has been proposed by the International Society for Cellular Therapy to be used to define an MSC [7]. These criteria include (i) adherence to plastic, (ii) capacity to differentiate to osteoblasts, adipocytes and chondroblasts and (iii) expression of the surface markers CD105 (endoglin), CD73 (ecto 5'-nucleotidase) and CD90 (Thy-1) and lack of the surface markers CD45 (pan-leukocyte marker), CD34 (marker for primitive haematopoietic progenitors and endothelial cells), CD14 and CD11 (markers for monocytes and macrophages), CD79α and CD19 (markers for B-cells) and HLA-DR (provided that MSCs are not stimulated by factors, such as IFN-γ). To isolate human (h)MSCs from bone marrow aspirates cells are grown in culture plastic ware to separate plastic adherent hMSCs from the other non-adherent bone marrow cells. For the verification of the hMSC characteristics, the plastic-adherent cells are tested for their ability to differentiate to osteoblasts, adipocytes and chondroblasts and examined for the expression or lack of expression of the above mentioned markers by FACS analysis [8]. In addition to bone marrow, a variety of other tissues, such as human adipose, can be used as a source for isolating hMSCs [9]. Interestingly, pericytes show characteristics of MSCs [10]. Pericytes isolated from skeletal muscles or non-muscle tissues have the potential to differentiate to osteobasts, adipocytes and chondroblasts and express typical MSC markers.

2. IMMUNOMODULATORY EFFECTS OF MSCs

There is growing evidence that MSCs modulate the activities of immune cells (reviewed in [11]). Immune cells of both types of immunity, innate and adaptive, are affected by MSCs (Table 1). Of the innate immunity, antigen-presenting dendritic cells (DCs), type I interferon-expression plasmacytoid dendritic cells (pDCs), anti-tumor acting natural killer (NK) cells and anti-bacterial acting neutrophils are targets of MSCs. Of the adaptive immunity, B-cells and different types of T-cells are susceptible to MSCs. Dendritic cells are important for antigen presentation. MSCs have been shown to block the maturation of monocytes to mature dendritic cells [12,13] suggesting that antigen presentation and, hence, immune responses are suppressed by MSCs. Also the expression levels of a number of cytokines in DCs are altered by MSCs [14]. Interestingly, while the secretion of the anti-inflammatory interleukin-10 is upregulated, the expression of the pro-inflammatory tumor necrosis factor is reduced [14,15] supporting the notion that MSCs have the potential to act immunosuppressive. MSCs' interference with the immune system is continued on the level of T-cells. First, as a consequence of MSCs negative effect of DC maturation the number of T-cells activated by DC-dependent antigen presentation decline. Second, MSCs inhibit the proliferation of activated T-cells [16-19] by arresting them in the G1 phase [20]. The G1 arrest was accompanied by downregulation of cyclin D2 and upregulation of $p27^{kip1}$. In addition, in response to MSCs, a shift in the T-helper cell population from pro-inflammatory T_H1 to anti-inflammatory T_H2 cells and an expansion of suppressive regulatory $CD4^+$ T-cells are observed [14,51] which may reduce T-helper cell-dependent B-cell response and hence antibody production. This may further contribute to the immunosuppressive effect of MSCs. In respect to the immune response to tumor cells, it is striking that MSCs inhibit the activity of $CD8^+$ cytotoxic T-cells [22] as well as the proliferation of cytotoxic NK-cells [14,23,24]. Hence, MSCs attack anti-tumor effector cells of both the adaptive and innate immune system and may therefore reduce the ability of the immune system to recognize and eliminate tumor cells. It is interesting that MSCs can also be targeted NK cells as MSCs express low levels of MHC class I molecules [25]. In the presence of interferon γ which increases the expression level of the MHC class I molecules, MSCs are more protected against NK-mediating cytotoxicity [25]. The balance between MSCs and NK cells and hence the extent of the cytotoxic effect of NK cells on tumor cells may therefore be dependent upon the level of certain cytokines. The effect of MSCs on immune cells seems to be accomplished by direct cell-cell contact and by soluble factors that are secreted by MSCs. Among these MSC-released factors are prostaglandin E2, interleukin-6, indoleamine 2,3-dioxygenase (IDO) and sHLA-G5 [14,21,23,26]. The expression of CD90 seems to be important for the immunosuppressive activity of MSCs, as downregulation of CD90 resulted in loss of the inhibitory effect of MSCs on the proliferation of PHA-stimulated peripheral blood lymphocytes [27,28]. This was accompanied by reduced secretion of sHLA-G und interleukin-10.

3. MSCs AND INJURIES

Inflammation seems to attract MSCs [31]. MSCs have been suggested to "sense" injuries as they enter wounds to contribute to wound healing [32-37]. By using bioluminescent imaging, Kidd et al. showed that, when injected to injured mice, MSCs expressing the firefly luciferase were predominantly visible in wounds, whereas, in non-injured mice, MSCs were found in lungs, liver and spleen [38]. Facilitated wound healing by MSCs could be demonstrated, when the lungs of mice were injured by bleomycin. MSCs that colonized the injured lung differentiated to specific lung epithelium-like cell phenotypes and suppressed inflammation and collagen deposition [32,39]. Intravenously delivered MSCs into rats have been shown to ameliorate recovery from middle cerebral artery occlusion (MCAO)-evoked stroke [34,40]. This was accompanied by the presence of MSCs in the ischemic hemisphere. Differentiation of MSCs to cells expressing neuronal markers have also been observed [40]. The notion that MSCs are able to differentiate to neurons has been supported by experiments with MSCs derived from umbilical cord blood [41-43]. However, whether MSCs are in fact able to transdifferentiate into neurons is a matter of debate, since MSCs have been shown to spontaneously fuse with other cells [44,45]. MSCs have also been reported to enter lesions of chronic rejection in rats with cardiac grafts or to invade infarcted myocards where they differentiate to fibroblasts or even to cardiomyocytes [37,46,47]. In the presence of MSCs, rats showed better recovery from kidney damage (mesangiolysis) [48]. The regenerated glomeruli contained MSC-derived glomerular cells. Also, ischemically injured renal tubules in mice could be repaired by MSCs which differentiated to tubular epithelial cells [49,50]. In diabetic mice, intracardically infused or intravenously injected MSCs increased the number of pancreatic islets and insulin production [51,52]. Some of the pancreatic islets contained hMSC-derived insulin-producing cells.

Table 1. Effects of MSCs on immune cells

type of immunity	cell type	function	effects of MSCs	MSC-released factor(s) involved	references
innate	dendritic cells (DCs), plasmacytoid DCs (pDCs)	antigen-presenting, expression of type I interferon	impairment of antigen-presenting function, inhibition of tumor necrosis factor production, increased expression of anti-inflammatory cytokine IL-10	prostaglandin E2	[12-14]
innate	natural killer cells (NKs)	anti-viral and anti-tumor effector activities	inhibition of cytotoxic effects, anti-proliferative, inhibition of interferon γ production	prostaglandin E2	[14, 23, 24]
innate	neutrophils	defense against bacteria	inhibition of respiratory burst activity and apoptosis	interleukin-6	[26]
adaptive	T-cells	several effector functions	anti-proliferative, increased survival of quiescent cells, decreased interferon γ production, decreased cytotoxicity as mediated by cytotoxic T-cells (CTL)	prostaglandin E2 / sHLA-GS / indoleamine 2,3-dioxygenase (IDO)	[14, 16-22]
adaptive	B-cells	antibody productions	controversial, maybe anti-proliferative		[20, 29, 30]

The apparent plasticity of MSCs and their ability to predominantly colonizes wounds have fueled the hope that MSCs are ideal tools for tissue regeneration [31]. In particular, MSCs may be useful agents to treat neurological disorders and spinal cord injury [53] as well as the infarcted myocardium [35,54,55]. MSCs can potentially also be used as vehicles to administer drugs to sites of injuries. E.g., BDNF (brain-derived neurotrophic factor) expressing MSCs have been injected into rats to improve recovery from stroke [34]. Similarly, insulin-producing MSCs have been administered to mice to treat diabetes [56]. However, this enthusiasm has recently been dampened by the observation that hMSC frequently undergo spontaneous malignant transformation *in vitro* [57]. The transformed hMSCs were shown to trigger the development of lung cancer in mice. In addition, hMSCs can be transformed into sarcoma cells [58-60]. Whether hMSCs injected in humans for therapeutic uses will also transform and induce cancer is not yet know.

4. MSCs AND CANCER

MSCs are also attracted to tumors [38,61,62]. E.g., luciferase-loaden MSCs specifically accumulated in breast cancer xenografts in mice [38]. Tumors can be assumed to be wounds that never heal [63]. It is, therefore, thought that MSCs "mistake" tumors for normal wounds, probably as a result of similar inflammatory signals that are released by wounds and tumors [64]. A number of studies support this hypothesis. When prostate Capan-1 cancer cells were injected into SCID (severe combined immunodeficient) mice whose bone marrow was replaced by bone marrow from beta-galactosidase transgenic mice, X-gal positive cells were identified in the tumor [65]. The X-gal positive cells were mostly fibroblasts and to a lesser extent endothelial cells suggesting that X-gal positive MSCs entered the tumor and differentiated into various stromal cells. In a similar way, bone marrow of a GFP-positive mouse was transplanted into a GFP-negative mouse with pancreatic insulinoma. GFP-positive cells were found within the tumor [66]. Of the myofibroblasts in the tumor, 25% were GFP positive and, hence, derived from the donor bone marrow.

The ability to trace and invade tumors may make MSCs a good tool for delivering anti-tumor drugs to the tumors. A number of studies have been undertaken to analyze this interesting possibility. In these studies, MSCs loaded with chemokines, cytokines or oncolytic viruses were injected into tumor-bearing mice. In one study, MSCs was engineered to express the immunostimulatory chemokine CX3CL1. It was found that CX3CL1-expressing MSCs inhibited lung metastasis formation by B16.F10 murine melanoma and C26 murine colon carcinoma cells [62]. Likewise, the growth of malignant human A375SM melanoma cells in mice was decreased when mice were injected with hMSCs expressing interferon β [61]. Also, TRAIL (TNF-related apoptosis inducing ligand) expressing hMSCs inhibited growth of DLD-1 colorectal cancer cells and U87 glioma cells in mouse xenografts [67, 68]. Another study showed that interleukin-2 overexpressing rat MSCs home to tumors formed by 9L gliomas and reduce their growth [69]. Fritz et al. transfected murine MSCs with the uPA (urokinase plasminogen activator) inhibitor hATF, an amino-terminal fragment of uPA, and administered these cells to mice to successfully treat bone lesions as induced by metastatic prostate cancer cells [70]. Two groups used hMSCs as vehicles to specifically deliver the oncolytic Delta24-RGD or CRAd adenovirus to glioma xenografts formed by U87MG or U251-V121 glioma cells [71,72]. These adenovirus-infected hMSCs entered the tumors and induced tumor growth inhibition or even elimination. Another interesting approach is the use of MSCs for localized chemotherapy. hMSCs were forced to express cytosine deaminase (CD), a prodrug activating enzyme that converts 5-fluorocytosine (5-FC) into the commonly used drug 5-fluorouracil (5-FU), and injected into mice bearing gastric cancer xenografts [73]. When these mice were systemically treated with 5-FC, tumor volume significantly decreased compared to the control group which did not receive hMSCs. In contrast to CD-expressing hMSCs, control hMSCs had no effect on tumor growth suggesting that the hMSC-CD-dependent conversion of 5-FC to 5-FU was required for the tumor-inhibiting effect.

Even if not loaded with anti-tumor drugs, MSCs are capable of interfering with tumor progression, as they are able to directly interact with tumor cells and to expose tumor cells to the many chemokines and cytokines they secret. Among the factors that they secret are interleukins, such as IL-6 and IL-8, other cytokines, such as TGFβ (transforming growth factor β) 1 and 2 [74] and chemokines, such als CCL2, CCL5 and CXCL12 (SDF-1 = stromal cell derived factor 1). hMSC-derived CCL5 (Rantes) may play an important role in breast cancer metastasis. When hMSCs and MDA-MB-231 breast cancer cells were subcutaneously co-injected into mice, MSCs stimulated breast cancer cells to metastasize to lung, an effect that could be mimicked by CCL5 [75]. Knock-down of the CCL5 receptor CCR in MDA-MB-231 cells abrogated the response of these cells to hMSCs suggesting that the MDA-MB-231/hMSC communication depended upon the interaction of CCL5 with CCR5. Effects of hMSCs on other types of breast cancer cells have also been reported. hMSCs have been found to promote the motility of MCF-7 cells [76], which, in contrast to the mesenchymal MDA-MB-231 cells, are epithelial-like breast cancer cells. As such they produce E-cadherin which causes these cells to form tight cell-cell contacts. Hence, the E-cadherin based cell-cell interaction needs to be interrupted to allow movement of MCF-7 cells. Consequently, E-cadherin expression in MCF-7 cells grown in conventional two-dimensional adherent cultures was found to be downregulated in the presence of MSCs [77,78]. In three-dimensional spheroid cultures, hMSCs caused the MCF-7 cell-cell contacts to be become less tight which was accompanied by E-cadherin shedding (removal of the extracellular E-cadherin domain) [76]. E-cadherin shedding in MCF-7 cells was demonstrated to be dependent on the metalloprotease ADAM10 (a disintegrin and metalloprotease 10). As inhibition of this enzyme by the specific inhibitor GI254023X blocked hMSC-induced motility of MCF-7 cells it is likely that hMSCs interfered with the activity of ADAM10 to increase the migratory activity of MCF-7. Unlike the effect of hMSCs on the metastasic activity of MDA-MB-231 cells, the hMSC effect on the migratory activity of MCF-7 cells could not be mimicked by CCL5 suggesting that hMSCs affect the behavior of mesenchymal and epithelial-like breast cancer cells by different factors. Besides migration, hMSCs have also been shown to increase breast cancer growth *in vivo* and *in vitro* [79, 80]. In SCID/beige mice, hMSCs allowed estrogen-receptor α (ERα)-expressing MCF-7 cells to grow independently of estrogen [79]. Interestingly, this was accompanied by an increased level of the progesterone receptor. These data may indicate that hMSCs play a role in the development of resistance towards anti-estrogens which are used to treat breast cancer patients with ERα-positive breast cancer. In three-dimensional *in vitro* cultures, hMSCs were found to promote the growth of MCF-7 cells and a number of other ERα-positive breast cancer cells (T47D, BT474 and ZR-75-1) [80]. It is noteworthy that the growth of the fast-growing MDA-MB-231 cells were not affected by hMSCs. Likewise, the effect of hMSCs on the migration of the fast-migrating MDA-MB-231 cells was much weaker than on slow-migrating MCF-7 cells [76]. It seems, therefore, that aggressive MDA-MB-231 cells already reached their limits in regard to their migratory and proliferative activities so that hMSCs are not able to further enhance them. In contrast, the metastatic potential of MDA-MB-231 cells may not be fully exploited and, hence, can be further increased by MSCs via CCL5.

MSCs also affect other types of cancer. Yu et al. showed that MSCs isolated from adipose tissues stimulated tumor growth when injected together with the lung cancer cell line H460 or the human glioblastoma-astrocytoma cell line U87MG in nude mice [81]. In tissue culture experiments, hMSCs stimulated the proliferation of H460 or U87MG cells suggesting that the effect of hMSCs on tumor growth was direct. Also indirect effects of MSCs on tumor expansion has been described. Djouad et al. showed that B16 melanoma cells, that were able to form tumors in immunocompetent syngeneic mice, failed to do so in allogeneic mice [82]. Tumor growth by B16 cells could be rescued in allogeneic mice, if MSCs were co-injected along with the B16 cancer cells. It is thought that, in the allogenic mice, the immunosuppressive activity of the MSCs prevented clearance of the tumor cells by the host immune system. Djouad and co-workers also demonstrated that Renca adenocarcinoma cells grew faster in mice when co-injected with MSCs [83], although, *in vitro* co-culture experiments, MSCs failed to affect the growth rate of Renca cells. Again it is believed that MSCs stimulated tumor growth *in vivo* by inhibiting the immune response.

Some studies show that MSCs can also act inhibitory on tumor growth. When Maestroni et al. compared the ability of Lewis lung carcinoma or B16 melanoma to form tumors in mice in the presence vs. absence of MSCs they found that, in the presence of bone marrow stroma, tumor formation was attenuated [84]. Similarly, when rat colon carcinoma cells entrapped in a gelatin matrix were implanted into rats, the extent of tumor outgrowth was reduced when MSCs were present [85]. Also the growth of gliomas in Fisher 344 rats was reported to be negatively modulated by MSCs [69].

Another study showed that hMSCs intravenously injected into athymic nude mice bearing Kaposi sarcomas entered the tumors and inhibited their growth [86]. This growth-inhibitory effect of hMSCs was accompanied by a decrease in the activity of AKT in the tumor cells suggesting that hMSCs induced an inhibition of the PI3K/AKT pathway. In support of this notion, overexpression of a constitutively active form of AKT rendered the Kaposi sarcoma cells resistant to hMSCs. The hMSC effect on the Kaposi sarcoma cells seems to be mediated by direct cell-cell contact as antibodies against E-cadherin prevented hMSC from modulating the tumor cell activity. Qiao et al found that, when hMSCs were injected together with H7402 or HepG2 hepatoma cells into SCID mice, the onset of tumor formation was delayed [87]. The anti-tumor effect of hMSCs was confirmed by tissue culture experiments demonstrating that hMSCs decreased proliferation and increased apoptosis by reducing the expression of pro-apoptotic proteins.

Cancer cells have also been shown to act back on MSCs. MDA-MB-231 and to a lesser extent MCF-7 breast cancer cells were found to stimulate the migratory activity of hMSCs in the Boyden chamber [76]. This effect could be mimicked by conditioned medium derived from these breast cancer cell lines. In addition, hMSCs were found to move towards and enter MCF-7 spheroids. Three MDA-MB-231 derived factors, the chemokine MCP-1 (CCL-2), cyclophilin B and hepatoma-derived growth factor (HDGF), have been shown to be able to stimulate hMSC migration [88,89]. Of these, MCP-1 are also secreted by the T47D breast cancer cell line as well as by primary breast cancer-derived stromal and epithelial cells [89]. Hence, breast cancer cells in general may be able to enhance the migratory activity of hMSCs. Also conditioned medium (CM) from B85 human colorectal cancer cells stimulated the migration of hMSCs [90]. Comparative cDNA microarray analyses of the hMSC exposed to CM from B85 cells and bone marrow revealed that the expression of 104 genes were upregulated in response to B85-CM. These genes included a number of genes coding for chemokines, such as SDF-1 (CXCL-12) and MCP-1. Interestingly, knock-down of SDF-1 in hMSCs abrogated the stimulatory effect of B85-CM. This suggests that factor(s) secreted by B85 colorectal cancer cells stimulated an SDF-1 dependent autocrine loop in hMSCs causing these cells to move faster.

CONCLUSIONS

There is striking evidence that MSCs are attracted to wounds and facilitate wound healing by downregulating the inflammatory response and by differentiating to those cell types that are required to restore the function of the injured tissue. Given their imazing plasticity MSCs may generally function as "repair cells" that quickly adopt to the needs of the tissue to which they have been recruited. In terms of cancer, this need may be the recruitment of cells that promote proliferation and migration and inhibit apoptosis. In fact, exposed to tumor-conditioned medium, MSCs have been found to differentiate to carcinoma-associated fibroblasts (CAFs) that are known to be involved in cancer progression [91]. Cancer may also "use" MSCs as a shield against the attack by the immune system. And, since exposure of cancer to anti-cancer drugs have been shown to result in an increase of a population of cells that express stem cell markers [92], MSCs may also help cancer cells to survive drug attacks as MSCs are drug-resistant [93]. The similarity of MSCs with cancer stem cells (CSCs) has even led to the discussion of whether, in certain cancers, CSCs are MSCs [94]. On the other hand, their tropism for cancers makes MSCs an ideal tool for delivering anti-cancer drugs to many types of cancers and may help to develop more specific strategies for cancer treatment.

REFERENCES

[1] Friedenstein, A. J., Piatetzky, S., II & Petrakova, K. V. (1966) Osteogenesis in transplants of bone marrow cells. *J Embryol Exp Morphol, 16*, 381-390.

[2] Friedenstein, A. & Kuralesova, A. I. (1971) Osteogenic precursor cells of bone marrow in radiation chimeras. *Transplantation, 12*, 99-108.

[3] Caplan, A. I. (1991) Mesenchymal stem cells. *J Orthop Res., 9*, 641-650.

[4] Friedenstein, A. J., Chailakhyan, R. K., Latsinik, N. V., Panasyuk, A. F. & Keiliss-Borok, I. V. (1974) Stromal cells responsible for transferring the microenvironment of the hemopoietic tissues. Cloning in vitro and retransplantation in vivo. *Transplantation, 17*, 331-340.

[5] Wexler, S. A., Donaldson, C., Denning-Kendall, P., Rice, C., Bradley, B. & Hows, J. M. (2003) Adult bone marrow is a rich source of human mesenchymal 'stem' cells but umbilical cord and mobilized adult blood are not. *Br J Haematol, 121*, 368-374.

[6] Phinney, D. G. (2002) Building a consensus regarding the nature and origin of mesenchymal stem cells. *J Cell Biochem Suppl, 38*, 7-12.

[7] Dominici, M., Le Blanc, K., Mueller, I., Slaper-Cortenbach, I., Marini, F., Krause, D., Deans, R., Keating, A., Prockop, D. & Horwitz, E. (2006) Minimal criteria for defining multipotent mesenchymal stromal cells. The International Society for Cellular Therapy position statement. *Cytotherapy, 8*, 315-317.

[8] Beyer Nardi, N. & da Silva Meirelles, L. (2006) Mesenchymal stem cells: isolation, in vitro expansion and characterization. *Handb Exp Pharmacol*, 249-282.

[9] Zuk, P. A., Zhu, M., Mizuno, H., Huang, J., Futrell, J. W., Katz, A. J., Benhaim, P., Lorenz, H. P. & Hedrick, M. H. (2001) Multilineage cells from human adipose tissue: implications for cell-based therapies. *Tissue Eng, 7*, 211-228.

[10]Crisan, M., Yap, S., Casteilla, L., Chen, C. W., Corselli, M., Park, T. S., Andriolo, G., Sun, B., Zheng, B., Zhang, L., Norotte, C., Teng, P. N., Traas, J., Schugar, R., Deasy, B. M., Badylak, S., Buhring, H. J., Giacobino, J. P., Lazzari, L., Huard, J. & Peault, B. (2008) A perivascular origin for mesenchymal stem cells in multiple human organs. *Cell Stem Cell, 3*, 301-313.

[11]Uccelli, A., Moretta, L. & Pistoia, V. (2008) Mesenchymal stem cells in health and disease. *Nat Rev Immunol, 8*, 726-736.

[12]Jiang, X. X., Zhang, Y., Liu, B., Zhang, S. X., Wu, Y., Yu, X. D. & Mao, N. (2005) Human mesenchymal stem cells inhibit differentiation and function of monocyte-derived dendritic cells. *Blood, 105*, 4120-4126.

[13]Ramasamy, R., Fazekasova, H., Lam, E. W., Soeiro, I., Lombardi, G. & Dazzi, F. (2007) Mesenchymal stem cells inhibit dendritic cell differentiation and function by preventing entry into the cell cycle. *Transplantation, 83*, 71-76.

[14]Aggarwal, S. & Pittenger, M. F. (2005) Human mesenchymal stem cells modulate allogeneic immune cell responses. *Blood, 105*, 1815-1822.

[15]Beyth, S., Borovsky, Z., Mevorach, D., Liebergall, M., Gazit, Z., Aslan, H., Galun, E. & Rachmilewitz, J. (2005) Human mesenchymal stem cells alter antigen-presenting cell maturation and induce T-cell unresponsiveness. *Blood, 105*, 2214-2219.

[16]Bartholomew, A., Sturgeon, C., Siatskas, M., Ferrer, K., McIntosh, K., Patil, S., Hardy, W., Devine, S., Ucker, D., Deans, R., Moseley, A. & Hoffman, R. (2002) Mesenchymal stem cells suppress lymphocyte proliferation in vitro and prolong skin graft survival in vivo. *Exp Hematol, 30*, 42-48.

[17]Di Nicola, M., Carlo-Stella, C., Magni, M., Milanesi, M., Longoni, P. D., Matteucci, P., Grisanti, S. & Gianni, A. M. (2002) Human bone marrow stromal cells suppress T-lymphocyte proliferation induced by cellular or nonspecific mitogenic stimuli. *Blood, 99*, 3838-3843.

[18]Rasmusson, I., Ringden, O., Sundberg, B. & Le Blanc, K. (2005) Mesenchymal stem cells inhibit lymphocyte proliferation by mitogens and alloantigens by different mechanisms. *Exp Cell Res, 305*, 33-41.

[19]Krampera, M., Glennie, S., Dyson, J., Scott, D., Laylor, R., Simpson, E. & Dazzi, F. (2003) Bone marrow mesenchymal stem cells inhibit the response of naive and memory antigen-specific T cells to their cognate peptide. *Blood, 101*, 3722-3729.

[20]Glennie, S., Soeiro, I., Dyson, P. J., Lam, E. W. & Dazzi, F. (2005) Bone marrow mesenchymal stem cells induce division arrest anergy of activated T cells. *Blood, 105*, 2821-2827.

[21]Selmani, Z., Naji, A., Zidi, I., Favier, B., Gaiffe, E., Obert, L., Borg, C., Saas, P., Tiberghien, P., Rouas-Freiss, N., Carosella, E. D. & Deschaseaux, F. (2008) Human leukocyte antigen-G5 secretion by human mesenchymal stem cells is required to suppress T lymphocyte and natural killer function and to induce CD4+CD25highFOXP3+ regulatory T cells. *Stem Cells, 26*, 212-222.

[22]Rasmusson, I., Ringden, O., Sundberg, B. & Le Blanc, K. (2003) Mesenchymal stem cells inhibit the formation of cytotoxic T lymphocytes, but not activated cytotoxic T lymphocytes or natural killer cells. *Transplantation, 76*, 1208-1213.

[23]Spaggiari, G. M., Capobianco, A., Abdelrazik, H., Becchetti, F., Mingari, M. C. & Moretta, L. (2008) Mesenchymal stem cells inhibit natural killer-cell proliferation,

cytotoxicity, and cytokine production: role of indoleamine 2,3-dioxygenase and prostaglandin E2. *Blood, 111*, 1327-1333.

[24] Sotiropoulou, P. A., Perez, S. A., Gritzapis, A. D., Baxevanis, C. N. & Papamichail, M. (2006) Interactions between human mesenchymal stem cells and natural killer cells. *Stem Cells, 24*, 74-85.

[25] Spaggiari, G. M., Capobianco, A., Becchetti, S., Mingari, M. C. & Moretta, L. (2006) Mesenchymal stem cell-natural killer cell interactions: evidence that activated NK cells are capable of killing MSCs, whereas MSCs can inhibit IL-2-induced NK-cell proliferation. *Blood, 107*, 1484-1490.

[26] Raffaghello, L., Bianchi, G., Bertolotto, M., Montecucco, F., Busca, A., Dallegri, F., Ottonello, L. & Pistoia, V. (2008) Human mesenchymal stem cells inhibit neutrophil apoptosis: a model for neutrophil preservation in the bone marrow niche. *Stem Cells, 26*, 151-162.

[27] Campioni, D., Lanza, F., Moretti, S., Ferrari, L. & Cuneo, A. (2008) Loss of Thy-1 (CD90) antigen expression on mesenchymal stromal cells from hematologic malignancies is induced by in vitro angiogenic stimuli and is associated with peculiar functional and phenotypic characteristics. *Cytotherapy, 10*, 69-82.

[28] Campioni, D., Rizzo, R., Stignani, M., Melchiorri, L., Ferrari, L., Moretti, S., Russo, A., Bagnara, G. P., Bonsi, L., Alviano, F., Lanzoni, G., Cuneo, A., Baricordi, O. R. & Lanza, F. (2009) A decreased positivity for CD90 on human mesenchymal stromal cells (MSCs) is associated with a loss of immunosuppressive activity by MSCs. *Cytometry B Clin Cytom, 76*, 225-230.

[29] Corcione, A., Benvenuto, F., Ferretti, E., Giunti, D., Cappiello, V., Cazzanti, F., Risso, M., Gualandi, F., Mancardi, G. L., Pistoia, V. & Uccelli, A. (2006) Human mesenchymal stem cells modulate B-cell functions. *Blood, 107*, 367-372.

[30] Traggiai, E., Volpi, S., Schena, F., Gattorno, M., Ferlito, F., Moretta, L. & Martini, A. (2008) Bone marrow-derived mesenchymal stem cells induce both polyclonal expansion and differentiation of B cells isolated from healthy donors and systemic lupus erythematosus patients. *Stem Cells, 26*, 562-569.

[31] Brooke, G., Cook, M., Blair, C., Han, R., Heazlewood, C., Jones, B., Kambouris, M., Kollar, K., McTaggart, S., Pelekanos, R., Rice, A., Rossetti, T. & Atkinson, K. (2007) Therapeutic applications of mesenchymal stromal cells. *Semin Cell Dev Biol, 18*, 846-858.

[32] Rojas, M., Xu, J., Woods, C. R., Mora, A. L., Spears, W., Roman, J. & Brigham, K. L. (2005) Bone marrow-derived mesenchymal stem cells in repair of the injured lung. *Am J Respir Cell Mol Biol, 33*, 145-152.

[33] Natsu, K., Ochi, M., Mochizuki, Y., Hachisuka, H., Yanada, S. & Yasunaga, Y. (2004) Allogeneic bone marrow-derived mesenchymal stromal cells promote the regeneration of injured skeletal muscle without differentiation into myofibers. *Tissue Eng, 10*, 1093-1112.

[34] Kurozumi, K., Nakamura, K., Tamiya, T., Kawano, Y., Kobune, M., Hirai, S., Uchida, H., Sasaki, K., Ito, Y., Kato, K., Honmou, O., Houkin, K., Date, I. & Hamada, H. (2004) BDNF gene-modified mesenchymal stem cells promote functional recovery and reduce infarct size in the rat middle cerebral artery occlusion model. *Mol Ther, 9*, 189-197.

[35] Barbash, I. M., Chouraqui, P., Baron, J., Feinberg, M. S., Etzion, S., Tessone, A., Miller, L., Guetta, E., Zipori, D., Kedes, L. H., Kloner, R. A. & Leor, J. (2003) Systemic

delivery of bone marrow-derived mesenchymal stem cells to the infarcted myocardium: feasibility, cell migration, and body distribution. *Circulation, 108*, 863-868.

[36] Mahmood, A., Lu, D., Lu, M. & Chopp, M. (2003) Treatment of traumatic brain injury in adult rats with intravenous administration of human bone marrow stromal cells. *Neurosurgery, 53*, 697-702.

[37] Wu, G. D., Nolta, J. A., Jin, Y. S., Barr, M. L., Yu, H., Starnes, V. A. & Cramer, D. V. (2003) Migration of mesenchymal stem cells to heart allografts during chronic rejection. *Transplantation, 75*, 679-685.

[38] Kidd, S., Spaeth, E., Dembinski, J. L., Dietrich, M., Watson, K., Klopp, A., Battula, V. L., Weil, M., Andreeff, M. & Marini, F. C. (2009) Direct evidence of mesenchymal stem cell tropism for tumor and wounding microenvironments using in vivo bioluminescent imaging. *Stem Cells, 27*, 2614-2623.

[39] Ortiz, L. A., Gambelli, F., McBride, C., Gaupp, D., Baddoo, M., Kaminski, N. & Phinney, D. G. (2003) Mesenchymal stem cell engraftment in lung is enhanced in response to bleomycin exposure and ameliorates its fibrotic effects. *Proc Natl Acad Sci U S A, 100*, 8407-8411.

[40] Chen, J., Li, Y., Wang, L., Zhang, Z., Lu, D., Lu, M. & Chopp, M. (2001) Therapeutic benefit of intravenous administration of bone marrow stromal cells after cerebral ischemia in rats. *Stroke, 32*, 1005-1011.

[41] Park, K. S., Jung, K. H., Kim, S. H., Kim, K. S., Choi, M. R., Kim, Y. & Chai, Y. G. (2007) Functional expression of ion channels in mesenchymal stem cells derived from umbilical cord vein. *Stem Cells, 25*, 2044-2052.

[42] Li, G. R., Sun, H., Deng, X. & Lau, C. P. (2005) Characterization of ionic currents in human mesenchymal stem cells from bone marrow. *Stem Cells, 23*, 371-38.

[43] Tondreau, T., Lagneaux, L., Dejeneffe, M., Massy, M., Mortier, C., Delforge, A. & Bron, D. (2004) Bone marrow-derived mesenchymal stem cells already express specific neural proteins before any differentiation. *Differentiation, 72*, 319-326.

[44] Krabbe, C., Zimmer, J. & Meyer, M. (2005) Neural transdifferentiation of mesenchymal stem cells--a critical review. *Apmis, 113*, 831-844.

[45] Wislet-Gendebien, S., Hans, G., Leprince, P., Rigo, J. M., Moonen, G. & Rogister, B. (2005) Plasticity of cultured mesenchymal stem cells: switch from nestin-positive to excitable neuron-like phenotype. *Stem Cells, 23*, 392-402.

[46] Toma, C., Pittenger, M. F., Cahill, K. S., Byrne, B. J. & Kessler, P. D. (2002) Human mesenchymal stem cells differentiate to a cardiomyocyte phenotype in the adult murine heart. *Circulation, 105*, 93-98.

[47] Wang, J. S., Shum-Tim, D., Chedrawy, E. & Chiu, R. C. (2001) The coronary delivery of marrow stromal cells for myocardial regeneration: pathophysiologic and therapeutic implications. *J Thorac Cardiovasc Surg, 122*, 699-705.

[48] Ito, T., Suzuki, A., Imai, E., Okabe, M. & Hori, M. (2001) Bone marrow is a reservoir of repopulating mesangial cells during glomerular remodeling. *J Am Soc Nephrol,* 12, 2625-2635.

[49] Lin, F., Cordes, K., Li, L., Hood, L., Couser, W. G., Shankland, S. J. & Igarashi, P. (2003) Hematopoietic stem cells contribute to the regeneration of renal tubules after renal ischemia-reperfusion injury in mice. *J Am Soc Nephrol, 14*, 1188-1199.

[50]Kale, S., Karihaloo, A., Clark, P. R., Kashgarian, M., Krause, D. S. & Cantley, L. G. (2003) Bone marrow stem cells contribute to repair of the ischemically injured renal tubule. *J Clin Invest, 112*, 42-49.

[51]Lee, R. H., Seo, M. J., Reger, R. L., Spees, J. L., Pulin, A. A., Olson, S. D. & Prockop, D. J. (2006) Multipotent stromal cells from human marrow home to and promote repair of pancreatic islets and renal glomeruli in diabetic NOD/scid mice. *Proc Natl Acad Sci U S A, 103*, 17438-17443.

[52]Hess, D., Li, L., Martin, M., Sakano, S., Hill, D., Strutt, B., Thyssen, S., Gray, D. A. & Bhatia, M. (2003) Bone marrow-derived stem cells initiate pancreatic regeneration. *Nat Biotechnol, 21*, 763-770.

[53]Phinney, D. G. & Isakova, I. (2005) Plasticity and therapeutic potential of mesenchymal stem cells in the nervous system. *Curr Pharm Des, 11*, 1255-1265.

[54]Amado, L. C., Saliaris, A. P., Schuleri, K. H., St John, M., Xie, J. S., Cattaneo, S., Durand, D. J., Fitton, T., Kuang, J. Q., Stewart, G., Lehrke, S., Baumgartner, W. W., Martin, B. J., Heldman, A. W. & Hare, J. M. (2005) Cardiac repair with intramyocardial injection of allogeneic mesenchymal stem cells after myocardial infarction. *Proc Natl Acad Sci U S A, 102*, 11474-11479.

[55]Itescu, S., Schuster, M. D. & Kocher, A. A. (2003) New directions in strategies using cell therapy for heart disease. *J Mol Med, 81*, 288-296.

[56]Xu, J., Lu, Y., Ding, F., Zhan, X., Zhu, M. & Wang, Z. (2007) Reversal of diabetes in mice by intrahepatic injection of bone-derived GFP-murine mesenchymal stem cells infected with the recombinant retrovirus-carrying human insulin gene. *World J Surg, 31*, 1872-1882.

[57]Rosland, G. V., Svendsen, A., Torsvik, A., Sobala, E., McCormack, E., Immervoll, H., Mysliwietz, J., Tonn, J. C., Goldbrunner, R., Lonning, P. E., Bjerkvig, R. & Schichor, C. (2009) Long-term cultures of bone marrow-derived human mesenchymal stem cells frequently undergo spontaneous malignant transformation. *Cancer Res, 69*, 5331-5339.

[58]Burns, J. S., Abdallah, B. M., Schroder, H. D. & Kassem, M. (2008) The histopathology of a human mesenchymal stem cell experimental tumor model: support for an hMSC origin for Ewing's sarcoma? *Histol Histopathol, 23*, 1229-1240.

[59]Li, N., Yang, R., Zhang, W., Dorfman, H., Rao, P. & Gorlick, R. (2009) Genetically transforming human mesenchymal stem cells to sarcomas: changes in cellular phenotype and multilineage differentiation potential. *Cancer, 115*, 4795-4806.

[60]Riggi, N., Suva, M. L., Suva, D., Cironi, L., Provero, P., Tercier, S., Joseph, J. M., Stehle, J. C., Baumer, K., Kindler, V. & Stamenkovic, I. (2008) EWS-FLI-1 expression triggers a Ewing's sarcoma initiation program in primary human mesenchymal stem cells. *Cancer Res, 68*, 2176-2185.

[61]Studeny, M., Marini, F. C., Champlin, R. E., Zompetta, C., Fidler, I. J. & Andreeff, M. (2002) Bone marrow-derived mesenchymal stem cells as vehicles for interferon-beta delivery into tumors. *Cancer Res, 62*, 3603-3608.

[62]Xin, H., Kanehira, M., Mizuguchi, H., Hayakawa, T., Kikuchi, T., Nukiwa, T. & Saijo, Y. (2007) Targeted delivery of CX3CL1 to multiple lung tumors by mesenchymal stem cells. *Stem Cells, 25*, 1618-1626.

[63]Dvorak, H. F. (1986) Tumors: wounds that do not heal. Similarities between tumor stroma generation and wound healing. *N Engl J Med, 315*, 1650-1659.

[64]Kidd, S., Spaeth, E., Klopp, A., Andreeff, M., Hall, B. & Marini, F. C. (2008) The (in) auspicious role of mesenchymal stromal cells in cancer: be it friend or foe. *Cytotherapy,* *10,* 657-667.

[65]Ishii, G., Sangai, T., Oda, T., Aoyagi, Y., Hasebe, T., Kanomata, N., Endoh, Y., Okumura, C., Okuhara, Y., Magae, J., Emura, M., Ochiya, T. & Ochiai, A. (2003) Bone-marrow-derived myofibroblasts contribute to the cancer-induced stromal reaction. *Biochem Biophys Res Commun, 309,* 232-240.

[66]Direkze, N. C., Hodivala-Dilke, K., Jeffery, R., Hunt, T., Poulsom, R., Oukrif, D., Alison, M. R. & Wright, N. A. (2004) Bone marrow contribution to tumor-associated myofibroblasts and fibroblasts. *Cancer Res, 64,* 8492-8495.

[67]Luetzkendorf, J., Mueller, L. P., Mueller, T., Caysa, H., Nerger, K. & Schmoll, H. J. (2009) Growth-inhibition of colorectal carcinoma by lentiviral TRAIL-transgenic human mesenchymal stem cells requires their substantial intratumoral presence. *J Cell Mol Med,* Epub ahead of print.

[68]Menon, L. G., Kelly, K., Yang, H. W., Kim, S. K., Black, P. M. & Carroll, R. S. (2009) Human bone marrow-derived mesenchymal stromal cells expressing S-TRAIL as a cellular delivery vehicle for human glioma therapy. *Stem Cells, 27,* 2320-2330.

[69]Nakamura, K., Ito, Y., Kawano, Y., Kurozumi, K., Kobune, M., Tsuda, H., Bizen, A., Honmou, O., Niitsu, Y. & Hamada, H. (2004) Antitumor effect of genetically engineered mesenchymal stem cells in a rat glioma model. *Gene Ther, 11,* 1155-1164.

[70]Fritz, V., Noel, D., Bouquet, C., Opolon, P., Voide, R., Apparailly, F., Louis-Plence, P., Bouffi, C., Drissi, H., Xie, C., Perricaudet, M., Muller, R., Schwarz, E. & Jorgensen, C. (2008) Antitumoral activity and osteogenic potential of mesenchymal stem cells expressing the urokinase-type plasminogen antagonist amino-terminal fragment in a murine model of osteolytic tumor. *Stem Cells, 26,* 2981-2990.

[71]Yong, R. L., Shinojima, N., Fueyo, J., Gumin, J., Vecil, G. G., Marini, F. C., Bogler, O., Andreeff, M. & Lang, F. F. (2009) Human bone marrow-derived mesenchymal stem cells for intravascular delivery of oncolytic adenovirus Delta24-RGD to human gliomas. *Cancer Res, 69,* 8932-8940.

[72]Sonabend, A. M., Ulasov, I. V., Tyler, M. A., Rivera, A. A., Mathis, J. M. & Lesniak, M. S. (2008) Mesenchymal stem cells effectively deliver an oncolytic adenovirus to intracranial glioma. *Stem Cells, 26,* 831-841.

[73]You, M. H., Kim, W. J., Shim, W., Lee, S. R., Lee, G., Choi, S., Kim, D. Y., Kim, Y. M., Kim, H. & Han, S. U. (2009) Cytosine deaminase-producing human mesenchymal stem cells mediate an antitumor effect in a mouse xenograft model. *J Gastroenterol Hepatol,* *24,* 1393-1400.

[74]Parekkadan, B., van Poll, D., Suganuma, K., Carter, E. A., Berthiaume, F., Tilles, A. W. & Yarmush, M. L. (2007) Mesenchymal stem cell-derived molecules reverse fulminant hepatic failure. *PLoS On., 2,* e941.

[75]Karnoub, A. E., Dash, A. B., Vo, A. P., Sullivan, A., Brooks, M. W., Bell, G. W., Richardson, A. L., Polyak, K., Tubo, R. & Weinberg, R. A. (2007) Mesenchymal stem cells within tumour stroma promote breast cancer metastasis. *Nature, 449,* 557-563.

[76]Dittmer, A., Hohlfeld, K., Lutzkendorf, J., Muller, L. P. & Dittmer, J. (2009) Human mesenchymal stem cells induce E-cadherin degradation in breast carcinoma spheroids by activating ADAM10. *Cell Mol Life Sci, 66,* 3053-3065.

[77] Hombauer, H. & Minguell, J. J. (2000). Selective interactions between epithelial tumour cells and bone marrow mesenchymal stem cells. *Br J Cancer, 82,* 1290-1296.

[78] Fierro, F. A., Sierralta, W. D., Epunan, M. J. & Minguell, J. J. (2004) Marrow-derived mesenchymal stem cells: role in epithelial tumor cell determination. *Clin Exp Metastasis, 21,* 313-319.

[79] Rhodes, L. V., Muir, S. E., Elliott, S., Guillot, L. M., Antoon, J. W., Penfornis, P., Tilghman, S. L., Salvo, V. A., Fonseca, J. P., Lacey, M. R., Beckman, B. S., McLachlan, J. A., Rowan, B. G., Pochampally, R. & Burow, M. E. (2009) Adult human mesenchymal stem cells enhance breast tumorigenesis and promote hormone independence. *Breast Cancer Res Treat,* Epub ahead of print.

[80] Sasser, A. K., Mundy, B. L., Smith, K. M., Studebaker, A. W., Axel, A. E., Haidet, A. M., Fernandez, S. A. & Hall, B. M. (2007) Human bone marrow stromal cells enhance breast cancer cell growth rates in a cell line-dependent manner when evaluated in 3D tumor environments. *Cancer Lett, 254,* 255-264.

[81] Yu, J. M., Jun, E. S., Bae, Y. C. & Jung, J. S. (2008) Mesenchymal stem cells derived from human adipose tissues favor tumor cell growth in vivo. Stem Cells De., 17, 463-473.

[82] Djouad, F., Plence, P., Bony, C., Tropel, P., Apparailly, F., Sany, J., Noel, D. & Jorgensen, C. (2003) Immunosuppressive effect of mesenchymal stem cells favors tumor growth in allogeneic animals. *Blood, 102,* 3837-3844.

[83] Djouad, F., Bony, C., Apparailly, F., Louis-Plence, P., Jorgensen, C. & Noel, D. (2006) Earlier onset of syngeneic tumors in the presence of mesenchymal stem cells. *Transplantation, 82,* 1060-1066.

[84] Maestroni, G. J., Hertens, E. & Galli, P. (1999) Factor(s) from nonmacrophage bone marrow stromal cells inhibit Lewis lung carcinoma and B16 melanoma growth in mice. *Cell Mol Life Sci, 55,* 663-667.

[85] Ohlsson, L. B., Varas, L., Kjellman, C., Edvardsen, K. & Lindvall, M. (2003) Mesenchymal progenitor cell-mediated inhibition of tumor growth in vivo and in vitro in gelatin matrix. *Exp Mol Pathol, 75,* 248-255.

[86] Khakoo, A. Y., Pati, S., Anderson, S. A., Reid, W., Elshal, M. F., Rovira, II, Nguyen, A. T., Malide, D., Combs, C. A., Hall, G., Zhang, J., Raffeld, M., Rogers, T. B., Stetler-Stevenson, W., Frank, J. A., Reitz, M. & Finkel, T. (2006) Human mesenchymal stem cells exert potent antitumorigenic effects in a model of Kaposi's sarcoma. *J Exp Med, 203,* 1235-1247

[87] Qiao, L., Xu, Z., Zhao, T., Zhao, Z., Shi, M., Zhao, R. C., Ye, L. & Zhang, X. (2008) Suppression of tumorigenesis by human mesenchymal stem cells in a hepatoma model. *Cell Res, 18,* 500-507.

[88] Lin, S. Y., Yang, J., Everett, A. D., Clevenger, C. V., Koneru, M., Mishra, P. J., Kamen, B., Banerjee, D. & Glod, J. (2008) The isolation of novel mesenchymal stromal cell chemotactic factors from the conditioned medium of tumor cells. *Exp Cell Res, 314,* 3107-3117.

[89] Dwyer, R. M., Potter-Beirne, S. M., Harrington, K. A., Lowery, A. J., Hennessy, E., Murphy, J. M., Barry, F. P., O'Brien, T. & Kerin, M. J. (2007) Monocyte chemotactic protein-1 secreted by primary breast tumors stimulates migration of mesenchymal stem cells. *Clin Cancer Res, 13,* 5020-5027.

[90]Menon, L. G., Picinich, S., Koneru, R., Gao, H., Lin, S. Y., Koneru, M., Mayer-Kuckuk, P., Glod, J. & Banerjee, D. (2007) Differential gene expression associated with migration of mesenchymal stem cells to conditioned medium from tumor cells or bone marrow cells. *Stem Cells, 25*, 520-528.

[91]Mishra, P. J., Humeniuk, R., Medina, D. J., Alexe, G., Mesirov, J. P., Ganesan, S., Glod, J. W. & Banerjee, D. (2008) Carcinoma-associated fibroblast-like differentiation of human mesenchymal stem cells. *Cancer Res, 68*, 4331-4339.

[92]Levina, V., Marrangoni, A. M., DeMarco, R., Gorelik, E. & Lokshin, A. E. (2008) Drug-selected human lung cancer stem cells: cytokine network, tumorigenic and metastatic properties. *PLoS One, 3*, e3077.

[93]Mueller, L. P., Luetzkendorf, J., Mueller, T., Reichelt, K., Simon, H. & Schmoll, H. J. (2006) Presence of mesenchymal stem cells in human bone marrow after exposure to chemotherapy: evidence of resistance to apoptosis induction. *Stem Cell, 24*, 2753-2765.

[94]Jorgensen, C. (2009) Link between cancer stem cells and adult mesenchymal stromal cells: implications for cancer therapy. *Regen Med, 4*, 149-152.

In: Cancer Stem Cells
Editor: Melissa E. Jordan, pp. 79-94

ISBN: 978-1-61668-971-1
© 2010 Nova Science Publishers, Inc.

Chapter IV

WNT SIGNALING IN COLON CANCER STEM CELLS

Tianxin Yu, Xi Chen and Chunming Liu[*]
University of Kentucky, Lexington, KY 40506, USA.

ABSTRACT

Colorectal cancer is the second leading cause of cancer-related death in the United States. Among many gene mutations associated with colorectal cancer, mutation of APC (adenomatous polyposis coli) or β-catenin, which activates Wnt signaling, represents the initiation step of colon tumorigenesis. Wnt signaling is known to play multiple roles in early development and formation of human cancers. In addition, Wnt signaling also regulates the self-renewal and differentiation of adult stem cells. Recently, cancer stem cells have emerged as an exciting new concept in cancer research. However, many challenging questions have also arisen. What is the definition of a cancer stem cell? Where do such cells originate and what are the markers for these cells? What's the genetic and epigenetic machinery that regulate the homeostasis of this cell population? What is the mechanism underlying the process of cancer stem cell-involved tumorigenesis? In this review, we will discuss the development and trends in the field of cancer stem cell research, with emphasis on colon cancer stem cells. Since Wnt signaling is involved in both intestinal stem cells and colon cancers, we will first discuss the mechanisms of the Wnt signal transduction pathway, and then discuss the roles of Wnt signaling in normal intestine and in colon cancer. Finally, we will discuss the challenges and opportunities in colon cancer stem cell research.

[*] Correspondence concerning this article should be addressed to: Chunming Liu, Markey Cancer Center and the Department of Molecular and Cellular Biochemistry, University of Kentucky, Lexington, KY 40506. E-mail: chunming.liu@uky.edu.

WNT SIGNALING PATHWAY

The Wnt gene was first identified as a preferential insertion site for the Murine Mammary Tumor Virus, resulting in overexpression of the Wnt-1 protein and the formation of mammary tumors [1]. Wnts are secreted glycoproteins. In human and mouse genomes, nineteen Wnt genes have been found. Each individual Wnt protein may have similar or drastically different functions. Some activate the canonical Wnt pathway, whereas others activate the non-canonical pathway, including the PCP pathway, and/or the Ca^{2+} pathway [2,3]. Wnt signaling is one of the major signaling pathways that controls cell proliferation and differentiation, and it also regulates the homeostasis of many tissues [4-6]. Deregulation of Wnt signaling plays a vital role in tumorigenesis [7,8].

The canonical pathway is also called the Wnt/β-catenin pathway. The central task of canonical Wnt signaling is to regulate β-catenin. β-catenin is a multifunctional protein depending on cellular localization. When on the cell membrane, it binds E-cadherin and regulates cell adhesion, whereas when in the nucleus, it binds TCF/LEF and regulates gene transcription. The level of cytoplasmic β-catenin is tightly controlled by the Axin degradation complex (Figure 1A). Axin is a scaffold protein; it interacts with APC, GSK-3, Casein Kinase Iα (CKIα) and β-catenin through different domains. In the absence of Wnt, β-catenin is sequentially phosphorylated by CKIα and GSK-3 within the Axin complex [9,10]. Phosphorylated β-catenin is recognized by β-Trcp, a component of E3 ubiquitin ligase complex, for ubiquitination [11-15]. Poly-ubiquitinated β-catenin is then degraded by the proteasome (Figure 1A). β-catenin phosphorylation is also regulated by Protein phosphatase 2A (PP2A). The specificity of PP2A-mediated β-catenin dephosphorylation is regulated by PR55α, a regulatory subunit of PP2A [16]. Whether β-catenin ubiquitination is regulated by a deubiquitinase is currently unknown.

In the presence of Wnt, Wnt binds to the receptor Frizzled (Fz) [17,18] and co-receptor Lrp5/6 (low-density-lipoprotein receptor-related proteins 5 and 6) [19-21] (Figure 1B). Fz receptors are seven trans-membrane repeat proteins that contain an extra-cellular N-terminal cysteine-rich domain (CRD) and an intra-cellular tail domain [22,23]. Binding of Wnt induces structural changes in the receptor that result in recruitment of Dvl to the cytoplasmic tail of Fz through its intra-cellular domain [24-27]. Fz can also activate signaling through heterotrimeric G proteins [28,29]. Lrp5/6 are single transmembrane proteins; binding of Wnt induces phosphorylation of Lrp5/6, creating a docking site for Axin [30], which is an inhibitory downstream component of the Wnt pathway. Recruitment of Axin to the co-receptor inhibits its function, and leads to stabilization of β-catenin by releasing it from the destruction complex [31] (Figure 1B).

Stabilized β-catenin translocates into the nucleus. In the nucleus, β-catenin interacts with the TCF family of transcription factors, which includes TCF-1, lymphoid enhancer factor-1 (LEF-1), TCF-3, and TCF-4 [32,33]. In the absence of β-catenin, TCF/LEF family members bind co-repressors such as CtBP [34], HDAC1 [35,36], and Groucho/TLE [37-39] and repress transcription (Figure 1A). When Wnt signaling is activated, β-catenin binds TCF/LEF and recruits co-activators through its N- and C-terminal transactivation domains, and subsequently activates downstream genes (Figure 1B). The C-terminus of β-catenin contains a strong transactivation domain [32,40,41]. This transactivation domain recruits p300/CBP which is required for Wnt signaling [40,42]. p300 and CBP are paralogous transcriptional coactivators; they acetylate nearby histones, thereby loosening chromatin in order to facilitate binding of other transcription factors [43,44]. The N-terminal transactivation domain of β-catenin directly associates with BCL9/Legless, which in turn recruits the transcriptional co-activator Pygopus [45-48] (Figure 1B). Pygopus contains a plant homeodomain (PHD). The PHD domain of ING (inhibitor of growth) can interact with tri-methylated histone H3, and is thought to regulate epigenetic modifications on target genes [49].

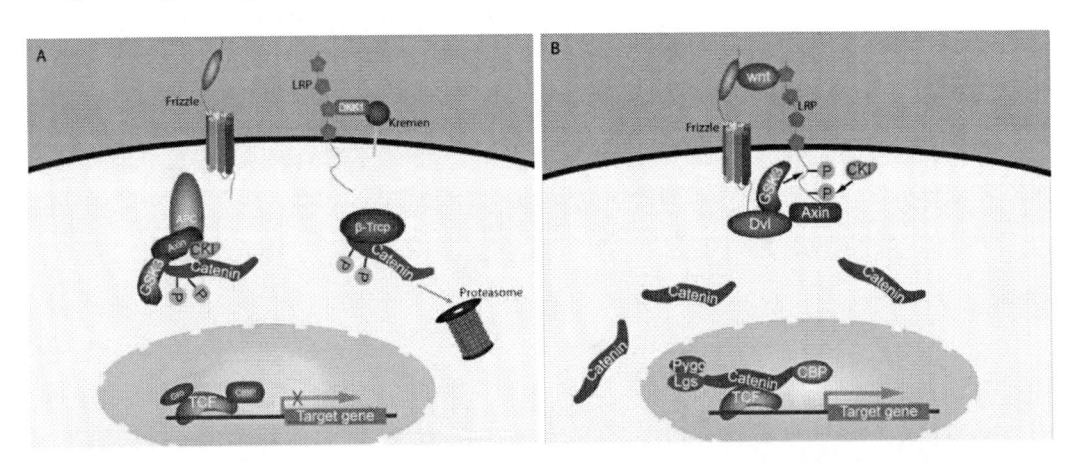

Figure 1. Wnt Signaling Pathway. (A) In the absence of Wnt, β-catenin is phosphorylated by the Axin destruction complex consisting of Axin, APC, GSK3 and CKIα. Phosphorylated β-catenin is recognized by β-Trcp for ubiquitination and proteasome degradation. In the nucleus, TCF recruits co-repressors such as CtBP and Groucho (Gro) to inhibit transcription. (B) Wnt binds to its receptor Frizzled and co-receptor LRP5/6. Wnt stimulates LRP5/6 phosphorylation and recruitment of Axin to LRP5/6, leading to release of β-catenin from the destruction complex. Stablized β-catenin enters the nucleus, binds to TCF, and recruits co-activators such as Pygopus (Pygo), Legless (Lgs) and P300/CBP to activate target gene expression.

WNT SIGNALING IN THE INTESTINE

The intestine is a tube-like organ. The luminal surface of the gut is covered by a continuous sheet of epithelial cells (Figure 2A). In the epithelium of the small intestine, this sheet folds into finger-like protrusions that extend into the lumen, called villi. In between each villus, the epithelial sheet additionally invaginates inward to form the crypts of Lieberkühn [50]. The colonic epithelium has no villi, but consists entirely of crypts. Intestinal stem cells are located at the bottom of the crypts. Crypt stem cells produce transit-amplifying cells that ultimately differentiate into enterocytes, goblet cells, and enteroendocrine cells (Figure 2B). In the small intestine, transit-amplifying cells additionally differentiate into Paneth cells [50,51]. Enterocytes are the most abundant cell type of the intestine, and perform the primary absorptive function of the intestine. Goblet cells secrete mucins that protect the luminal surface. Enteroendocrine cells are located throughout the crypt-villus axis and secrete intestinal hormones. Paneth cells are found at the bottom of crypts and release lysozyme as well as other anti-microbial molecules. With the exception of Paneth cells, terminally differentiated cells migrate along the crypt-villi axis and are shed into lumen after 3-5 days [51].

Wnt signaling is the major player in regulating cell fate along the crypt-villus axis [52-54]. Since TCF4-deficient mice lack proliferating cells in the intestinal crypts [54], Wnt signaling is known to be essential for self-renewal of intestine stem cells, and the bottom of the crypt is thought to be a stem cell niche in which Wnt plays a vital role controlling the differentiation, migration and proliferation of the epithelial stem cells [55]. Overexpression of Dkk1, a Wnt inhibitor, in the intestine causes loss of crypt and secretory cell lineages [56]. APC is a negative regulator of β-catenin and the major tumor suppressor in colorectal cancer. Deletion of APC in the mouse intestine activates Wnt signaling and results in expansion of the crypts [57]. As a well-established target of Wnt, MYC deletion in the intestine rescues the defects in proliferation and migration in APC$^{-/-}$ mice [58]. In addition, expression of the Wnt agonist R-spondin1 in mice induces crypt cell proliferation [59]. These data further suggest that Wnt signaling plays essential roles in maintaining the stem cell compartment and regulating cell proliferation and differentiation in the intestine.

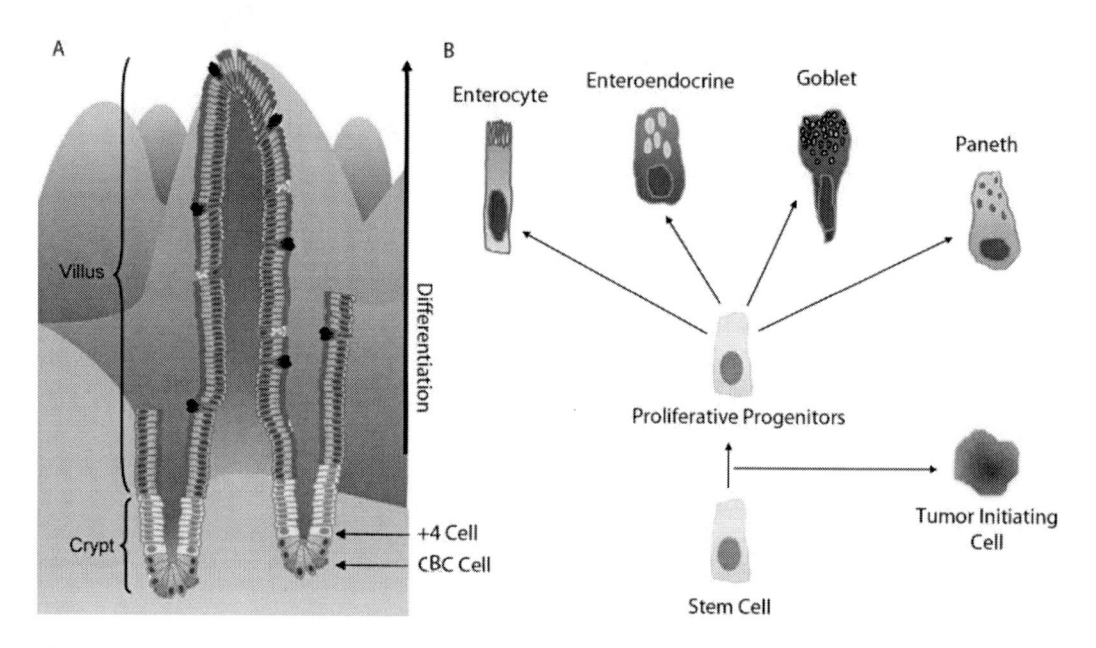

Figure 2. Wnt signaling in the intestine. (A) Structure of the intestine. The epithelium of the small intestine is composed of the crypt and villus. Stem cells (+4 and CBCs) are located at the bottom of crypts. Self-renewal and differentiation of the stem cells are regulated by Wnt signaling. (B) Lineage of intestinal stem cells. Intestinal stem cells produce transit-amplifying cells, which ultimately differentiate into enterocytes, goblet cells, enteroendocrine cells and Paneth cells. Tumor initiating cells likely originate from stem cells or transit-amplifying cells containing APC or β-catenin mutations.

WNT SIGNALING IN COLON CANCER

Aberrant Wnt signaling was first linked to colon cancer by the observation that FAP patients had a mutation in the *APC* gene [60-63]. In addition, APC mutations have been found in more than 80% of sporadic colon cancer. These APC mutants contain C-terminal truncations. Since the Axin-binding domain and part of the β-catenin-binding domains are missing, these APC mutants are unable to regulate β-catenin phosphorylation, ubiquitination or degradation [64]. This allows β-catenin to accumulate and results in constitutively active Wnt signaling [65,66]. The APC$^{min/+}$ mouse model provided clear evidence showing the role of mutant APC in initiation of formation of tumors in the intestine [67,68]. Moreover, conditional deletion of the *APC* gene in the adult mouse intestine results in a "crypt progenitor-like" phenotype with altered patterns of proliferation and differentiation [57,69], which eventually leads to the formation of tumors [70].

In sporadic colorectal tumors that retain wild-type *APC*, mutations are frequently found in the β-catenin (*CTNNB1*) [66,71] or Axin2 gene [72]. Mutations of the β-catenin gene prevent β-catenin phosphorylation by CKIα or GSK-3, and prevent β-Trcp-mediated ubiquitination/degradation [9]. These mutations result in chronic activation of Wnt signaling that ultimately lead to colon cancer. As an example, targeted deletion of the N-terminus of β-catenin in the intestinal epithelium of mice produces thousands of adenomatous polyps within weeks [73]. Moreover, in a mouse model of colitis-associated colorectal carcinoma, using 1,2-dimethylhydrazine and dextran sulfate sodium, mice develop dysplastic lesions and invasive colorectal cancer that strongly stains for β-catenin in the nuclei [74].

Although, APC and β-catenin mutations are the initiating step of colonic tumorigenesis [8], down-regulation of other tumor suppressor genes may also contribute to the development of colon cancer. For example, Krüppel like factor 4 (KLF4), interacts with β-catenin to repress Wnt signaling and inhibit tumor growth [75]. KLF$^{+/-}$/APC$^{Min/+}$ mice developed, on average, 59% more intestinal adenomas than Apc$^{Min/+}$ mice [76]. In addition, it is important to further analyze the cross-talk between Wnt signaling and other signaling pathways, such as PTEN/Akt, Notch, BMP and Hedgehog in the tumorigenesis of colon cancer as well as other cancers.

INTESTINAL STEM CELLS

Intestinal stem cells are located in the bottom of crypts (Figure 2A). Hierarchies of stem cell models suggest that there are 4 to 6 stem cells per crypt, which decide the ultimate pattern of the entire crypt [77]. Due to the lack of specific markers, the exact position of these cells within the crypts is still unclear. Currently, there are two models for intestinal stem cells: the +4 label-retaining cells (LRC) model and the crypt columnar base cells (CBC) model [77,78].

Since the relative "quiescent" status is thought to be one of the characters of stem cells [79], DNA label retention is used as a marker for "stemness" [80]. The +4 LRC model is based on the results of DNA label retention experiments. Long-term BrdU and ^{3}H-thymidine label-retaining cells are located at the +4 position, just above the crypt base columnar and Paneth cells at the base of the crypt [51]. These cells have the quiescent or slow cycling character [51,81]. Additional evidence suggests that these +4 cells indeed have stem cell activity [82]. The neural RNA-binding protein Musashi-1, which has been proposed as a stem cell marker of human colon epithelium, is expressed in the +4 cells as well as CBC cells [83,84]. Several other stem cell markers such as Sox4 [85], phosphorylated PTEN, phosphorylated AKT and AKT-phosphorylated β-catenin (S552) [86], are also localized in the +4 cells. S552-phosphorylated β-catenin is associated with its nuclear localization. These observations support the notion that the +4 cells are potential intestinal stem cells. However, the label retention property of the stem cells does not address the functional characteristics of these cells. Thus, functional evidence is lacking to fully support the +4 LRC model. In addition, there are about 16 cells around the +4 position; the exact position of +4 LRCs in the intestine is not well defined [77,78].

By analyzing Wnt target genes, Lgr5 (or Grp49) was identified as a novel intestinal stem cell marker. Lgr5 (leucine-rich-repeat-containing G-protein-coupled receptor 5) encodes an orphan G-protein-coupled receptor with a leucine-rich extracellular domain [87]. Lgr5 was identified as a Wnt target gene in a micro-array study [88]. *In situ* hybridization and Lrg5-EGFP knock-in studies suggest that Lgr5 is expressed the crypt columnar base cells (CBC) which are intermingled with the Paneth cells [89]. Lineage-tracing experiments with an inducible Cre knock-in allele and the Rosa26-lacZ reporter strain demonstrated that these CBC cells are cable of maintaining epithelial self-renewal over long periods of time and generate all of the major differentiated cell types, thus strongly suggesting that the CBCs are intestinal stem cells and the Lgr5 is a marker for these cells [89,90]. When Lrg5$^+$ cells were isolated from the crypt and sorted with the GFP marker, a single Lgr5$^+$ cell was shown to generate a crypt-villus structure [91]. These data further support that Lgr5 is a specific marker for intestinal stem cells. The current barrier to use Lgr5 as a stem cell marker is the lack of a specific antibody that recognizes the extracellular domain of Lrg5.

Following the discovery of Lgr5, the stem cell transcription profile was analyzed using sorted Lrg5 stem cells. Among the genes tested by in situ hybridization, olfactomedin-4 (Olfm4) and achaete scute-like-2 (Ascl2) have been identified as novel stem cell markers that are expressed in Lrg5 stem cells [92,93]. Olfm4 is a secreted protein with unknown function. An Olfm4 family member, ONT1, acts as a BMP antagonist in Xenopus [94]. Ascl2 is a basic helix-loop-helix transcription factor. Expression of Ascl2 induces ectopic crypts on the villi; deletion of Ascl2 gene in the small intestine results in loss of Lgr5 stem cells, suggesting that Ascl2 plays a key role in regulating intestinal stem cells [93]. As Lgr5, Ascl2 is a Wnt target gene, while Olfm4 is not, implying that these cells are regulated by multiple signaling pathways [92,93].

Using similar lineage-tracing methods described above [89,90], Bmi1 was identified as another intestinal stem cell marker [95]. Bmi1 belongs to the polycomb group (PcG) gene family, which functions in gene silencing through chromatin modifications. Bmi1 was initially identified as an oncogene that regulates cell proliferation and transformation [96,97]. Later it was found to play an important role in hematopoiesis and development of the nervous systems [98]. Bmi1 is also crucial for self-renewal of stem cells and cancer initiation [99-101]. The role of Bmi1 in controlling cell proliferation and self-renewal might be through its function as a polycomb group (PcG) protein , which facilitates histone modification and regulates gene silencing [102-104]. Although it was originally reported that Bmi1 is expressed in the +4 cells in the intestine, Van de Flier et al. reported that Bmi1 expression is enriched in Lgr5 cells, suggesting that these two stem cell markers may be express in overlapping cells in the intestine [92]. Again, the exact position of +4 LRCs requires further refinement.

Prominin1 (Prom1 or CD133) is a five-transmembrane-domain-containing glycoprotein. It has been proposed as a marker for cancer stem cells, including colon cancer stem cells [105,106]. To determine if Prom1 is a marker for normal intestinal stem cells, lineage-tracing experiments were performed by two groups [107,108]. Zhu et al. reported that expression of Prom1 overlaps with Lgr5 expression in the small intestine; YFP-labeled Prom1 cells remained present at 60 days and gave rise to four differentiated cell types [108]. However,

Snippert et al. demonstrated that Prom1 expression is not restricted to the CBCs, but rather is also detected in transit-amplifying progenitor cells [107]. Snippert et al. further demonstrated the stem cell tracing should be analyzed quantitatively. Most of the Prom1-YFP tracing is initiated in the transit-amplifying cells, which can only last for a few days, whereas about 10% of tracing is initiated in the stem cells, which can last 60 days [107]. In contrast, the frequency of long-term tracing in Lgr5 cells is much higher [89]. This also raises a concern of the stem cell tracing technique: it can only determine if a gene is expressed in the stem cells but it cannot give a definitive answer as to whether this gene is a stem cell-specific gene.

Recently, doublecortin and Ca^{2+}/calmodulin-dependent kinase-like-1 (DCAMKL-1) was identified as a putative intestinal stem cell marker, which specifically marks the quiescent cells in the lower two-thirds of the intestinal crypt epithelium and occasionally marks CBCs [109]. DCAMKL-1 is a microtubule-associated kinase expressed in post-mitotic neurons [110]. Using Gene Ontology (GO) term enrichment analysis, DCAMKL-1 was found to be expressed in comparison with gastric epithelial progenitor and whole stomach libraries [111]. It was later found to be expressed in gastric stem cells [112]. Most frequently, DCAMKL-1 was found at or near position +4; much less frequently, it was localized in CBC cells [109]. Using conjugated anti-DCAMKL-1 antibody, which targets the extracellular C-terminal epitope, epithelial stem cells from mouse small intestine were labeled and isolated by FACS. Sorted cells were grown in suspension culture for further analysis. It was demonstrated that the resulting spheroids in suspension culture have proliferation capacity and are positive for stem cell markers and progenitor cell markers [109]. It has been proposed that DCAMKL-1 marks the quiescent stem cells and Lgr5 marks the cycling stem cells in the intestine. However, another group demonstrated only 21% of the DCAMKL-1 cells were localized in the crypts, while about 50% were localized on villi and 29% were localized in the crypt-villus junction. This group found that these cells also express Cox-1 and Cox-2, markers for tuft cells. Thus, DCAMKL-1 cells are probably tuft cells rather than stem cells [113]. Tuft cells are also called brush cells; the function of these cells is currently not known. It will be interesting to investigate the lineage of tuft cells in the intestine. Despite the interesting properties of DCAMKL-1 cells in *in vitro* cultures, the role of DCAMKL-1 in stem cells has yet to be determined.

COLON CANCER STEM CELLS

Since Wnt signaling plays essential roles in both normal intestinal stem cells and colon cancers, it was hypothesized that colon cancer is initiated from intestinal stem cells or progenitor cells [88] (Figure 2B). Lgr5 is a Wnt target gene as well as a stem cell marker; deletion of APC genes in Lgr5 cells leads to rapid transformation of these cells [114]. In contrast, deletion of APC in non-stem cells fails to induce transformation [114]. In these Wnt signaling-induced adenomas, the expression of Lgr5-EGFP was restricted to a small population of cells, suggesting that stem cells or progenitor cells are maintained in these tumors, thus strongly supporting the cancer stem cell concept [114].

Like many other types of stem cells, cancer stem cells are basically defined by the ability to self-renew and the capability of generating differentiated cells. In addition, two other characteristics of cancer stem cells differ from other stem cells: 1) the potential of transformation toward adenomas, i.e., the ability to give rise to heterogeneous progeny of cells, and to maintain diverse and specialized progression [115], and 2) the ability to 'escape' from normal cell cycle regulation and enter into the tumorigenic status, which is parallel to the difference in property between embryonic carcinoma and normal embryonic stem cells [116]. In the small intestine, transformed cells are originally and mainly located at the bottom of the crypt, which is also considered to be the main location of cells that give rise to intestinal cancer [114].

The major challenge in the field of colon cancer stem cells is one characterized by the lack of a widely accepted specific cancer stem cell marker. Two groups independently reported the identification of a colorectal cancer stem cell based on the surface marker CD133 (Prom1) [105-106]. Purified CD133$^+$ cells grew exponentially *in vitro* for long periods of time as undifferentiated tumor spheres. Limiting dilution analysis suggested that the tumor initiating cells enriched more than 200-fold in CD133$^+$ cells [105,106]. However, as discussed above, CD133 (Prom1) is not likely a specific marker for normal intestinal stem cells, and whether it is a specific marker for colon cancer stem cell is also questionable [117]. Shmelkov et al. demonstrated that CD133$^-$ and CD133$^+$ cells were equally capable of tumor initiation, butthe metastatic CD133$^-$ cells form more aggressive tumors in the xenograft model [117]. Clearly, other markers for colon cancer stem cells need to be identified and characterized.

Markers such as epithelial cell adhesion molecule (EpCAM) and CD44 have been used to isolate human colorectal cancer stem cells in a reproducible and consistent way. The isolated population was studied and demonstrated to have a certain gene expression profile, though variable, indicating correlation among expression of other stem cell markers such as CD44, CD133 and CD166 [107,108,118,119]. The normal intestinal stem cell markers, such as Lgr5, Bmi1 and DCAMKL-1, are also potential markers for colon cancer stem cells. In addition to its expression in intestinal stem cells and adenomas, Lrg5 is also expressed in the ovarian and hepatocellular carcinomas [120,121]. Further analysis of Lgr5 as a marker for cancer stem cells, particularly stem cells from human colon cancer, requires a specific antibody for immunohistochemistry and flow cytometry.

SUMMARY

Constitutive activation of Wnt/β-catenin signaling is a hallmark of colorectal cancer. Moreover, this signal transduction event also governs intestinal stem cell identity and tissue homeostasis. The concept of cancer stem cells implies that stem cells are the culprit of cancer origin and progression. The findings that Lgr5 is a stem cell marker and a Wnt target gene substantiate the importance of Wnt signaling in stem cell biology. Lgr5, together with other intestinal stem cell markers, provides surrogate index to track the role of the Wnt pathway in intestinal stem cells and in tumorigenesis. Stem cells usually reside in a specialized niche. Communication between the niche and stem cell, such as through Wnt signaling, plays a critical role in stem cell self-renewal and differentiation. It is of great interest to investigate how cancer stem cells abduct the normal stroma for cancer growth. *In vitro* culture of a single Lgr5+ cell is able to recapitulate the basic organization of intestine epithelia. The requirement of Wnt and Notch signaling highlights the importance of these two pathways in regulating intestinal stem cells. This *in vitro* model will greatly facilitate research on intestinal stem cell biology and extend our understanding of the role of stem cells in colon cancer initiation and progression.

Because of its roles in colon cancer and stem cells, Wnt signaling becomes a very attractive target for colon cancer prevention and therapeutics. It is expected that inhibiting Wnt signaling would inhibit colon cancer stem cells. From high throughput screenings, several small molecular inhibitors targeting the Wnt pathway have been identified. For example, CPG049090 inhibits the β-catenin/TCF interaction; IGC-001 inhibits the interaction of β-catenin/CBP [122,123]; XAV939 and IWRs stabilize Axin [124,125]. Wnt signaling is required for both tumorigenesis and stem cell self-renewal; how to inhibit cancer stem cells but not normal intestinal stem cells will be an exciting but challenging question.

ACKNOWLEDGMENTS

We thank Drs. B. Mark Evers and Nathan Vanderford for critically reading this manuscript and Donna A. Gilbreath for helping with the figures. C.L. is supported by R01 DK071976 from the NIH.

REFERENCES

[1]   Nusse R, Varmus HE. Many tumors induced by the mouse mammary tumor virus contain a provirus integrated in the same region of the host genome. *Cell* 1982; 31 (1):99-109.

[2]   Clevers H. Wnt/beta-catenin signaling in development and disease. *Cell* 2006; 127 (3):469-480.

[3]   Logan CY, Nusse R. The Wnt signaling pathway in development and disease. *Annu Rev Cell Dev Biol* 2004; 20:781-810.

[4]   Czyz J, Wobus A. Embryonic stem cell differentiation: the role of extracellular factors. *Differentiation* 2001; 68 (4-5):167-174.

[5]   Malhotra S, Kincade PW. Wnt-related molecules and signaling pathway equilibrium in hematopoiesis. *Cell Stem Cell* 2009; 4 (1):27-36.

[6]   Wodarz A, Nusse R. Mechanisms of Wnt signaling in development. *Annu Rev Cell Dev Biol* 1998; 14:59-88.

[7]   Giles RH, van Es JH, Clevers H. Caught up in a Wnt storm: Wnt signaling in cancer. *Biochim Biophys Acta* 2003; 1653 (1):1-24.

[8]   Kinzler KW, Vogelstein B. Lessons from hereditary colorectal cancer. *Cell* 1996; 87 (2):159-170.

[9]   Liu C, Li Y, Semenov M *et al.* Control of beta-catenin phosphorylation/degradation by a dual-kinase mechanism. *Cell* 2002; 108 (6):837-847.

[10] Amit S, Hatzubai A, Birman Y *et al.* Axin-mediated CKI phosphorylation of beta-catenin at Ser 45: a molecular switch for the Wnt pathway. *Genes Dev* 2002; 16 (9):1066-1076.

[11] Hart M, Concordet JP, Lassot I *et al.* The F-box protein beta-TrCP associates with phosphorylated beta-catenin and regulates its activity in the cell. *Curr Biol* 1999; 9 (4):207-210.

[12] Jiang J, Struhl G. Regulation of the Hedgehog and Wingless signalling pathways by the F-box/WD40-repeat protein Slimb. *Nature* 1998; 391 (6666):493-496.

[13] Liu C, Kato Y, Zhang Z *et al.* beta-Trcp couples beta-catenin phosphorylation-degradation and regulates Xenopus axis formation. *Proc Natl Acad Sci U S A* 1999; 96 (11):6273-6278.

[14] Spencer E, Jiang J, Chen ZJ. Signal-induced ubiquitination of IkappaBalpha by the F-box protein Slimb/beta-TrCP. *Genes Dev* 1999; 13 (3):284-294.

[15] Winston JT, Strack P, Beer-Romero P *et al.* The SCFbeta-TRCP-ubiquitin ligase complex associates specifically with phosphorylated destruction motifs in IkappaBalpha and beta-catenin and stimulates IkappaBalpha ubiquitination in vitro. *Genes Dev* 1999; 13 (3):270-283.

[16] Zhang W, Yang J, Liu Y *et al.* PR55 alpha, a regulatory subunit of PP2A, specifically regulates PP2A-mediated beta-catenin dephosphorylation. *J Biol Chem* 2009; 284 (34):22649-22656.

[17] Bhanot P, Brink M, Samos CH *et al.* A new member of the frizzled family from Drosophila functions as a Wingless receptor. *Nature* 1996; 382 (6588):225-230.

[18] Yang-Snyder J, Miller JR, Brown JD, Lai CJ, Moon RT. A frizzled homolog functions in a vertebrate Wnt signaling pathway. *Curr Biol* 1996; 6 (10):1302-1306.

[19] Pinson KI, Brennan J, Monkley S, Avery BJ, Skarnes WC. An LDL-receptor-related protein mediates Wnt signalling in mice. *Nature* 2000; 407 (6803):535-538.

[20] Tamai K, Semenov M, Kato Y *et al.* LDL-receptor-related proteins in Wnt signal transduction. *Nature* 2000; 407 (6803):530-535.

[21] Wehrli M, Dougan ST, Caldwell K *et al.* arrow encodes an LDL-receptor-related protein essential for Wingless signalling. *Nature* 2000; 407 (6803):527-530.

[22] Dann CE, Hsieh JC, Rattner A *et al.* Insights into Wnt binding and signalling from the structures of two Frizzled cysteine-rich domains. *Nature* 2001; 412 (6842):86-90.

[23] Hsieh JC, Rattner A, Smallwood PM, Nathans J. Biochemical characterization of Wnt-frizzled interactions using a soluble, biologically active vertebrate Wnt protein. *Proc Natl Acad Sci U S A* 1999; 96 (7):3546-3551.

[24] Umbhauer M, Djiane A, Goisset C *et al.* The C-terminal cytoplasmic Lys-thr-X-X-X-Trp motif in frizzled receptors mediates Wnt/beta-catenin signalling. *Embo J* 2000; 19 (18):4944-4954.

[25] Wong HC, Bourdelas A, Krauss A *et al.* Direct binding of the PDZ domain of Dishevelled to a conserved internal sequence in the C-terminal region of Frizzled. *Mol Cell* 2003; 12 (5):1251-1260.

[26] Rothbacher U, Laurent MN, Deardorff MA *et al.* Dishevelled phosphorylation, subcellular localization and multimerization regulate its role in early embryogenesis. *Embo J* 2000; 19 (5):1010-1022.

[27] Axelrod JD, Miller JR, Shulman JM, Moon RT, Perrimon N. Differential recruitment of Dishevelled provides signaling specificity in the planar cell polarity and Wingless signaling pathways. *Genes Dev* 1998; 12 (16):2610-2622.

[28] Katanaev VL, Ponzielli R, Semeriva M, Tomlinson A. Trimeric G protein-dependent frizzled signaling in Drosophila. *Cell* 2005; 120 (1):111-122.

[29] Liu X, Rubin JS, Kimmel AR. Rapid, Wnt-induced changes in GSK3beta associations that regulate beta-catenin stabilization are mediated by Galpha proteins. *Curr Biol* 2005; 15 (22):1989-1997.

[30] Mao J, Wang J, Liu B *et al.* Low-density lipoprotein receptor-related protein-5 binds to Axin and regulates the canonical Wnt signaling pathway. *Mol Cell* 2001; 7 (4):801-809.

[31] Tamai K, Zeng X, Liu C *et al.* A mechanism for Wnt coreceptor activation. *Mol Cell* 2004; 13 (1):149-156.

[32] van de Wetering M, Cavallo R, Dooijes D *et al.* Armadillo coactivates transcription driven by the product of the Drosophila segment polarity gene dTCF. *Cell* 1997; 88 (6):789-799.

[33] Brunner E, Peter O, Schweizer L, Basler K. pangolin encodes a Lef-1 homologue that acts downstream of Armadillo to transduce the Wingless signal in Drosophila. *Nature* 1997; 385 (6619):829-833.

[34] Brannon M, Brown JD, Bates R, Kimelman D, Moon RT. XCtBP is a XTcf-3 co-repressor with roles throughout Xenopus development. *Development* 1999; 126 (14):3159-3170.

[35] Billin AN, Thirlwell H, Ayer DE. Beta-catenin-histone deacetylase interactions regulate the transition of LEF1 from a transcriptional repressor to an activator. *Mol Cell Biol* 2000; 20 (18):6882-6890.

[36] Kioussi C, Briata P, Baek SH *et al.* Identification of a Wnt/Dvl/beta-Catenin --> Pitx2 pathway mediating cell-type-specific proliferation during development. *Cell* 2002; 111 (5):673-685.

[37] Cavallo RA, Cox RT, Moline MM *et al.* Drosophila Tcf and Groucho interact to repress Wingless signalling activity. *Nature* 1998; 395 (6702):604-608.

[38] Roose J, Molenaar M, Peterson J *et al.* The Xenopus Wnt effector XTcf-3 interacts with Groucho-related transcriptional repressors. *Nature* 1998; 395 (6702):608-612.

[39] Levanon D, Goldstein RE, Bernstein Y *et al.* Transcriptional repression by AML1 and LEF-1 is mediated by the TLE/Groucho corepressors. *Proc Natl Acad Sci U S A* 1998; 95 (20):11590-11595.

[40] Hecht A, Vleminckx K, Stemmler MP, van Roy F, Kemler R. The p300/CBP acetyltransferases function as transcriptional coactivators of beta-catenin in vertebrates. *Embo J* 2000; 19 (8):1839-1850.

[41] Cox RT, Pai LM, Kirkpatrick C, Stein J, Peifer M. Roles of the C terminus of Armadillo in Wingless signaling in Drosophila. *Genetics* 1999; 153 (1):319-332.

[42] Takemaru KI, Moon RT. The transcriptional coactivator CBP interacts with beta-catenin to activate gene expression. *J Cell Biol* 2000; 149 (2):249-254.

[43] Ogryzko VV, Schiltz RL, Russanova V, Howard BH, Nakatani Y. The transcriptional coactivators p300 and CBP are histone acetyltransferases. *Cell* 1996; 87 (5):953-959.

[44] Goldman PS, Tran VK, Goodman RH. The multifunctional role of the co-activator CBP in transcriptional regulation. *Recent Prog Horm Res* 1997; 52:103-119; discussion 119-120.

[45] Belenkaya TY, Han C, Standley HJ *et al.* pygopus Encodes a nuclear protein essential for wingless/Wnt signaling. *Development* 2002; 129 (17):4089-4101.

[46] Kramps T, Peter O, Brunner E *et al.* Wnt/wingless signaling requires BCL9/legless-mediated recruitment of pygopus to the nuclear beta-catenin-TCF complex. *Cell* 2002; 109 (1):47-60.

[47] Parker DS, Jemison J, Cadigan KM. Pygopus, a nuclear PHD-finger protein required for Wingless signaling in Drosophila. *Development* 2002; 129 (11):2565-2576.

[48] Thompson B, Townsley F, Rosin-Arbesfeld R, Musisi H, Bienz M. A new nuclear component of the Wnt signalling pathway. *Nat Cell Biol* 2002; 4 (5):367-373.

[49] Soliman MA, Riabowol K. After a decade of study-ING, a PHD for a versatile family of proteins. *Trends Biochem Sci* 2007; 32 (11):509-519.

[50] Crosnier C, Stamataki D, Lewis J. Organizing cell renewal in the intestine: stem cells, signals and combinatorial control. *Nat Rev Genet* 2006; 7 (5):349-359.

[51] Marshman E, Booth C, Potten CS. The intestinal epithelial stem cell. *Bioessays* 2002; 24 (1):91-98.

[52] Reya T, Clevers H. Wnt signalling in stem cells and cancer. *Nature* 2005; 434 (7035):843-850.

[53] Batlle E, Henderson JT, Beghtel H *et al*. Beta-catenin and TCF mediate cell positioning in the intestinal epithelium by controlling the expression of EphB/ephrinB. *Cell* 2002; 111 (2):251-263.

[54] Korinek V, Barker N, Moerer P *et al*. Depletion of epithelial stem-cell compartments in the small intestine of mice lacking Tcf-4. *Nat Genet* 1998; 19 (4):379-383.

[55] Pardal R, Clarke MF, Morrison SJ. Applying the principles of stem-cell biology to cancer. *Nat Rev Cancer* 2003; 3 (12):895-902.

[56] Pinto D, Gregorieff A, Begthel H, Clevers H. Canonical Wnt signals are essential for homeostasis of the intestinal epithelium. *Genes Dev* 2003; 17 (14):1709-1713.

[57] Sansom OJ, Reed KR, Hayes AJ *et al*. Loss of Apc in vivo immediately perturbs Wnt signaling, differentiation, and migration. *Genes Dev* 2004; 18 (12):1385-1390.

[58] Sansom OJ, Meniel VS, Muncan V *et al*. Myc deletion rescues Apc deficiency in the small intestine. *Nature* 2007; 446 (7136):676-679.

[59] Kim KA, Kakitani M, Zhao J *et al*. Mitogenic influence of human R-spondin1 on the intestinal epithelium. *Science* 2005; 309 (5738):1256-1259.

[60] Groden J, Thliveris A, Samowitz W *et al*. Identification and characterization of the familial adenomatous polyposis coli gene. *Cell* 1991; 66 (3):589-600.

[61] Kinzler KW, Nilbert MC, Su LK *et al*. Identification of FAP locus genes from chromosome 5q21. *Science* 1991; 253 (5020):661-665.

[62] Nishisho I, Nakamura Y, Miyoshi Y *et al*. Mutations of chromosome 5q21 genes in FAP and colorectal cancer patients. *Science* 1991; 253 (5020):665-669.

[63] Powell SM, Zilz N, Beazer-Barclay Y *et al*. APC mutations occur early during colorectal tumorigenesis. *Nature* 1992; 359 (6392):235-237.

[64] Yang J, Zhang W, Evans PM *et al*. Adenomatous polyposis coli (APC) differentially regulates beta-catenin phosphorylation and ubiquitination in colon cancer cells. *J Biol Chem* 2006; 281 (26):17751-17757.

[65] Korinek V, Barker N, Morin PJ *et al*. Constitutive transcriptional activation by a beta-catenin-Tcf complex in APC-/- colon carcinoma. *Science* 1997; 275 (5307):1784-1787.

[66] Morin PJ, Sparks AB, Korinek V *et al*. Activation of beta-catenin-Tcf signaling in colon cancer by mutations in beta-catenin or APC. *Science* 1997; 275 (5307):1787-1790.

[67] Moser AR, Pitot HC, Dove WF. A dominant mutation that predisposes to multiple intestinal neoplasia in the mouse. *Science* 1990; 247 (4940):322-324.

[68] Su LK, Kinzler KW, Vogelstein B *et al.* Multiple intestinal neoplasia caused by a mutation in the murine homolog of the APC gene. *Science* 1992; 256 (5057):668-670.

[69] Andreu P, Colnot S, Godard C *et al.* Crypt-restricted proliferation and commitment to the Paneth cell lineage following Apc loss in the mouse intestine. *Development* 2005; 132 (6):1443-1451.

[70] Shibata H, Toyama K, Shioya H *et al.* Rapid colorectal adenoma formation initiated by conditional targeting of the Apc gene. *Science* 1997; 278 (5335):120-123.

[71] Munemitsu S, Albert I, Rubinfeld B, Polakis P. Deletion of an amino-terminal sequence beta-catenin in vivo and promotes hyperphosporylation of the adenomatous polyposis coli tumor suppressor protein. *Mol Cell Biol* 1996; 16 (8):4088-4094.

[72] Liu W, Dong X, Mai M *et al.* Mutations in AXIN2 cause colorectal cancer with defective mismatch repair by activating beta-catenin/TCF signalling. *Nat Genet* 2000; 26 (2):146-147.

[73] Harada N, Tamai Y, Ishikawa T *et al.* Intestinal polyposis in mice with a dominant stable mutation of the beta-catenin gene. *Embo J* 1999; 18 (21):5931-5942.

[74] Wang JG, Wang DF, Lv BJ, Si JM. A novel mouse model for colitis-associated colon carcinogenesis induced by 1,2-dimethylhydrazine and dextran sulfate sodium. *World J Gastroenterol* 2004; 10 (20):2958-2962.

[75] Zhang W, Chen X, Kato Y *et al.* Novel cross talk of Kruppel-like factor 4 and beta-catenin regulates normal intestinal homeostasis and tumor repression. *Mol Cell Biol* 2006; 26 (6):2055-2064.

[76] Ghaleb AM, McConnell BB, Nandan MO *et al.* Haploinsufficiency of Kruppel-like factor 4 promotes adenomatous polyposis coli dependent intestinal tumorigenesis. *Cancer Res* 2007; 67 (15):7147-7154.

[77] van der Flier LG, Clevers H. Stem cells, self-renewal, and differentiation in the intestinal epithelium. *Annu Rev Physiol* 2009; 71:241-260.

[78] Scoville DH, Sato T, He XC, Li L. Current view: intestinal stem cells and signaling. *Gastroenterology* 2008; 134 (3):849-864.

[79] Tumbar T, Guasch G, Greco V *et al.* Defining the epithelial stem cell niche in skin. *Science* 2004; 303 (5656):359-363.

[80] Kiel MJ, He S, Ashkenazi R *et al.* Haematopoietic stem cells do not asymmetrically segregate chromosomes or retain BrdU. *Nature* 2007; 449 (7159):238-242.

[81] Potten CS, Owen G, Booth D. Intestinal stem cells protect their genome by selective segregation of template DNA strands. *J Cell Sci* 2002; 115 (Pt 11):2381-2388.

[82] Bjerknes M, Cheng H. The stem-cell zone of the small intestinal epithelium. III. Evidence from columnar, enteroendocrine, and mucous cells in the adult mouse. *Am J Anat* 1981; 160 (1):77-91.

[83] Nishimura S, Wakabayashi N, Toyoda K, Kashima K, Mitsufuji S. Expression of Musashi-1 in human normal colon crypt cells: a possible stem cell marker of human colon epithelium. *Dig Dis Sci* 2003; 48 (8):1523-1529.

[84] Imai T, Tokunaga A, Yoshida T *et al.* The neural RNA-binding protein Musashi1 translationally regulates mammalian numb gene expression by interacting with its mRNA. *Mol Cell Biol* 2001; 21 (12):3888-3900.

[85] Van der Flier LG, Sabates-Bellver J, Oving I *et al.* The Intestinal Wnt/TCF Signature. *Gastroenterology* 2007; 132 (2):628-632.

[86] He XC, Zhang J, Tong WG *et al.* BMP signaling inhibits intestinal stem cell self-renewal through suppression of Wnt-beta-catenin signaling. *Nat Genet* 2004; 36 (10):1117-1121.

[87] Hsu SY, Liang SG, Hsueh AJ. Characterization of two LGR genes homologous to gonadotropin and thyrotropin receptors with extracellular leucine-rich repeats and a G protein-coupled, seven-transmembrane region. *Mol Endocrinol* 1998; 12 (12):1830-1845.

[88] van de Wetering M, Sancho E, Verweij C *et al.* The beta-catenin/TCF-4 complex imposes a crypt progenitor phenotype on colorectal cancer cells. *Cell* 2002; 111 (2):241-250.

[89] Barker N, van Es JH, Kuipers J *et al.* Identification of stem cells in small intestine and colon by marker gene Lgr5. *Nature* 2007; 449 (7165):1003-1007.

[90] Barker N, van de Wetering M, Clevers H. The intestinal stem cell. *Genes Dev* 2008; 22 (14):1856-1864.

[91] Sato T, Vries RG, Snippert HJ *et al.* Single Lgr5 stem cells build crypt-villus structures in vitro without a mesenchymal niche. *Nature* 2009; 459 (7244):262-265.

[92] van der Flier LG, Haegebarth A, Stange DE, van de Wetering M, Clevers H. OLFM4 is a robust marker for stem cells in human intestine and marks a subset of colorectal cancer cells. *Gastroenterology* 2009; 137 (1):15-17.

[93] van der Flier LG, van Gijn ME, Hatzis P *et al.* Transcription factor achaete scute-like 2 controls intestinal stem cell fate. *Cell* 2009; 136 (5):903-912.

[94] Inomata H, Haraguchi T, Sasai Y. Robust stability of the embryonic axial pattern requires a secreted scaffold for chordin degradation. *Cell* 2008; 134 (5):854-865.

[95] Sangiorgi E, Capecchi MR. Bmi1 is expressed in vivo in intestinal stem cells. *Nat Genet* 2008; 40 (7):915-920.

[96] Haupt Y, Alexander WS, Barri G, Klinken SP, Adams JM. Novel zinc finger gene implicated as myc collaborator by retrovirally accelerated lymphomagenesis in E mu-myc transgenic mice. *Cell* 1991; 65 (5):753-763.

[97] Jacobs JJ, Scheijen B, Voncken JW *et al.* Bmi-1 collaborates with c-Myc in tumorigenesis by inhibiting c-Myc-induced apoptosis via INK4a/ARF. *Genes Dev* 1999; 13 (20):2678-2690.

[98] van der Lugt NM, Domen J, Linders K *et al.* Posterior transformation, neurological abnormalities, and severe hematopoietic defects in mice with a targeted deletion of the bmi-1 proto-oncogene. *Genes Dev* 1994; 8 (7):757-769.

[99] Valk-Lingbeek ME, Bruggeman SW, van Lohuizen M. Stem cells and cancer; the polycomb connection. *Cell* 2004; 118 (4):409-418.

[100] Lessard J, Sauvageau G. Bmi-1 determines the proliferative capacity of normal and leukaemic stem cells. *Nature* 2003; 423 (6937):255-260.

[101] Kang MK, Kim RH, Kim SJ *et al.* Elevated Bmi-1 expression is associated with dysplastic cell transformation during oral carcinogenesis and is required for cancer cell replication and survival. *Br J Cancer* 2007; 96 (1):126-133.

[102] Wei J, Zhai L, Xu J, Wang H. Role of Bmi1 in H2A ubiquitylation and Hox gene silencing. *J Biol Chem* 2006; 281 (32):22537-22544.

[103] Wang H, Wang L, Erdjument-Bromage H *et al.* Role of histone H2A ubiquitination in Polycomb silencing. *Nature* 2004; 431 (7010):873-878.

[104] Rajasekhar VK, Begemann M. Concise review: roles of polycomb group proteins in development and disease: a stem cell perspective. *Stem Cells* 2007; 25 (10):2498-2510.

[105] O'Brien CA, Pollett A, Gallinger S, Dick JE. A human colon cancer cell capable of initiating tumour growth in immunodeficient mice. *Nature* 2007; 445 (7123):106-110.

[106] Ricci-Vitiani L, Lombardi DG, Pilozzi E *et al*. Identification and expansion of human colon-cancer-initiating cells. *Nature* 2007; 445 (7123):111-115.

[107] Snippert HJ, van Es JH, van den Born M *et al*. Prominin-1/CD133 marks stem cells and early progenitors in mouse small intestine. *Gastroenterology* 2009; 136 (7):2187-2194 e2181.

[108] Zhu L, Gibson P, Currle DS *et al*. Prominin 1 marks intestinal stem cells that are susceptible to neoplastic transformation. *Nature* 2009; 457 (7229):603-607.

[109] May R, Sureban SM, Hoang N *et al*. Doublecortin and CaM Kinase-like-1 and Leucine-Rich-Repeat-Containing G-Protein-Coupled Receptor Mark Quiescent and Cycling Intestinal Stem Cells, Respectively. *Stem Cells* 2009; 27 (10):2571-2579.

[110] Lin PT, Gleeson JG, Corbo JC, Flanagan L, Walsh CA. DCAMKL1 encodes a protein kinase with homology to doublecortin that regulates microtubule polymerization. *J Neurosci* 2000; 20 (24):9152-9161.

[111] Giannakis M, Stappenbeck TS, Mills JC *et al*. Molecular properties of adult mouse gastric and intestinal epithelial progenitors in their niches. *J Biol Chem* 2006; 281 (16):11292-11300.

[112] Giannakis M, Chen SL, Karam SM, Engstrand L, Gordon JI. Helicobacter pylori evolution during progression from chronic atrophic gastritis to gastric cancer and its impact on gastric stem cells. *Proc Natl Acad Sci U S A* 2008; 105 (11):4358-4363.

[113] Gerbe F, Brulin B, Makrini L, Legraverend C, Jay P. DCAMKL-1 expression identifies Tuft cells rather than stem cells in the adult mouse intestinal epithelium. *Gastroenterology* 2009; 137 (6):2179-2180; author reply 2180-2171.

[114] Barker N, Ridgway RA, van Es JH *et al*. Crypt stem cells as the cells-of-origin of intestinal cancer. *Nature* 2009; 457 (7229):608-611.

[115] Dalerba P, Cho RW, Clarke MF. Cancer stem cells: models and concepts. *Annu Rev Med* 2007; 58:267-284.

[116] Chambers I, Smith A. Self-renewal of teratocarcinoma and embryonic stem cells. *Oncogene* 2004; 23 (43):7150-7160.

[117] Shmelkov SV, Butler JM, Hooper AT *et al*. CD133 expression is not restricted to stem cells, and both CD133+ and CD133- metastatic colon cancer cells initiate tumors. *J Clin Invest* 2008; 118 (6):2111-2120.

[118] Dalerba P, Dylla SJ, Park IK *et al*. Phenotypic characterization of human colorectal cancer stem cells. *Proc Natl Acad Sci U S A 2007*; 104 (24):10158-10163.

[119] Takaishi S, Okumura T, Tu S *et al*. Identification of gastric cancer stem cells using the cell surface marker CD44. *Stem Cells* 2009; 27 (5):1006-1020.

[120] McClanahan T, Koseoglu S, Smith K *et al*. Identification of overexpression of orphan G protein-coupled receptor GPR49 in human colon and ovarian primary tumors. *Cancer Biol Ther* 2006; 5 (4):419-426.

[121] Yamamoto Y, Sakamoto M, Fujii G *et al*. Overexpression of orphan G-protein-coupled receptor, Gpr49, in human hepatocellular carcinomas with beta-catenin mutations. *Hepatology* 2003; 37 (3):528-533.

[122] Emami KH, Nguyen C, Ma H *et al.* A small molecule inhibitor of beta-catenin/CREB-binding protein transcription [corrected]. *Proc Natl Acad Sci U S A* 2004; 101 (34):12682-12687.

[123] Lepourcelet M, Chen YN, France DS *et al.* Small-molecule antagonists of the oncogenic Tcf/beta-catenin protein complex. *Cancer Cell* 2004; 5 (1):91-102.

[124] Chen B, Dodge ME, Tang W *et al.* Small molecule-mediated disruption of Wnt-dependent signaling in tissue regeneration and cancer. *Nat Chem Biol* 2009; 5 (2):100-107.

[125] Huang SM, Mishina YM, Liu S *et al.* Tankyrase inhibition stabilizes axin and antagonizes Wnt signalling. *Nature* 2009; 461 (7264):614-620.

In: Cancer Stem Cells
Editor: Melissa E. Jordan, pp. 95-101

ISBN: 978-1-61668-971-1
© 2010 Nova Science Publishers, Inc.

Chapter V

STEM CELLS IN HEAD AND NECK CANCER: A KEY TO THE FUTURE?

Chiara Bianchini[1], Andrea Ciorba[1], Roberta Piva[2], Stefano Pelucchi[1] and Antonio Pastore[1]

[1]ENT Department, University Hospital of Ferrara, Italy;
[2]Department of Biochemistry and Molecular Biology, University of Ferrara, Italy.

ABSTRACT

The biology of stem cells and their properties have already been recognized as integral to tumour pathogenesis in several types of cancer. A role for stem cells has been demonstrated, so far, for the hematopoietic system diseases, as well as for several solid tumours such as breast, brain and lung cancer. There is a rising interest in the field of oncology in order to understand if cancer stem cells can play a key role also in the pathogenesis of head and neck tumours. It is likely that cancer stem cells are a minor population of tumour cells that possess the stem cell property of self-renewal. The evidence that the development of a tumour comes from a small number of cells with stem-like characteristic, could bring to the identification of therapies against these cellular targets, fundamental for maintenance and progression of the lesion. This new model for cancer will have significant implications for the way we will study and treat tumours.

Head and neck cancer is still the sixth most common cancer type worldwide. Disappointingly, despite significant advances in surgical and other treatments that enhance quality of life, survival rates have only moderately improved during the last 20 years.

Aim of this chapter is to discuss among this new model of cancerogenesis.

INTRODUCTION

Understanding the biological mechanisms of cancer development and spreading, represents a primary purpose in order to eradicate the disease. In the last years, the existence as well as the pathological meaning of cancer stem cells has been matter of discussion and a large number of articles have been published about the role that these cells play in the development and maintenance of the tumours. Cancer stem cells are neoplastic cells which have stem features such as self-renewal, high migration capacity, drug resistance, high proliferation abilities.

The existence of cancer stem cells has been supported by numerous researches. In specific tumor models such as acute myeloid leukemia, it has been demonstrated that definite cellular subsets express antigenic markers similar to hematopoietic stem cells, showing clonogenic activity (Lapidot et al. T, 1994; Bonnet D et al, 1997; Graziano A et al 2008). Nonetheless, it has been reported that cells with staminal properties (such as high proliferation rate, ability of expansion and growth in tissue environments different from the original one) could reside also in solid tumours built by heterogeneous cellular populations (Reya et al., 2001; Graziano A et al 2008).

Particularly, it seems to be evidence of stem-like cells within solid tumors of brain, lung, breast, ovarian, prostate, colon cancer and also larynx (Dontu G et al., 2005; Graziano A et al 2008; Ferrandina G et al 2009; Li CY et al, 2009; McDonald SA, et al 2009; Tirino V, et al 2009; Ailles L et al 2009; Wei XD et al 2009). Therefore, the development of a tumour seems related to the growth and to the spreading of a small cluster of cells with stem-like characteristic. In the future, only the comprehension of the biology of these cell types could provide specific therapeutic targets, in order to hamper cancer progression.

Head and neck cancer is still the sixth most common cancer type worldwide. Disappointingly, despite significant advances in surgical and other treatments that enhance quality of life, survival rates have only moderately improved during the last 20 years (Braakhuis BJ et al 2005; Forastiere A et al 2001). Moreover, head and neck cancer has a severe impact on patients' quality of life and the significant morbidity subsequent to treatment often require long term multidisciplinary care (Bianchini C et al 2008).

CONCERNING STEM CELLS AND CANCER CELLS

One key feature of cancer cells is their unlimited cell division capacity, reminiscent of the self-renewing proliferation of stem cells. However, there are differences that set cancer cells apart from stem cells. Firstly, the self-renewing mechanism in stem cells responds to a feedback system that senses the number of mature cells and regulates the rate of division, whereas in cancer cells this feedback mechanism is disrupted. Secondly, high-grade tumour cells lack the ability to properly differentiate into mature cells, suggesting aberrant differentiation programs. Thus, only understanding the molecular differences between stem cells and cancer cells may help provide us with new insights into the mechanism of tumorogenesis (Bianchini C et al 2008; Cabanillas R et al 2009; Graziano A et al 2008; Zhou ZT et al 2008).

At the molecular level, some recent studies have evidenced that maintenance of stem cells and tumour cells may involve some common pathways (Pardal R et al 2005). One example is the polycomb gene bmi-1. In mice, this gene was recently shown to be essential for maintaining both the hematopoietic stem cell state as well as the leukemic activity (Lessard J, et al 2003). Also Wnt signaling cascade as well as sonic hedgehog (Shh) have been reported to be involved in both neoplastic tissue/cell maintenance and tumorigenesis (Polakis P 2000; Reya T el al 2003; Watkins DN et al 2003).

ISOLATION OF CANCER STEM CELLS TO STUDY THE BIOLOGY OF THE TUMOUR

So far, rare subpopulations of cancer stem cells have been identified for leukemia and other solid tumours (Lapidot et al. T, 1994; Bonnet D et al, 1997). Within these tumours, these rare fractions of cancer stem cells are in large part responsible for maintaining the tumour mass, as they have the capacity to self-renew and to generate a high number of progeny via differentiation program.

Recent studies of cell lines derived from oral squamous cell carcinoma indicate the presence of subpopulations of cells with phenotypic and behavioral characteristics corresponding to both normal epithelial stem cells and to cells capable of initiating tumours in vivo (Costea et al., 2006; Chiou SH et al 2008).

Recently, also in human laryngeal tumours, chinese investigators have characterized a cluster of CD 133+ stem cells of the Hep-2 cell line, suggesting that this subset population could own a strong selected tumorigenic ability (Wei XD et al 2009). A population of highly malignant cells in a head and neck squamous cell carcinoma cell line has also been established from primary head and neck tumours using sequential rounds of xenotransplantation. These cells named SASVO3, possess enhanced tumorigenic ability both in vitro and in vivo; it has been reported that SASVO3 cells exhibits properties of cancer stem cells, including increased abilities of sphere-forming, potential of transplanted tumor growth and elevated expression of stem cell markers such as Bmi1 (Chen CY et al 2009).

CANCER PROGRESSION: A "STAMINAL" POINT OF VIEW

For cancer development it has been proposed that, a stem cell acquires one (or more) genetic alterations, and forms an area in the mucosal epithelium with genetically altered daughter cells. As cancer stem cells escape the normal control mechanisms and gain growth advantage, the patch starts to expand developing a malignant clone (Bianchini C et al 2008).

Hirata offered a specific point of view concerning this topic. In his papers he supports the idea that carcinoma progression originates in the "hetero-duplication mitosis" that divides non-maturable stem cells into two different types of daughter cells: maturable and non-maturable cancerous stem cells. The divided nonmaturable daughter stem cell, repeats the original mitosis while reproducing the above two types of daughter stem cells, thus continuing hetero-duplication mitotic progression of the cancer. The maturable daughter cells become terminally mature cancer cells (Hirata Y 1999).

The application of these stem cell concepts could explain many important neoplastic features including the clonal origin and heterogeneity of tumours, the occasional formation of tumours from the transit amplifying cells or progenitor cells, the formation of precancerous ''patches'' as well as the concept of "field cancerization". Slaughter firstly proposed this term in order to describe a situation in which: (1) oral cancer develops in multifocal areas of precancerous change; (2) histologically abnormal tissue surrounds the tumour; (3) oral cancer often consists of multiple independent lesions that sometimes coalesce; and (4) the persistence of abnormal tissue after surgery may explain second primary tumours and local recurrences (Slaughter DP et al 1953). Since the Slaughter proposal, within head and neck cancers, many investigators have found cancer cells associated to genetic alterations in tumour adjacent macroscopically normal tissue and surgical margins (Braakhuis BJ et al 2005). Analyses of loss of heterozygosity, microsatellite instability, chromosomal instability and mutations in the p53 gene have been used to detect these alterations and to identify a "field at risk" (Bianchini C et al 2008; Braakhuis BJ et al 2005; Hittelman WN, 2001; Cheng ZG, 2009).

These observations may lead to consider that also head and neck tumours should originate from aberrant stem cells, and that carcinogenesis should be considered as a multistep process, in which an accumulation of genetic and epigenetic alterations forms the basis for the progression from a normal cell to a cancer one.

GENE EXPRESSION AND MARKERS OF HEAD AND NECK CANCER STEM CELLS

Understanding the molecular biology of cancer stem cells would help not only in identifying the mechanism of tumorogenesis, but could also offer the possibility to detect cellular indicators of malignant conversion and progression, thus helping in early identification of cancer stem cells in a specific tissue. This could represent a powerful tool for early diagnosis of particular interest for clinical practice.

So far, only very few "staminal markers" have been identified in head and neck tumours (see also Table 1). Particularly in head and neck squamous cell carcinomas, cells expressing specific antigens, such as the surface CD 44+, as well as high levels of nuclear BMI1, have been reported to be capable of initiating tumor growth and to be involved in the spreading (Ailles L et al 2009). Also Aldehyde dehydrogenase 1 (ALDH1) has been considered as a marker for cancer stem cells. Even if the role of ALDH1 in head and neck squamous cell carcinoma has yet to be determined, it has been reported that ALDH1+ cells displayed radioresistance and represented a reservoir for tumor growth (Chen YC et al 2009; Clay MR et al 2010). In the same way, also in nasopharyngeal cell lines at least two genes, gp96 and GDF15, have been described to be involved in radioresistance as it has been reported that knockdown of these genes enhances radiosensitivity (Chang JT et al 2007).

Sterz CM et al, using immunohistochemical analysis, found antigens CD44 and MMP-9 to co-localize tumour cells at the invasive front within head and neck squamous cell carcinomas; particularly at the western blot analysis they pointed to a role of a MMP-9 positive basal-cell-like cell layer in the process of HNSCC invasiveness (Sterz CM et al, 2009).

Table 1. Putative markers in Head and Neck Cancers

Markers	Tumour Type	References
CD 133+	Squamous Cell Carcinoma	Wei XD et al 2009
CD 44+	Squamous Cell Carcinoma	Ailles L et al 2009
ALDH1	Squamous Cell Carcinoma	Chen YC et al 2009; Clay MR et al 2010
MPP-9	Squamous Cell Carcinoma	Sterz CM et al, 2009
GDF 15	Nasopharyngeal Carcinoma	Chang JT et al 2007

CONCLUSIONS

It is likely that stem cell biology already had an impact in the cancer research field since it seems increasingly evident that cancer can be considered a stem-cell disorder. The stem-cell model for cancer probably could have an impact also on the identification of future therapeutic targets.

Particularly, in a near future, among head and neck tumours will be necessary to (1) further elucidate the critical molecular events involved in head and neck carcinogenesis, and (2) identify possible cellular/molecular markers or cellular site of intervention.

ACKNOWLEDGMENT

The oncological project of the ENT Clinic and of the Molecular Biology Section at the University of Ferrara is also supported by a grant for scientific research from the CARIFE Foundation and by a grant for scientific research from the University of Ferrara and the Emilia Romagna Region.

REFERENCES

Ailles L, Prince M. Cancer stem cells in head and neck squamous cell carcinoma. *Methods Mol Biol.* 2009;568:175-93.

Bianchini C, Ciorba A, Pelucchi S, Piva R, Pastore A. Head and neck cancer: the possible role of stem cells. *Eur Arch Otorhinolaryngol.* 2008 Jan;265(1):17-20.

Bonnet D, Dick JE. 1997. Human acute myeloid leukemia is organized as a hierarchy that originates from a primitive hematopoietic cell. *Nat Med 3*:730–737.

Braakhuis BJ, Leemans CR, BrakenhoV RH (2005) Expanding fields of genetically altered cells in head and neck squamous carcinogenesis. *Semin Cancer Biol 15*:113–120

Cabanillas R, Llorente JL. The Stem Cell Network model: clinical implications in cancer. *Eur Arch Otorhinolaryngol.* 2009 Feb;266(2):161-70.

Chang JT, Chan SH, Lin CY, Lin TY, Wang HM, Liao CT, Wang TH, Lee LY, Cheng AJ. Differentially expressed genes in radioresistant nasopharyngeal cancer cells: gp96 and GDF15. *Mol Cancer Ther.* 2007 Aug;6(8):2271-9.

Chen CY, Chiou SH, Huang CY, Jan CI, Lin SC, Tsai ML, Lo JF. Distinct population of highly malignant cells in a head and neck squamous cell carcinoma cell line established by xenograft model. *J Biomed Sci.* 2009 Nov 16;16:100.

Chen YC, Chen YW, Hsu HS, Tseng LM, Huang PI, Lu KH, Chen DT, Tai LK, Yung MC, Chang SC, Ku HH, Chiou SH, Lo WL. Aldehyde dehydrogenase 1 is a putative marker for cancer stem cells in head and neck squamous cancer. *Biochem Biophys Res Commun.* 2009 Jul 31;385(3):307-13.

Chen ZG. The cancer stem cell concept in progression of head and neck cancer. *J Oncol.* 2009;2009:894064. Epub 2009 Dec 3.

Chiou SH, Yu CC, Huang CY, Lin SC, Liu CJ, Tsai TH, Chou SH, Chien CS, Ku HH, Lo JF. Positive correlations of Oct-4 and Nanog in oral cancer stem-like cells and high-grade oral squamous cell carcinoma. *Clin Cancer Res.* 2008 Jul 1;14(13):4085-95.

Clay MR, Tabor M, Owen JH, Carey TE, Bradford CR, Wolf GT, Wicha MS, Prince ME. Single-marker identification of head and neck squamous cell carcinoma cancer stem cells with aldehyde dehydrogenase. *Head Neck.* 2010 Jan 13.

Costea DE, Tsinkalovsky O, Vintermyr OK, Johannessen AC, Mackenzie IC. 2006. Cancer stem cells—new and potentially important targets for the therapy of oral squamous cell carcinoma. *Oral Dis 12*:443–454.

Dontu G, Liu S, Wicha MS. 2005. Stem cells in mammary development and carcinogenesis: Implications for prevention and treatment. *Stem Cell Rev 1*:207–213.

Ferrandina G, Martinelli E, Petrillo M, Prisco MG, Zannoni G, Sioletic S, Scambia G. CD133 antigen expression in ovarian cancer. *BMC Cancer.* 2009 Jul 7;9(1):221.

Forastiere A, Koch W, Trotti A, Sidransky D (2001) Medical progress–head and neck cancer. *N Engl J Med 345*:1890–1900

Graziano A, d'Aquino R, Tirino V, Desiderio V, Rossi A, Pirozzi G. The stem cell hypothesis in head and neck cancer. *J Cell Biochem.* 2008 Feb 1;103(2):408-12.

Hirata Y (1999) Progression of cancer. Med Hypotheses 52(6):51–13

Hittelman WN (2001) Genetic instability in epithelial tissues at risk for cancer. *Ann N Y Acad Sci 952*:1–12

Lapidot T, Sirard C, Vormoor J, Murdoch B, Hoang T, Caceres-Cortes J, Minden M, Paterson B, Caligiuri MA, Dick JE. 1994. A cell initiating human acute myeloid leukaemia after transplantation into SCIDmice. *Nature 367*:645–648.

Lessard J, Sauvageau G (2003) Bmi-1 determines the proliferative capacity of normal and leukaemic stem cells. *Nature 423*(6937):255–260

Li CY, Li BX, Liang Y, Peng RQ, Ding Y, Xu DZ, Zhang X, Pan ZZ, Wan DS, Zeng YX, Zhu XF, Zhang XS. Higher percentage of CD133+ cells is associated with poor prognosis in colon carcinoma patients with stage IIIB. *J Transl Med.* 2009 Jul 7;7(1):56.

McDonald SA, Graham TA, Schier S, Wright NA, Alison MR. Stem cells and solid cancers. *Virchows Arch.* 2009 Jul;455(1):1-13. Epub 2009 Jun 5.

Pardal R, Molofsky AV, He S, Morrison SJ (2005) Stem cell selfrenewal and cancer stem cells proliferation are regulated by common networks that balance the activation of proto-oncogenes and tumor suppressors. *Cold Spring Harb Symp Quant Biol 70*:177–185.

Polakis P (2000) Wnt signaling and cancer. *Genes Dev 14*(15):1837–1851

Reya T, Morrison SJ, Clarke MF, Weissman IL. 2001. Stem cells, cancer, and cancer stem cells. *Nature 414*:105–111.

Reya T, Duncan AW, Ailles L, Domen J, Scherer DC, Willert K, Hintz L, Nusse R, Weissman IL (2003) A role for wnt signalling in self-renewal of haematopoietic stem cells. *Nature 423*(6938):409–414

Slaughter DP, Southwick HW, Smejkal W (1953) "Field cancerization" in oral stratified squamous epithelium. *Cancer 6*:963–968

Sterz CM, Kulle C, Dakic B, Makarova G, Böttcher MC, Bette M, Werner JA, Mandic R. A basal-cell-like compartment in head and neck squamous cell carcinomas represents the invasive front of the tumor and is expressing MMP-9. *Oral Oncol.* 2010 Feb;46(2):116-22.

Tirino V, Camerlingo R, Franco R, Malanga D, La Rocca A, Viglietto G, Rocco G, Pirozzi G. The role of CD133 in the identification and characterisation of tumour-initiating cells in non-small-cell lung cancer. *Eur J Cardiothorac Surg.* 2009 May 21.

Watkins DN, Berman DM, Burkholder SG, Wang B, Beachy PA, Baylin SB (2003) Hedgehog signalling within airway epithelial progenitors and in small-cell lung cancer. *Nature 422*(6929):313– 317

Wei XD, Zhou L, Cheng L, Tian J, Jiang JJ, Maccallum J. In vivo investigation of CD133 as a putative marker of cancer stem cells in Hep-2 cell line. *Head Neck.* 2009 Jan;31(1):94-101.

Zhou ZT, Jiang WW. Cancer stem cell model in oral squamous cell carcinoma. *Curr Stem Cell Res Ther.* 2008 Jan;3(1):17-20.

In: Cancer Stem Cells
Editor: Melissa E. Jordan, pp. 103-124

ISBN: 978-1-61668-971-1
© 2010 Nova Science Publishers, Inc.

Chapter VI

REGULATION OF CANCER STEM CELLS BY THE NOTCH SIGNALING PATHWAY: BASIC MECHANISMS AND CLINICAL IMPLICATIONS[1]

Min-Hua Zheng[‡], Yi-Yang Hu[≠], Luo-An Fu, and Hua Han[*]
Fourth Military Medical University, Xi'an, China

1. GENERAL REVIEW OF CANCER STEM CELLS (CSCs)

1.1. History of CSC Research

Although the relationship between cancer and embryonic development was revealed more than one century ago [1], the concept of CSCs was discovered only recently through two aspects of biological progress. One is the discovery of stem cells in the hematopoietic system in the 1960s [2], which was further investigated by Spangrude et al. who purified the hematopoietic stem cells (HSCs) from mouse bone marrow (BM) with the use of a variety of phenotypic markers, and confirmed the biological properties of HSCs by in vitro and in vivo studies [3]. The second is that in 1977–1978, Fidler et al. and Kripke et al. reported that subpopulation of cells derived from the B16 melanoma differ greatly in their ability to produce lung colonies. This indicates that the parental tumor is composed of heterogeneous clones of cells that differ in their biological behavior, such as the ability to form metastasis [4, 5].

[1] This work was supported by grants from the Natural Science Foundation of China (30973370) and the Ministry of Science and Technology of China (2006AA02A111, 2009CB521706).
‡ These authors contributed equally to this study.
≠ These authors contributed equally to this study.
* For correspondence: Hua Han, Department of Medical Genetics and Developmental Biology, Fourth Military Medical University, Chang-Le Xi Street #17, Xi'an 710032, China, Tel. +86-29-84774487, e-mail, huahan@fmmu.edu.cn.

These studies led to the first pioneering discovery of CSCs in 1994 by Lapidot and Dick, who identified a leukemic CSC capable of initiating human acute myeloid leukemia (AML) after transplantation into an immunodeficient mouse [6]. Subsequent studies have confirmed the existence of stem cell-like cancer cells or CSCs in other types of leukemia, and more importantly, in solid tumors. These tumor cells with strong potentials for self-renewal and multi-lineage differentiation have been recognized as critical cell populations responsible for tumor initiation and growth, metastasis, and drug- and radiation-resistance.

1.2. CSCs in Hematopoietic Malignancies

CSCs in leukemia are also called leukemic stem cells (LSCs) or leukemia-initiating cells. These cells hold at least some surface markers of normal HSCs, and maintain the key HSC properties of self-renewal and differentiation potentials. Thus, AML stem cells are identified by the $CD34^+CD38^-$ phenotype and the ability to initiate histologically similar leukemia in NOD/SCID mice [7]. LSCs have been documented for nearly all AML subtypes and are phenotypically described as $CD34^+/CD38^-$. The interleukin (IL)-3 receptor alpha chain (CD123) was strongly expressed in $CD34^+/CD38^-$ cells from primary AML specimens. Conversely, normal BM-derived $CD34^+/CD38^-$ cells showed virtually no detectable expression of CD123, indicating that CD123 represents a unique marker for primitive AML stem cells [8]. Moreover, AML stem cells are negative for c-kit expression; in contrast, HSC is positive for c-kit expression. In most AML patients, AML stem cells reside in a quiescent cell cycle state, analogous to their normal HSC counterparts [9]. Pten, a tumour suppressor in adult hematopoietic cells, regulates the proliferation of both HSCs and AML stem cells. It promoted HSC proliferation, leading to HSC depletion cell-autonomously and preventing HSCs from stably reconstituting in irradiated mice. On the other hand, conditional depletion of *Pten* leads to the myeloproliferative disease within days and transplantable leukemia within weeks [10].

Using the same thinking, investigators have demonstrated that CSCs exist in other leukemia including chronic myeloid leukemia (CML) and acute lymphoblast leukemia (ALL). Similar to LSCs in AML, the immunophenotype of CML stem cells is $CD34^+/CD38^-$ as well [11]. Considerable interest has focused on the observation that CML stem cells show a reduced or absent dependence on growth factors for their survival. Studies on human CMLs have identified LSCs that also demonstrate a quiescent phenotype, as AML stem cells [12]. In normal mouse HSCs, the process of self-renewal involves the β-catenin-signaling pathway. CML stem cells also depend on that pathway. Jamieson et al. revealed that activation of β-catenin in CML granulocyte-macrophage progenitors appears to enhance the self-renewal activity and leukemic potential of these cells [13].

1.3. CSCs in Solid Tumors

Al-Hajj et al. were the first to identify and prospectively isolate a subpopulation of $CD44^-$ $CD24^{-/low}lin^-$ cells, which was responsible for the propagation of tumors from eight of nine human metastatic breast cancer specimens. Their research also showed that as few as 100 cells with this phenotype were able to initiate tumors upon transplantation into immune-deficient NOD/SCID mice. The tumorigenic subpopulation of tumor cells could be serially passaged, each time generating new tumors containing additional CD44$^-$CD24$^{-/low}$lin$^-$ tumorigenic cells as well as diverse mixed populations of nontumorigenic cells present in the initial tumor. Thus, these breast tumors seem to originate from a low-frequency tumorigenic cell that is phenotypically and functionally distinct from the bulk tumor cells. These breast tumorigenic cells appear to fulfill the criteria of true stem cells and can be defined as CSCs [14].

A similar finding was subsequently made in human brain tumors. Singh et al. purified CSCs from human brain tumors of different phenotypes that possess a marked capacity for proliferation, self-renewal, and differentiation. The increased self-renewal capacity of the brain tumor stem cells (BTSCs) was highest from the most aggressive clinical samples of medulloblastoma, compared with other low-grade gliomas. Most interestingly, the BTSC was exclusively isolated with the cell fraction expressing the neural stem cells (NSCs) surface marker CD133. Moreover, these isolated CD133$^+$ cells could differentiate in culture into tumor cells similar to the tumor cell types from the patients [15]. The further study by Singh et al. showed that injection of as few as 100 CD133$^+$ cells produced a tumor that could be serially transplanted and phenotypically resembled the patients' original tumors. In contrast, the injection of 10^5 CD133$^-$ cells did not cause a tumor [16]. Besides CD133, markers such as BMI-1, nestin, Sox2, Musashi, SSEA-1 (CD15), and activated Notch signaling pathway have also been suggested to identify the glioma CSC [17]. In addition, the characteristics of CSCs, such as self-renewal, differentiation, and the ability to recapitulate tumors were also found in other brain tumors [18, 19].

Similarly, the subpopulation of tumor cells with CSC characteristics was soon found in other solid tumors, such as melanomas (CD20$^+$), prostate cancer (CD44$^+$α2β1$^+$CD133$^+$), colorectal cancer (CD133$^+$), and pancreatic cancer (CD44$^+$EpCam$^+$CD24$^+$) [20-23]. The identification of tumor initiating cells in various types of tumors provides new insights into human tumor pathogenesis. It gives strong supports for the CSC hypothesis as the basis for many solid tumors, meanwhile indicating a previously unidentified cellular target for more effective cancer therapies.

2. THE NOTCH SIGNALING PATHWAY

2.1. The Components of the Notch Signaling Pathway

The Notch gene was first uncovered by Morgan in 1914, with its name derived from the notching wing phenotype in *Drosophila* mutants carrying mutations in the Notch locus. In 1985, Artavanis-Tsakonas et al. successfully cloned the gene, which encodes a large single-pass type I transmembrane receptor [24,25]. Mammals have four Notch receptors, which have the extracellular domain (ECD) containing tandem epidermal growth factor (EGF)-like repeats mediating interactions with ligands, a transmembrane domain (TMD), and the intracellular domain (NICD) composed of a RAM (RBP-J association molecule), nuclear localization signals (NLS), an ankyrin repeats (ANK), transactivation domain (TAD), and a PEST region involved in protein degradation [26].

The core Notch signaling pathway is evolutionarily highly conserved. The canonical Notch signaling pathway mainly comprises receptors, ligands, transcriptional complex components in the nucleus, and downstream genes, with a growing roster of regulatory molecules. Notch signaling is initiated upon ligand binding by receptors between neighboring cells. The two major classes of Notch ligands in *Drosophila* are Delta and Serrate, while they give rise to five ligands in mammals as Delta-like (Dll)1/3/4 and Jagged1/2, respectively. Like Notch receptors, all of the ligands are single-pass type I transmembrane proteins, with a specific DSL domain as a putative Notch-binding surface. Ligand binding triggers a series of proteolytic events in TMD executed by the γ-secretase, resulting in the release of NICD from the membrane and its translocation into the nucleus [26].

The signal-induced transcriptional activation complex, recruited by NICD, mainly comprises the DNA-binding protein RBP-J (also termed CBF1), and mastermind-like (MAML) protein [26]. This protein complex, in turn, directs the assembly of additional co-activators that drive target gene expression. Although RBP-J has been generally accepted as the major effector of Notch pathway, we note here that RBP-J-independent non-canonical Notch signaling has also been reported [27].

In spite of numerous RBP-J binding sites throughout the genome, until now, only the basic helix–loop–helix (bHLH) transcriptional repressors, for example, the enhancer of split (HES) family genes have been identified as canonical downstream effector genes [28]. In addition, some tissue specific downstream genes have been uncovered, such as Myc oncogene regulated by Notch in T lymphocytes [29]. Concerning the pleiotropic effects of Notch pathway, indeed, the whole spectrum of Notch transcriptional targets in genome has yet to be discovered.

2.2. The Regulation of the Notch Signaling Pathway

Productive Notch ligand-receptor binding depends on post-translational events, such as glycosylation of receptors mediated by OFUT-1 and Fringe. Many of the EGF repeats in Notch receptors can be fucosylated by the fucosyltransferase OFUT-1. In cells expressing Fringe, the fucose is extended by the glycosyltransferase activity of Fringe, altering the ability of specific ligands to activate Notch. For example, Fringe-modified receptors favor binding of Delta instead of Jagged family of Notch ligands [30].

The half-time of Notch and DSL proteins on membrane is decided by the endocytosis of receptors and ligands, executed mainly by ubiquitin E3 ligase such as Delex and Mindbomb, respectively. The E3 ubiquitin ligases shift receptor and ligand membrane trafficking toward endocytosis-mediated degradation or recycling. The endosomal sorting therefore is a key step to restrict the level of Notch activation. During Notch signal activation, NICD is phosphorylated on its TAD domain and targeted for proteasomal degradation by E3 ubiquitin ligase such as Fbw7, leading to attenuation of the signal. Mutations that stabilize NICD can cause T cell acute lymphoblastic leukemia in humans [28]. Another protein, Lethal Giant Discs (LGD), is also required to maintain Notch in the OFF state, for the change of LGD protein level results in ligand-independent Notch activation [31]. In addition, it should be noted that γ-secretase cleavage can also occur at the endosomal compartments, perhaps following mono-ubiquitination of NICD, leading to down regulation of Notch acitivity [28,31].

The local distribution and activation of Notch receptors on the cell membrane are controlled by some polarity proteins, for examples, Numb and Crumbs, and in that way results in regional specific Notch activity. Numb, only inherited by unique daughter cell after asymmetric cell division, can promote Notch endocytosis and degradation [28,31]. On the other hand, the apical polarity protein Crumbs appears to paly a role in restricting γ-secretase activity thus limiting the cellular area and extent of Notch activation [28,31].

Mammalian Notch recceptors are heterodimers formed by ECD and TMD/NICD through noncovalent interactions. The posttranslational single polypeptide of Notch receptor is cleavaged by protein convertases Furin at site 1 (S1) into ECD and TMD/NICD in the trans-Golgi compartment, and is then targeted to the cell surface as a heterodimer. On the binding of Notch ligands, Notch receptors are successively cleaved by a cell surface metalloprotease (ADAM10/ADAM17) at S2, releasing ECD and leaving approximately 12 amino acids of the TMD on the extracellular side, and subsequently by the presenilin complex that has a γ-secretase activity and cleaves within the membrane at S3 and S4. The latter cleavage releases NICD and a Nβ peptide. After these cleavages mediated by 3 enzyme complexes, the NICD is released from the membrane and translocates into the nucleus, with the Notch ECD transendocytosed into the signal-sending cell with the ligands, and the Nβ peptide on TMD entering the intercellular mesenchyma. Like Notch receptors, Notch ligands as type I transmembrane protein are also subject to extracelluar cleavage by ADAM protease followed by transmembrane domain cleavage by γ-secretase. Ligand processing may be important for its downregulation and membrane clearance. Alternatively, it could generate biologically soluble ligands that may acts as antagonists of Notch signaling [28,31].

In the absence of NICD, the DNA-binding protein RBP-J associates with corepressor (Co-R) proteins and histone deacetylases (HDACs) to repress its target promoters. In mammals, while RBP-J can form complexes with a series of ubiquitous corepressors, the MINT protein emerged as the critical repressor of Notch target genes [26,28]. The binding of NICD to RBP-J triggers an allosteric change that facilitates displacement of transcriptional repressors. The NICD/RBP-J interface is then recognized by MAML, and this ternary complex recruits coactivators (Co-A) such as histone acetylases (HATs), and chromatin-remodeling factors, to assemble an active transcriptional complex on target promoters [26,28,31].

3. THE REGULATION OF CSCS BY THE NOTCH SIGNALING PATHWAY

3.1. Roles of Notch Signaling in Normal Stem Cell Maintenance

Stem Cell Self-Renewal

Notch activation is essential for maintaining the self-renewal of diverse stem cells. In the hematopoietic system, the requirement of Notch signaling on HSC self-renewal is most prominent in adult-type HSC generation [32]. Duncan et al explored in situ the Notch activation in HSCs near the trabecular bone surface in BM, using mice harboring green fluorescence protein (GFP) as a reporter under the CSL binding sequence, indicating that Notch activity in HSCs contributes to inhibiting HSC differentiation [33]. Forced expression of a constitutively active form of Notch1 [34,35] or wild-type HES1 [36] potentially expands the murine HSCs and inhibits HSC differentiation. Soluble forms of Dll1 have been used to expand the number of cultured human HSCs, in the presence of hematopoietic cytokines [37,38]. However, to date, the HSC expansion degrees have not been robust enough to establish clinically applications. A recent work by Delaney et al indicates that high doses of immobilized Dll1-Fc treatment induce apoptosis of HSCs instead of triggering expansion [38]. In addition, it appears that diverse Notch ligands have different biologic effects on HSC expansion in vitro [32]. These issues raise the importance of the levels of Notch activity and the types of Notch ligands in promoting self-renewal of adult HSCs.

Notch activation can also promote NSC self-renewal. Conditional knockout of Notch1 [39] or RBP-J [40] in developing mouse brain resulted in depletion of NSCs and premature neurogenesis, indicating that this pathway is required for the maintenance and expansion of embryonic NSC pool. Moreover, Notch or RBP-J deletion in the mouse retina also leads to the exhausting of retinal progenitor cells (RPCs), a type of multipotent neural progenitor cells [41,42]. For adult NSCs, Andreu-Agulló at al recently demonstrated that Notch was active in astroglia-like NSCs (type B cell), but not in transit-amplifying progenitors (type C cell) of the subependymal zone in adult mice, and that the level of Notch transcriptional activity correlated with self-renewal [43]. In addition, in vitro analysis of self-renewal in neurospheres has implicated that Notch signaling can efficiently promote NSC expansion and potentially could be harnessed for transplantation-based brain repair [44].

Stem Cell Multipotency

Notch signaling has an important role in hematopoiesis as a mediator of cell fate determination. A number of studies demonstrate that Notch signaling inhibits myeloid differentiation from progenitor cells [45]. Further studies by Han et al revealed that when RBP-J is deleted, common lymphoid progenitor (CLP) cell mainly give rise to B-cells, instead of T-cells [46]. These results indicate that Notch-RBP-J signaling regulate the multipotency of CLP by promoting one cell fate while inhibiting another during binary choice. In the case of NSCs, Notch signal promotes astrocyte gila cell fate, while inhibiting neuronal and oligodendrocyte cell commitment [47]. For adult NSCs, it has been shown that Notch activity-high cells were substantially more multipotent than Notch activity-low cells [48]. In addition, RPCs are multipotent for seven neural cell types. On the deletion of Notch1 [41] or RBP-J [42], RPCs are biased to photoreceptor cell fate. The regulation of stem cell multipotency by Notch signaling might be a useful tool to induce specific cell types from stem cells for therapy. For example, Osakada et al recently reported that when blocking Notch signaling pathway, the ES cell derived RPC differentiate into Crx+ photoreceptor progenitors [49].

Stem Cell Niche

Tissue stem cells reside within specific microenvironment with defined anatomical location termed 'niches'. HSCs have Notch receptors on their membrane, and osteoblasts on the surfaces of trabecular bone express Notch ligand Jagged1 and have been identified as one of the BM HSC niches [50]. Using transgenic mice that express constitutive active parathyroid hormone receptor under the control of the collagen type-IV promoter, Calvi et al found that when Jagged1 is overexpressed in the osteoblasts, HSCs are increased. The authors argue that the increase in HSCs is a direct consequence of the increased osteoblastic niche area and Jagged1 overexpression in osteoblasts [51]. These results indicate that interactions between osteoblast-expressed Notch ligands such as Jagged1 and signal transmission to the Notch receptor-expressing HSCs might be one of the molecular mechanisms underlying the regulation of HSCs in the osteoblastic niches in BM.

The subventricular zone (SVZ) and the subgranular zone (SGZ) of the hippocampus region are the primary regions in which NSCs reside and support neurogenesis in the adult brain [52,53]. In both the SVZ and SGZ regions, endothelial cells (ECs) and the specialized basal lamina are essential components of the NSC niche. These ECs provide attachment for SVZ and SGZ astrocytes and generate a variety of signals that control stem cell self-renewal and lineage commitment [53,54]. In fact, angiogenesis and neurogenesis may be signal reciprocally co-regulated by factors including bFGF, VEGF, IGF-1 and Notch [52,53,55,56]. Notch signaling has been found to regulate the vascular formation. Mutant mice with disrupted Notch pathway components display various defects in blood vessel formation [55]. In addition, deletion of RBP-J has been shown to disturb the vascular homeostasis in mouse neural retina [57]. All these research works indicate that Notch signaling is potentially involved in NSCs niches by regulating adjacent vascular structures.

The maintenance of stem cells demands their exact location in the stem cell niches. Cell adhesion between adjacent stem cells contributes to meeting this requirement. In BM, adherens junction composed of cadherin and β-catenin formed between the osteoblasts and HSCs, which ensure the binding of multiple pairs of receptors and ligands [50]. Similarly, adherens junctions with cadherin and β-catenin are formed between NSCs at the lumen of the ventricle. When epithelial architecture and adherens junctions are disrupted, cell proliferation in the ventricular zone are also disturbed [50,58]. β-catenin may mediate the loss of growth control when adherens junctions are disrupted, because disruptions of adherens junctions may lead to misregulation and accumulation of cytoplasmic β-catenin, which in turn activates Wnt signaling in the NSC pool [59]. Adherens junction disturbance is seen in various Notch-interfered mouse models. In Notch1, RBP-J and Hes1-deleted mouse retina, the adherens junctions between RPCs are severely disturbed, indicating Notch function on the maintenance of adherens junctions [41,42].

3.2. Influence of the Notch Signaling in CSCs

CSCs are considered as the real driving force behind cancer growth, and the critical intrinsic reason for chemo- or radio- therapeutic resistance and cancer relapse. While self-renewal, CSCs retain the differentiation potential giving rise to non-self-renewing differentiated cancer cells that would constitute the bulk of the cancer tissue. CSCs share multiple characteristics with normal stem cells, and it seems that critical signaling pathways that govern stem cells during development such as Notch, Wnt, BMP and Hedgehog signaling pathways would also regulate CSCs. The genetic alteration of these signaling pathways would lead CSCs to become independent of growth signals or to resist antigrowth signals and would allow them to undergo uncontrolled proliferation and tumorigenesis [60]. At present, a growing amount of evidence has shown an association between Notch signaling alterations and cancer behaviors [29,61]. A few published reports further revealed that Notch signaling probably influence tumorigenesis by the regulation of CSCs, as we will review below from several aspects of CSC characteristics. Based on these research works, Notch signaling inhibitors are already tested in clinical trails with cancer patients [62].

CSC Self-Renewal and Multipotency

Notch signaling plays a central role in T-cell acute lymphoblastic leukaemia (TALL) pathogenesis. More than 50% of TALLs patients show activating mutations in Notch1 locus [63]. Besides them, up to 1% of TALL patients carry a chromosome translocation that leads to the expression of constitutively active Notch1 (N1ICD) [63-65]. Members of the Notch family have critical roles in keeping HSC in an undifferentiated state and may act as gatekeepers for factors governing self-renewal and lineage commitment, and factors preventing uncontrolled proliferation of HSCs and their transformation into LSCs [63,66]. Based on these findings, a clinical trial with the γ-secretase inhibitor (GSI) in patients with refractory TALL has been developed at present [67].

In brain tumors, markers such as CD133 have been used to identify rare cells bearing the unique ability to form tumor neurospheres [68]. A recent report shows that pharmacological inhibition of Notch signaling by GSI results in the depletion of a CD133$^+$ CSC population [69]. Down-regulation of Notch pathway has also been linked to cellular differentiation in both normal development and in neoplasms [29,47]. GSI in medulloblastoma cultures increased RNA levels of two markers of cerebellar neuronal differentiation, Tuj1 and GABRA6, in a dose-dependent fashion. During development, the GABRA6 expression is specifically found in cerebellar granule cells as they mature. Its induction suggests that the activated differentiation after Notch blockade in medulloblastoma cultures resembles the normal maturation of cerebellar granule neuron precursors. Further analysis revealed that Notch blockade suppressed expression of Hes1 and caused cell cycle exit, apoptosis, and differentiation in medulloblastoma cell lines [70]. Additionally, upon Notch inactivation, viable populations of better-differentiated cells continued to grow, but were unable to efficiently form soft-agar colonies or tumor xenografts, suggesting that a cell fraction required for tumor propagation had been depleted [70]. Interestingly, Notch signaling levels were higher in the stem-like cell fraction, providing a potential mechanism for their increased sensitivity to inhibition of this pathway. Nestin is another candidate of CSCs markers. Further observations demonstrated that apoptotic rates following Notch blockade were almost 10-fold higher in primitive nestin-positive cells as compared with nestin-negative ones. CSCs in brain tumors thus seem to be selectively vulnerable to Notch blocking agents, compared with none cancer stem-like cells [70].

Notch signaling is also involved in breast CSC self-renewal. Recently, it has been reported that residual breast tumors after chemo-therapy are enriched with CSCs with increased self-renewal capability due to the alteration of developmentally conserved signaling pathways such as Notch [67]. Similarly, Notch signaling protects breast tumors from drug-induced apoptosis in preclinical models [71]. Activation of Notch signaling has been observed in approximately 40% of breast tumor patients. In fact, Notch1 and Notch2 expression in breast tumor tissues have been associated with clinical prognosis [72]. Parr et al revealed that Notch1 expression was up-regulated, whereas Notch2 expression was downregulated in poorly differentiated breast tumors, compared with their expression in well-differentiated breast tumors, respectively [72]. Further evidence showed that high Jagged1 expression together with Notch1 in poorly differentiated breast tumors were associated with low overall survival [73]. It has also been shown that breast stem cells are enriched by selection of anoikis-resistant cells or cells expressing the membrane phenotype $ESA^+CD44^+CD24^{low}$. Using these breast cancer stem cell populations, Harrison et al found that Notch4 signaling activity was 8-fold higher in stem cell-enriched cell populations compared with differentiated cells, whereas Notch1 signaling activity was 4-fold lower in the stem cell-enriched cell populations. Pharmacologic or genetic inhibition of Notch1 or Notch4 reduced stem cell activity in vitro and reduced tumor formation in vivo, but Notch4 inhibition produced a more robust effect with a complete inhibition of tumor initiation observed [74].

CSC Metastasis

Balint et al reported that Notch activity could facilitate the metastasis of melanoma. In their study, the activation of Notch1 signaling is required for β-catenin-mediated human primary melanoma progression [75]. Accordingly, Liu et al further demonstrated that Notch1 signaling promotes primary melanoma invasion by up-regulating N-cadherin expression [76]. The N-cadherin and β-catenin-mediated adherens junctions enhanced the implantation of tumor cells into none primary tissues. In addition, Wang et al reported that Notch signaling plays a critical role in pancreatic cancer cell invasion. Their research showed that down-regulation of Notch1 reduced nuclear factor-κB (NF-κB) DNA-binding activity, and its target genes, such as vascular endothelial growth factor (VEGF) and matrix metalloproteinase-9 (MMP-9) expression [77]. Hu et al also showed that hepatocarcinoma growing under a Notch deficient environment had higher incidence of liver matastasis [78].

The mechanisms of Notch function on cancer stem cell metastasis are closely related with epithelium-mesenchymal transitions (EMT). EMT describes the differentiation switch between polarized epithelial cells and motile mesenchymal cells, and facilitates cell movements and generation of new tissues during embryogenesis. EMT contributes to tumor invasion and vascular intravasation during cancer metastasis. TGF-β signaling is a major inducer of EMT not only during embryonic development, but also during cancer progression in mouse models [79]. Timmerman et al reported that Notch promotes EMT during cardiac development and oncogenic transformation. In chicken and mice, the formation of heart valve and septa includes a prominent EMT process of intracardial cells which respond to Notch signaling in a sequential manner, therefore initiates expression of TGF-β2 in order to induce Snail expression and repress E-cadherin [80]. Interestingly, Zavadil et al demonstrated the inverse scenario that TGF-β signaling can induce expression of Notch ligands, such as Jagged-1, which activates Notch signaling, leading to EMT and epithelial cell cycle arrest in cell models in vitro [81]. In summary, Jagged1/Notch signaling mediates EMT in cancer metastasis with integration of TGF-β signaling.

Drug- and Radiation-Resistence

The resistence of CSCs to drug- and radiation-therapy is the main reason for cancer metastasis and relapse, thus becoming the main blockade of successful clinical treatment of cancers. Research works revealed that Notch activity also participates in drug- and radiation-resistence. In the chemotherapy of breast cancer, trastuzumab is an anti-HER2 inhibitor that is considered the first choice of treatment for ErBb2-positive breast tumors. A recent article showed that ErBb2 overexpression suppressed Notch1 activity in ErBb2-positive breast cancer models and this effect could be reversed by trastuzumab. In trastuzumab-resistant breast cancer models, Notch inhibition showed an additional anti-tumor effect. These results suggested that Notch signaling might play a role in the resistance to trastuzumab in breast cancer. This resistance may be prevented or reversed by the concomitant or subsequent inhibition of Notch pathway in breast cancer therapy [82].

Although radiotherapy is the most effective nonsurgical treatment for gliomas at present, gliomas are highly radioresistant and recurrence is nearly universal. Researchers from several laboratories suggest that CSCs contribute to radioresistance in gliomas and breast cancers [83,84]. Wang et al showed that inhibition of Notch pathway with GSI rendered the glioma stem cells more sensitive to radiation. GSI enhanced radiation-induced cell death and impaired clonogenic survival of glioma stem cells, but not non-stem glioma cells. Expression of the constitutively active NICD of Notch1 or Notch2 protected glioma stem cells against radiation. Moreover, knockdown of Notch1 or Notch2 sensitizes glioma stem cells to radiation and impaired xenograft tumor formation [83]. These results suggest a critical role of Notch signaling to regulate radio-resistance of glioma stem cells. Inhibition of Notch signaling are prospective to improve the outcome of current radio-therapy in glioma treatment.

3.3. The Mechanisms of Notch Signaling in the Regulation of CSCs

In fact, there is evidence that in the absence of other oncogenes, physiological activation of Notch signaling is necessary for differentiation programs in various mammalian cells. However, in coordination with other oncogenes, Notch activity seems to promote CSCs amplification in malignancy.

C-myc is a direct downstream genes of Notch pathway in TALL [85]. In addition, Gustafsson et al identified the protein binding of NICD and HIF1α in normal NSCs [86]. It has been demonstrated that HIF2α could activate downstream mitogen Oct4, which could accelerate cell proliferation, as an oncogene [87]. Therefore, it is possible that HIF2α which specifically expressed in glioma CSCs instead of none stem cell-like glioma cells, may also bind to NICD and subsequently transactivate Oct4 expression, which eventually lead to uncontrolled proliferation of CSCs. Kim et al show that hypoxia increases the expression of the stem cell gene Dll1 in neuronal tumor cells [88]. Inhibition of Dll1 enhances spontaneous differentiation, decreases clonogenicity, and reduces in vivo tumor growth. Overexpression of Dll1 inhibits differentiation and enhances tumorigenic potentials. The Dll1 cytoplasmic domain, especially Tyr339 and Ser355, is required for maintaining both clonogenicity and tumorigenicity [88].

Additionally, it has been suggested that Notch1 may mediate the tumorigenic effect of oncogenic RAS protein [89]. Gain of function mutations in RAS occurs in early breast cancer and plays a central role in breast tumorigenesis. Research by Weijzen et al showed that Notch1 was highly expressed in all RAS-positive breast cancer samples. In addition, down-regulation of Notch1 expression in RAS-transformed human breast cells led to a significant decrease in their proliferation. Moreover, the inhibition of RAS signaling also led to the blockade of Notch1 activation. Furthermore, the expression of oncogenic RAS led to higher levels of proteins involved in Notch signal activation [89]. Altogether, these results revealed that Notch receptor may be regulated by upstream oncogene Ras.

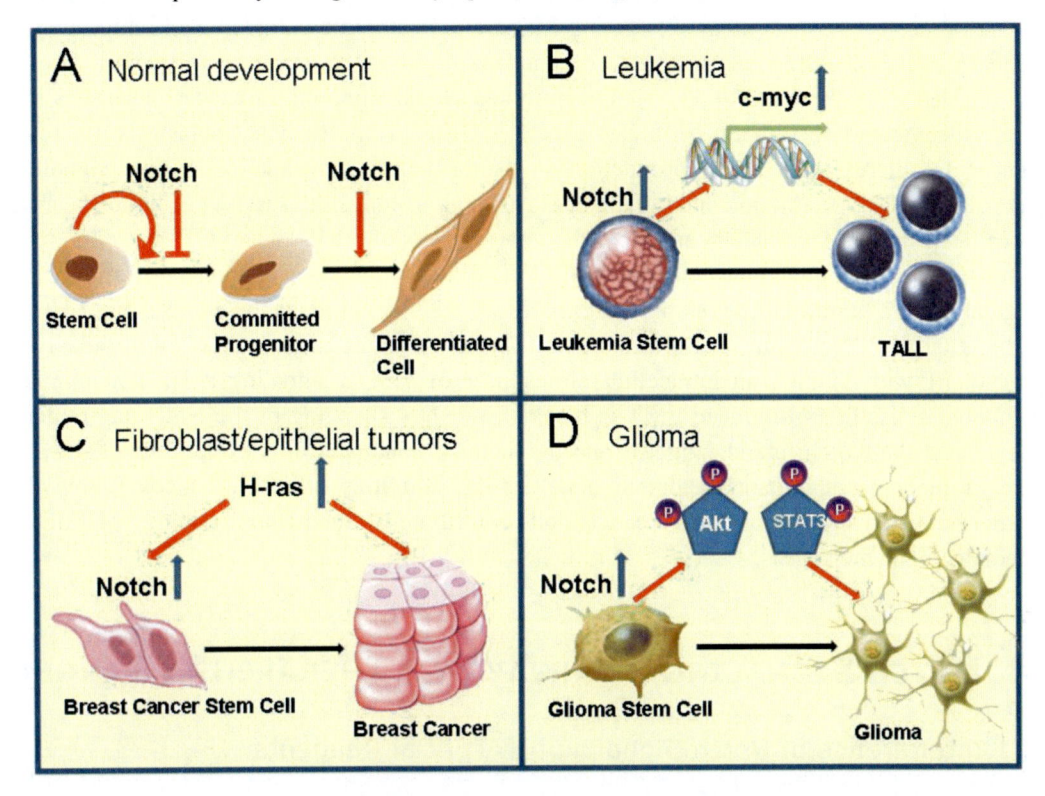

Figure 1. The mechanisms of Notch signaling in the regulation of CSCs. A. Physiological activation of Notch signaling is necessary for stem cell self-renewal, keeping stem cell uncommitted, and for terminal differentiation of certain cell types. B. In T-cell acute lymphoblastic leukemia (TALL) pathogenesis, the oncogene c-myc is a direct downstream genes of Notch pathway, which promote the uncontrolled proliferation of leukemia stem cells. C. The expression of oncogene H-ras in breast cancer leads to Notch signal activation, therefore results in overproduction of breast cancer stem cells. D. In glioma, Notch activation can reinforce the survival of glioma stem cells by enhancing Akt and STAT3 phosphorylation.

3.4. The Cross-Talk between Notch Signaling and Other Signaling

Rapid proliferation and high motility are hallmarks of both embryonic stem cells in development and CSCs in tumorigenesis. Wnt/Notch (Wntch) signaling promotes CSCs proliferation, similar effect with its function on developmental stem cells. Overexpression of β-catenin, a downstream activator of the WNT signaling pathway, expands the transplantable HSC pool in long-term cultures [90]. Furthermore, activation of WNT signaling also increases the expression of other transcription factors and cell cycle regulators important in HSC renewal, such as HoxB4 and Notch1 [33,90]. In addition, collaboration of Notch and Wnt signaling has also been seen in the initiation of liver cancer [91,92]. On the contrary, TGF-β signaling has inhibitory function on cell-cycle progress of CSCs, such as leukemia stem cells (LSCs) and glioma stem cells (GSCs) [93,94]. Moreover, positive or negative reciprocal regulation between the Notch pathway and the p53 pathway, varies with cancer cell types and cancer stages and co-regulates CSCs self-renewal and multi-potency [61]. Therefore, selective or combined targeting of more than a single pathway could improve the efficacy and reduce the toxicity of cancer therapies.

Evidence for the roles of TGF-β signaling and Notch signaling in cancer metastasis has been documented specifically in breast cancer. TGF-β promotes bone metastasis of breast cancer by increasing PTHrP production in tumor cells. Blockade of TGF-β signaling decreases PTHrP production and bone metastasis, and prolongs the survival of tumor-bearing mice [95]. In addition, TGF-β enhances the gene expression of IL11 and CTGF, which may contribute to osteolytic bone metastasis [96]. TGF-β and Notch signaling converge in the regulation of a number of developmental processes. TGF-β increases the expression of Hes1, a direct target of Notch, in several cell types [97]. TGF-β induces the interaction of the NICD of Notch1 with Smad3, an intracellular transducer of TGF-β signaling [97]. In mammary epithelial cells, TGF-β-induced EMT is blocked by RNA silencing of the Notch target gene Hey-1 and the Notch ligand Jagged1, and by chemical inactivation of Notch [98]. TGF-β is one of the most abundant factors in bone matrix, and it is critical to uncover how the autocrine Notch signaling in breast cancer cells contributes to the pathophysiology of TGF-β-mediated bone metastasis.

4. NOTCH SIGNALING PATHWAY AS A THERAPEUTIC TARGET

4.1 Interference of Notch Signaling by Artificial Reagents

Since the Notch signaling pathway plays a critical role in the initiation and development of cancer, it is plausible that targeting the Notch signaling steps, including receptor/ligand binding, release of NICD, interaction of NICD, downstream targets, or even the stability of NICD protein, may have antitumor effects. Currently, one of the emerging approaches for blocking Notch signaling is to suppress the proteolytic step that leads to the generation of NICD. Because the pivotal role of γ-secretase in Notch activation has been well shown, and GSI can prevent Notch receptor activation, several types of GSI have been tested for antitumor effects. An original GSI, IL-X (cbz-IL-CHO), was shown to have Notch1-dependent antineoplastic activity in Ras-transformed fibroblasts [89]. Tripeptide GSI (z-Leu-leu-Nle-CHO) was showed to suppress the growth of melanoma and Kaposi sarcoma in tumor cell lines and/or xenografts in mice [99,100]. Treatment with dipeptide GSI, N-[N-(3,5-difluorophenacetyl)-L-alanyl]-S-phenylglycine t-butyl ester (DAPT) also resulted in a marked reduction in medulloblastoma growth and induced G0-G1 cell cycle arrest and apoptosis in a TALL animal model [101,102]. Another GSI, dibenzazepine, inhibits epithelial cell proliferation and induce goblet cell differentiation in intestinal adenomas in APC knockout mice [103]. More recently, a phase I clinical trial for a Notch inhibitor, MK0752 (developed by Merck, Whitehouse Station, NJ), has been launched for relapsed or refractory TALL and advanced breast cancer patients (http://www.clinicaltrials.gov/ct/show/NCT00100152). Besides the evidence of GSI in directly inactivating Notch signaling on cancer cells, GSI may also suppress angiogenesis in solid tumors by interfering in the cross-talk between the tumor and vasculature through Notch signaling [104].

Although γ-secretase has been regarded as a promising target of Notch signal targeting therapeutics in cancer, there is still no systematic explaination of the detailed mechanism of GSI-induced tumor repression. In recent years, growing evidence has demonstrated that GSI can stimulate apoptosis or induce cell cycle arrest in solid tumor and hematopoietic cancers [100-103]. Loss of function of tumor suppressor genes may be an explanation for the development and progression of cancer. In colon cancer, the frequency of depletion or mutation of tumor suppressor APC is high, and this results in the oncogene-addicted survival of colon cancer cells. Notch activation is one of survival signals in these cancer cells. After the treatment of GSI, the ratio of spontaneous apoptosis of colon cancer cells is increased by the activation of caspase-3 [105]. In the meantime, in the study of GSI-induced repression of TALL cells, researchers observed that inhibition of Notch signaling engaged the Rb pathway and elicited cell cycle exit [106]. Taken together, γ-secretase is a promising target of Notch signal targeting therapeutics in cancer.

4.2. Targeting Notch Signaling to Deplete CSCs

Notch signaling participates in multiple aspects of tumor growth and anti-tumor responses of the hosts, such as tumor cell proliferation and survival, tumor angiogenesis and vasculogenesis, anti-tumor innate as well as adaptive immune responses, and so on [29,61,67]. Concerning the stemness of CSCs, researchers have started efforts to interfere CSCs through Notch signaling pathway. The most exciting concept would be the exhausting of CSCs by blocking Notch signaling, based on the finding that Notch signaling is essential for stem cell maintenance.

Fan et al blocked Notch pathway by GSIs to reduce neurosphere growth and clonogenicity in vitro. The putative CSC markers CD133, Nestin, BMI1, and OLIG2 were reduced following Notch blockade. Using in vitro and in vivo assays, these authors demonstrate that Notch pathway blockade depletes stem-like cells in glioblastoma cells, suggesting that GSIs may be useful as chemotherapeutic reagents to target CSCs in malignant gliomas [69]. Notch pathway inhibition appears to deplete stem-like cancer cells through reduced proliferation and increased apoptosis associated with decreased Akt and STAT3 phosphorylation [69]. Hoey et al developed selective anti-human and anti-mouse Dll4 antibodies. They found that each antibody inhibited tumor growth and that the combination of the two antibodies was more effective than either alone [107]. In addition to interfer the proliferation of tumor cells and neovasculogenesis, treatment with anti-human Dll4 reduced cancer stem cell frequency [107]. Zhen et al investigated the ability of As(2)O(3) to inhibit the formation of tumor in three different cell lines. Their results indicate the negative regulation of CSCs by As(2)O(3). In addition, a Western blot analysis revealed decreased levels of Notch1 and Hes1 proteins due to As(2)O(3) treatment [108]. The authors conclude that As(2)O(3) has a remarkable inhibitory effect on CSCs in glioma cell lines in vivo and in vitro; in addition, they determined that the mechanism of CSC inhibition involves the deregulation of Notch activation [108].

Radiotherapy represents the most effective nonsurgical treatments for gliomas. However, gliomas are highly radioresistant and recurrence is nearly universal. Inhibition of Notch pathway with GSI rendered the glioma stem cells more sensitive to radiation at clinically relevant doses [83]. In their study, GSI enhanced radiation-induced cell death and impaired clonogenic survival of glioma stem cells, but not non-stem glioma cells [83]. Moreover, knockdown of Notch1 or Notch2 sensitized glioma stem cells to radiation and impaired xenograft tumor formation [83]. These growing evidence indicated that the Notch signaling plays a critical role in the regulation of radioresistance of glioma stem cells, and demonstrated that inhibition of Notch signaling holds promise to improve the efficiency of current radiotherapy in glioma treatment. Interrogation of a possible role of the Notch signaling axis on tumor-radioresistance revealed a modest induction of Jagged-1 expression on the surface of nonadherent CSC-enriched cells after fractionated radiation as well as increases in the levels of activated Notch-1 in the culturemedia of CSC-enriched cells, indicating that altered activity in the Notch pathway may partially explain the apparent radioresistance present in the CSC fraction [109]. Moreover, HER2-negative tumors overexpress Notch1 and Notch3. Knockdown of Notch pathway resulted in sensitization of breast cancer cells to deionizing radiation, leading to cell death; the effect was more significant in stem marker CD44$^+$ than in CD44$^-$ cells, and more profound in the HER2-negative than in positive cancer cells [110]. This study indicates that inhibition of Notch signaling could antagonize survival signal of HER2-negative breast cancer-initiating cells carrying genomic damage, and suggests that targeted suppression of the Notch pathway may give the rationale for sensitizing HER2-negative cancer-initiating cells to a therapeutic approach.

It has been commonly accepted that CSCs contributes to the tumor angiogenesis. It is found that CSCs produce much higher levels of VEGF in both normoxic and hypoxic conditions than the non-CSC population, and this CSC-mediated VEGF production leads to amplified endothelial cell migration and tube formation in vitro [111]. A VEGF-overexpression glioma model has recently provided supportive evidence for this as well by showing that glioblastoma CSCs overexpressing VEGF produce larger, more vascular, and highly hemorrhagic tumors [112]. When it was supplemented the endothelial migration and tube-formation assays with the VEGF-blocking antibody bevacizumab (Avastin), the in vitro endothelial cell behaviors were blocked [111]. Moreover, in vivo administration of bevacizumab potently inhibited the growth, vascularity, and hemorrhage of xenografts derived from CSCs, whereas no effects were seen on xenografts from non-CSCs [111]. Recently, Han's group reported that general blockade of Notch signaling in tumor-bearing mice could lead to defective angiogenesis in tumors through inhibition of HIF activation [78].

In recent study, Alteria reported that in estrogen receptor (ER) positive breast cancer cells, GSI inhibited the growth of cancer cells in vitro and in vivo by the disrruption of Notch-survivin axis [113]. It may be envisioned for a role of survivin as a Notch target in clinically aggressive breast cancer. First, Notch-induced heightened survivin levels at mitosis may deregulate multiple mitotic checkpoints, and ultimately contribute to genetic instability and aneuploidy, in vivo. And this Notch-survivin axis may directly promote drug and radiation resistance [113]. This is consistent with the common notion that Notch signaling may play a important role in the chemotherapy and radiotherapy-resistence of CSCs. Higher survivin levels have been consistently linked to inhibition of apoptosis induced by DNA damaging agents. Furthermore, survivin may operate as a Notch-regulated cytoprotective and/or mitotic factor to promote long-term persistence of breast cancer "stem cells", potentially contributing to ductal carcinoma in situ, an idea consistent with the presence of survivin in "stemness" gene signatures, and its role in hematopoietic stem cell viability [113]. Anyway, growing evidence demonstrated that inhibition of Notch signaling in cancer cells may accelerate the repression of cancer by depletion of CSCs which survive mainly on the activation of Notch signaling. And it has been proposed for Notch, that γ-secretase inhibitors have been pursued as therapy for potential "Notch-addicted" tumors cell, especially CSCs.

5. PERSPECTIVES

The hypothesis that cancers arise from CSCs has changed the perspectives on new approaches to treating the disease such as CSC target therapies. Developmental signaling pathways such as Notch, BMPs, Wnt and Hedgehog play critical roles in controlling adult stem cells in homeostatic tissues. In fact, the Notch signaling pathway is a highly evolutionary conserved signaling pathway involved in proliferation and differentiation of embryonic and adult stem cells and also participates in cancer development. If we take into account the above information, it seems reasonable to consider these signaling pathway components as good targets for the development of new anticancer drugs. Currently, five clinical trials with GSI are underway in cancer patients (breast cancer, central nervous system cancer and leukaemia and lymphoma patients) [67]. Furthermore, pharmaceutical companies are also working on the development of new drugs against the Notch pathway. They are not only focusing on obtaining new GSI capable of simultaneously blocking all Notch isoforms, they are also looking for monoclonal antibodies against specific Notch receptors and ligands to reduce the treatment- associated toxicities. Further, clinical trials with these new anti-Notch agents in combination with current chemo- and radio- therapies are necessary to provide proof of the efficacy of CSC-targeted therapy in various tumour types.

REFERENCES

[1]   Cohnheim J, Congenitales, quergestreiftes muskelsarkon der nireren. *Virchows Arch* 1875; 65: 64.

[2]   Till JE, McCulloch EA. A direct measurement of the radiation sensitivity of normal mouse bone marrow cells. *Rad. Res.* 1961; 14: 213-222.

[3]   Spangrude GJ, Heimfeld S, Weissman IL. Purification and characterization of mouse hematopoietic stem cells. *Science.* 1988; 241: 58-62.

[4]   Fidler IJ, Kripke ML. Metastasis results from preexisting variant cells within a malignant tumor. *Science.* 1977; 197: 893-895.

[5]   Kripke ML, Gruys E, Fidler IJ. Metastatic heterogeneity of cells from an ultraviolet light-induced murine fibrosarcoma of recent origin. *Cancer Res.* 1978; 38: 2962-2967.

[6]   Lapidot T, Sirard C, Vormoor J, Murdoch B, Hoang T, Caceres-Cortes J, Minden M, Paterson B, Caligiuri MA, Dick JE. A cell initiating human acute myeloid leukaemia after transplantation into SCID mice. *Nature.* 1994; 367: 645-648.

[7]   Bonnet D, Dick JE. Human acute myeloid leukemia is organized as a hierarchy that originates from a primitive hematopoietic cell. *Nat Med.* 1997; 3: 730-737.

[8]   Jordan CT, Upchurch D, Szilvassy SJ, Guzman ML, Howard DS, Pettigrew AL, Meyerrose T, Rossi R, Grimes B, Rizzieri DA, Luger SM, Phillips GL. The interleukin-

3 receptor alpha chain is a unique marker for human acute myelogenous leukemia stem cells. *Leukemia*. 2000; 14: 1777-1784.

[9]   Guan Y, Gerhard B, Hogge DE. Detection, isolation, and stimulation of quiescent primitive leukemic progenitor cells from patients with acute myeloid leukemia (AML). *Blood*. 2003; 101: 3142-3149.

[10] Yilmaz OH, Valdez R, Theisen BK, Guo W, Ferguson DO, Wu H, Morrison SJ. Pten dependence distinguishes haematopoietic stem cells from leukaemia-initiating cells. *Nature*. 2006; 441: 475-482.

[11] Holyoake TL, Jiang X, Drummond MW, Eaves AC, Eaves CJ. Elucidating critical mechanisms of deregulated stem cell turnover in the chronic phase of chronic myeloid leukemia. *Leukemia*. 2002; 16: 549-558.

[12] Holyoake T, Jiang X, Eaves C, Eaves A. Isolation of a highly quiescent subpopulation of primitive leukemic cells in chronic myeloid leukemia. *Blood*. 1999; 94: 2056-64.

[13] Jamieson CH, Ailles LE, Dylla SJ, Muijtjens M, Jones C, Zehnder JL, Gotlib J, Li K, Manz MG, Keating A, Sawyers CL, Weissman IL. Granulocyte-macrophage progenitors as candidate leukemic stem cells in blast-crisis CML. *N Engl J Med*. 2004; 351: 657-67.

[14] Al-Hajj M, Wicha MS, Benito-Hernandez A, Morrison SJ, Clarke MF. Prospective identification of tumorigenic breast cancer cells. *Proc Natl Acad Sci*. 2003; 100: 3983-8.

[15] Singh SK, Clarke ID, Terasaki M, Bonn VE, Hawkins C, Squire J, Dirks PB. Identification of a cancer stem cell in human brain tumors. *Cancer Res*. 2003; 63: 5821-8.

[16] Singh SK, Hawkins C, Clarke ID, Squire JA, Bayani J, Hide T, Henkelman RM, Cusimano MD, Dirks PB. Identification of human brain tumour initiating cells. *Nature*. 2004; 432: 396-401.

[17] Park DM, Rich JN. Biology of glioma cancer stem cells. Mol Cells. 2009; 28: 7-12.

[18] Galli R, Binda E, Orfanelli U, Cipelletti B, Gritti A, De Vitis S, Fiocco R, Foroni C, Dimeco F, Vescovi A. Isolation and characterization of tumorigenic, stem-like neural precursors from human glioblastoma. *Cancer Res*. 2004; 64: 7011-21.

[19] Yuan X, Curtin J, Xiong Y, Liu G, Waschsmann-Hogiu S, Farkas DL, Black KL, Yu JS. Isolation of cancer stem cells from adult glioblastoma multiforme. *Oncogene*. 2004; 23: 9392-400.

[20] Fang D, Nguyen TK, Leishear K, Finko R, Kulp AN, Hotz S, Van Belle PA, Xu X, Elder DE, Herlyn M. A tumorigenic subpopulation with stem cell properties in melanomas. *Cancer Res*. 2005; 65: 9328-37.

[21] Collins AT, Berry PA, Hyde C, Stower MJ, Maitland NJ. Prospective identification of tumorigenic prostate cancer stem cells. *Cancer Res*. 2005; 65: 10946-51.

[22] Dalerba P, Dylla SJ, Park IK, Liu R, Wang X, Cho RW, Hoey T, Gurney A, Huang EH, Simeone DM, Shelton AA, Parmiani G, Castelli C, Clarke MF. Phenotypic characterization of human colorectal cancer stem cells. *Proc Natl Acad Sci U S A*. 2007; 104: 10158-63.

[23] Prince ME, Sivanandan R, Kaczorowski A, Wolf GT, Kaplan MJ, Dalerba P, Weissman IL, Clarke MF, Ailles LE. Identification of a subpopulation of cells with cancer stem cell properties in head and neck squamous cell carcinoma. *Proc Natl Acad Sci U S A*. 2007; 104: 973-8.

[24] Wharton KA, Yedvobnick B, Finnerty VG, Artavanis-Tsakonas S. opa: A novel family of transcribed repeats shared by the Notch locus and other developmentally regulated loci in D. melanogaster. *Cell.* 1985; 40(1): 55-62.

[25] Wharton KA, Johansen KM, Xu T, Artavanis-Tsakonas S. Nucleotide sequence from the neurogenic locus Notch implies a gene product that shares homology with proteins containing EGF-like repeats. *Cell.* 1985; 43(3 Pt 2): 567-81.

[26] Bray SJ. Notch signalling: a simple pathway becomes complex. *Nat. Rev. Mol. Cell Biol.* 2006; 7: 678-689.

[27] Martinez Arias A, Zecchini V, Brennan K. CSL-independent Notch signalling: a checkpoint in cell fate decisions during development? *Curr Opin Genet Dev.* 2002; 12(5): 524-33.

[28] Kopan R, Ilagan MX. The canonical Notch signaling pathway: unfolding the activation mechanism. *Cell.* 2009; 137: 216-233.

[29] Koch U, Radtke F. Notch and cancer: a double-edged sword. *Cell Mol Life Sci.* 2007; 64: 2746 – 2762.

[30] Haines N, Irvine KD. Glycosylation regulates Notch signalling. *Nat Rev Mol Cell Biol.* 2003; 4: 786–797.

[31] Ilagan MX, Kopan R. SnapShot: notch signaling pathway. *Cell.* 2007; 128(6): 1246.

[32] Chiba S. Notch signaling in stem cell systems. *Stem Cells.* 2006; 24(11): 2437-47.

[33] Duncan AW, Rattis FM, DiMascio LN, Congdon KL, Pazianos G, Zhao C, Yoon K, Cook JM, Willert K, Gaiano N, Reya T. Integration of Notch and Wnt signaling in hematopoietic stem cell maintenance. *Nat Immunol.* 2005; 6: 314 –322.

[34] Varnum-Finney B, Xu L, Brashem-Stein C, Nourigat C, Flowers D, Bakkour S, Pear WS, Bernstein ID. Pluripotent, cytokinedependent, hematopoietic stem cells are immortalized by constitutive Notch1 signaling. *Nat Med.* 2000; 6: 1278 –1281.

[35] Stier S, Cheng T, Dombkowski D, Carlesso N, Scadden DT. Notch1 activation increases hematopoietic stem cell self-renewal in vivo and favors lymphoid over myeloid lineage outcome. *Blood.* 2002; 99: 2369 –2378.

[36] Kunisato A, Chiba S, Nakagami-Yamaguchi E, Kumano K, Saito T, Masuda S, Yamaguchi T, Osawa M, Kageyama R, Nakauchi H, Nishikawa M, Hirai H. HES-1 preserves purified hematopoietic stem cells ex vivo and accumulates side population cells in vivo. *Blood.* 2003; 101: 1777–1783.

[37] Suzuki T, Yokoyama Y, Kumano K, Takanashi M, Kozuma S, Takato T, Nakahata T, Nishikawa M, Sakano S, Kurokawa M, Ogawa S, Chiba S. Highly efficient ex vivo expansion of human hematopoietic stem cells using Delta-Fc chimeric protein. *Stem Cells.* 2006; 24(11): 2456-65.

[38] Delaney C, Varnum-Finney B, Aoyama K, Brashem-Stein C, Bernstein ID. Dose-dependent effects of the Notch ligand Delta1 on ex vivo differentiation and in vivo marrow repopulating ability of cord blood cells. *Blood.* 2005; 106(8): 2693-9.

[39] Mason HA, Rakowiecki SM, Raftopoulou M, Nery S, Huang Y, Gridley T, Fishell G. Notch signaling coordinates the patterning of striatal compartments. *Development.* 2005; 132(19): 4247-58.

[40] Gao F, Zhang Q, Zheng MH, Liu HL, Hu YY, Zhang P, Zhang ZP, Qin HY, Feng L, Wang L, Han H, Ju G. Transcription factor RBP-J-mediated signaling represses the differentiation of neural stem cells into intermediate neural progenitors. *Mol Cell Neurosci.* 2009; 40(4): 442-50.

[41] Jadhav AP, Mason HA, Cepko CL. Notch1 inhibits photoreceptor production in the developing mammalian retina. *Development.* 2006; 133: 913-923.

[42] Zheng MH, Shi M, Pei Z, Gao F, Han H, Ding YQ. The transcription factor RBP-J is essential for retinal cell differentiation and lamination. *Mol Brain.* 2009; 2:38.

[43] Andreu-Agulló C, Morante-Redolat JM, Delgado AC, Fariñas I. Vascular niche factor PEDF modulates Notch-dependent stemness in the adult subependymal zone. *Nat Neurosci.* 2009; 12(12): 1514-23.

[44] Hitoshi S, Alexson T, Tropepe V, Donoviel D, Elia AJ, Nye JS, Conlon RA, Mak TW, Bernstein A, van der Kooy D. Notch pathway molecules are essential for the maintenance, but not the generation, of mammalian neural stem cells. *Genes Dev.* 2002; 16(7): 846–858.

[45] Radtke F, Wilson A, Ernst B, MacDonald HR. The role of Notch signaling during hematopoietic lineage commitment. *Immunol Rev.* 2002; 187: 65-74.

[46] Han H, Tanigaki K, Yamamoto N, Kuroda K, Yoshimoto M, Nakahata T, Ikuta K, Honjo T. Inducible gene knockout of transcription factor recombination signal binding protein-J reveals its essential role in T versus B lineage decision. Int Immunol. 2002; 14: 637-645.

[47] Louvi A, Artavanis-Tsakonas S. Notch signalling in vertebrate neural development. *Nat Rev Neurosci.* 2006; 7: 93-102.

[48] Mizutani K, Yoon K, Dang L, Tokunaga A, Gaiano N. Differential Notch signalling distinguishes neural stem cells from intermediate progenitors. *Nature.* 2007; 449: 351–355.

[49] Osakada F, Ikeda H, Mandai M, Wataya T, Watanabe K, Yoshimura N, Akaike A, Sasai Y, Takahashi M. Toward the generation of rod and cone photoreceptors from mouse, monkey and human embryonic stem cells. *Nat Biotech.* 2008; 26: 215-224.

[50] Li LH, Xie T. Stem cell niche: structure and function. *Annu Rev Cell Dev Biol.* 2005; 21: 605–31.

[51] Calvi LM, Adams GB, Weibrecht KW, Weber JM, Olson DP. Osteoblastic cells regulate the haematopoietic stem cell niche. *Nature.* 2003; 425: 841–46.

[52] Temple S. The development of neural stem cells. *Nature.* 2001; 414: 112–17.

[53] Doetsch F. A niche for adult neural stem cells. *Curr Opin Genet Dev.* 2003; 13: 543–50.

[54] Shen Q, Goderie SK, Jin L, Karanth N, Sun Y. Endothelial cells stimulate selfrenewal and expand neurogenesis of neural stem cells. *Science.* 2004; 304: 1338–40.

[55] Phng LK, Gerhardt H. Angiogenesis: a team effort coordinated by notch. *Dev Cell.* 2009; 16(2): 196-208.

[56] Aberg MA, Aberg ND, Palmer TD, Alborn AM, Carlsson-Skwirut C. IGF-I has a direct proliferative effect in adult hippocampal progenitor cells. *Mol Cell Neurosci.* 2003; 24: 23–40.

[57] Dou GR, Wang YC, Hu XB, Hou LH, Wang CM, Xu JF, Wang YS, Liang YM, Yao LB, Yang AG, Han H. RBP-J, the transcription factor downstream of Notch receptors, is essential for the maintenance of vascular homeostasis in adult mice. *FASEB J.* 2008; 22(5): 1606-17.

[58] Doetsch F. A niche for adult neural stem cells. *Cell.* 2003; 112: 535–548.

[59] Chenn A, Walsh CA. Regulation of cerebral cortical size by control of cell cycle exit in neural precursors. *Science.* 2002; 297(5580): 365-9.

[60] Rosen JM, Jordan CT. The increasing complexity of the cancer stem cell paradigm. *Science* 2009; 324: 1670-73.

[61] Paolo Dotto G. Notch tumor suppressor function. *Oncogene.* 2008; 27(38): 5115–5123.

[62] Miele L, Miao H, Nickoloff BJ. Notch signaling as a novel cancer therapeutic target. *Curr Cancer Drug Targets.* 2006; 6: 313–23.

[63] Ellisen LW, Bird J, West DC, Soreng AL, Reynolds TC, Smith SD, Sklar J. TAN-1, the human homolog of the Drosophila notch gene, is broken by chromosomal translocations in T lymphoblastic neoplasms. *Cell.* 1991; 66: 649–661.

[64] Weng AP, Ferrando AA, Lee W. Activating mutations of NOTCH1 in human T cell acute lymphoblastic leukemia. *Science.* 2004; 306: 269–271.

[65] Aster JC. Deregulated NOTCH signaling in acute T-cell lymphoblastic leukemia/lymphoma: new insights, questions, and opportunities. *Int J Hematol.* 2005; 82: 295–301.

[66] Pui JC, Allman D, Xu L, DeRocco S, Karnell FG, Bakkour S, Lee JY, Kadesch T, Hardy RR, Aster JC, Pear WS. Notch1 expression in early lymphopoiesis influences B versus T lineage determination. *Immunity.* 1999; 11: 299–308.

[67] Bolós V, Blanco M, Medina V, Aparicio G, Díaz-Prado S, Grande E. Notch signalling in cancer stem cells. *Clin Transl Oncol.* 2009; 11: 11-19.

[68] Liu G, Yuan X, Zeng Z, Tunici P, Ng H, Abdulkadir IR, Lu L, Irvin D, Black KL, Yu JS. Analysis of gene expression and chemoresistance of CD133+ cancer stem cells in glioblastoma. *Molecular Cancer.* 2006; 5: 67.

[69] Fan X, Khaki L, Zhu TS, Soules ME, Talsma CE, Gul N, Koh C, Zhang J, Li YM, Maciaczyk J, Nikkhah G, Dimeco F, Piccirillo S, Vescovi AL, Eberhart CG. Notch pathway blockade depletes CD133-positive glioblastoma cells and inhibits growth of tumor neurospheres and xenografts. *Stem Cells.* 2009; 28: 5-16.

[70] Fan X, Matsui W, Khaki L, Stearns D, Chun J, Li YM, Eberhart CG. Notch pathway inhibition depletes stem-like cells and blocks engraftment in embryonal brain tumors. *Cancer Res.* 2006; 66(15): 7445-52.

[71] Stylianou S, Clarke RB, Brennan K. Aberrant activation of notch signaling in human breast cancer. *Cancer Res.* 2006; 66: 1517–1525.

[72] Parr C, Watkins G, Jiang WG. The possible correlation of Notch-1 and Notch-2 with clinical outcome and tumour clinicopathological parameters in human breast cancer. *Int J Mol Med.* 2004; 14: 779–786.

[73] Reedijk M, Odorcic S, Chang L. High-level coexpression of JAG1 and NOTCH1 is observed in human breast cancer and is associated with poor overall survival. *Cancer Res.* 2005; 65: 8530–8537.

[74] Harrison H, Farnie G, Howell SJ, Rock RE, Stylianou S, Brennan KR, Bundred NJ, Clarke RB. Regulation of breast cancer stem cell activity by signaling through the Notch4 receptor. *Cancer Res.* 2010; 70(2): 709-18.

[75] Balint K, Xiao M, Pinnix CC, Soma A, Veres I, Juhasz I, Brown EJ, Capobianco AJ, Herlyn M, Liu ZJ. Activation of Notch1 signaling is required for beta-catenin-mediated human primary melanoma progression. *J Clin Invest.* 2005; 115(11): 3166-76.

[76] Liu ZJ, Xiao M, Balint K, Smalley KS, Brafford P, Qiu R, Pinnix CC, Li X, Herlyn M. Notch1 signaling promotes primary melanoma progression by activating mitogen-activated protein kinase/phosphatidylinositol 3-kinase-Akt pathways and up-regulating N-cadherin expression. *Cancer Res.* 2006; 66(8): 4183-90.

[77] Wang Z, Banerjee S, Li Y, Rahman KM, Zhang Y, Sarkar FH. Down-regulation of notch-1 inhibits invasion by inactivation of nuclear factor-kappaB, vascular endothelial growth factor, and matrix metalloproteinase-9 in pancreatic cancer cells. *Cancer Res.* 2006; 66(5): 2778-84.

[78] Hu XB, Feng F, Wang YC, Wang L, He F, Dou GR, Liang L, Zhang HW, Liang YM, Han H. Blockade of Notch signaling in tumor-bearing mice may lead to tumor regression, progression, or metastasis, depending on tumor cell types. *Neoplasia.* 2009; 11(1):32-8.

[79] Yang J, Weinberg RA. Epithelial-mesenchymal transition: at the crossroads of development and tumor metastasis. *Dev Cell.* 2008; 14(6): 818-29.

[80] Timmerman LA, Grego-Bessa J, Raya A, Bertrán E, Pérez-Pomares JM, Díez J, Aranda S, Palomo S, McCormick F, Izpisúa-Belmonte JC, de la Pompa JL. Notch promotes epithelialmesenchymal transition during cardiac development and oncogenic transformation. *Genes Dev.* 2004; 18: 99–115.

[81] Zavadil J, Cermak L, Soto-Nieves N, Böttinger EP. Integration of TGF-beta/Smad and Jagged1/Notch signalling in epithelial-to-mesenchymal transition. *EMBO J.* 2004; 23(5): 1155-65.

[82] Osipo C, Patel P, Rizzo P, Clementz AG, Hao L, Golde TE, Miele L. ErbB-2 inhibition activates Notch-1 and sensitizes breast cancer cells to a gamma-secretase inhibitor. *Oncogene.* 2008; 27: 5019–5032.

[83] Wang J, Wakeman TP, Lathia JD, Hjelmeland AB, Wang XF, White RR, Rich JN, Sullenger BA. Notch promotes radioresistance of glioma stem cells. *Stem Cells.* 2010; 28(1): 17-28.

[84] Phillips TM, McBride WH, Pajonk F. The response of CD24 –/low /CD44 + breast cancer–initiating cells to radiation. *J Natl Cancer Inst.* 2006; 98: 1777–85.

[85] Weng AP, Millholland JM, Yashiro-Ohtani Y, Arcangeli ML, Lau A, Wai C, Del Bianco C, Rodriguez CG, Sai H, Tobias J, Li Y, Wolfe MS, Shachaf C, Felsher D, Blacklow SC, Pear WS, Aster JC. c-Myc is an important direct target of Notch1 in T-cell acute lymphoblastic leukemia/lymphoma. *Genes Dev.* 2006; 20(15): 2096-109.

[86] Gustafsson MV, Zheng X, Pereira T, Gradin K, Jin S, Lundkvist J, Ruas JL, Poellinger L, Lendahl U, Bondesson M. Hypoxia requires notch signaling to maintain the undifferentiated cell state. *Dev Cell.* 2005; 9(5): 617-28.

[87] Keith B, Simon MC. Hypoxia-inducible factors, stem cells, and cancer. *Cell.* 2007; 129(3): 65-72.

[88] Kim Y, Lin Q, Zelterman D, Yun Z. Hypoxia-regulated delta-like 1 homologue enhances cancer cell stemness and tumorigenicity. *Cancer Res.* 2009; 69(24): 9271-80.

[89] Weijzen S, Rizzo P, Braid M, Vaishnav R, Jonkheer SM, Zlobin A, Osborne BA, Gottipati S, Aster JC, Hahn WC, Rudolf M, Siziopikou K, Kast WM, Miele L. Activation of Notch-1 signaling maintains the neoplastic phenotype in human Ras-transformed cells. *Nat Med.* 2002; 8: 979-986.

[90] Reya T, Duncan AW, Ailles L, Domen J, Scherer DC, Willert K, Hintz L, Nusse R, Weissman IL. A role for Wnt signalling in self-renewal of haematopoietic stem cells. *Nature.* 2003; 423(6938): 409-14.

[91] Reya T, Clevers H. Wnt signalling in stem cells and cancer. *Nature.* 2005; 434: 843-850.

[92] Mishra L, Banker T, Murray J, Byers S, Thenappan A, He AR, Shetty K, Johnson L, Reddy EP. Liver stem cells and hepatocellular carcinoma. *Hepatology*. 2009; 49(1): 318-29.

[93] Lin HK, Bergmann S, Pandolfi PP. Deregulated TGF-beta signaling in leukemogenesis. *Oncogene*. 2005; 24(37): 5693-700.

[94] Clark PA, Treisman DM, Ebben J, Kuo JS. Developmental signaling pathways in brain tumor-derived stem-like cells. *Dev Dyn*. 2007; 236(12): 3297-308.

[95] Yin JJ, Selander K, Chirgwin JM, Dallas M, Grubbs BG, Wieser R, Massagué J, Mundy GR, Guise TA. TGF-beta signaling blockade inhibits PTHrP secretion by breast cancer cells and bone metastases development. *J Clin Invest*. 1999; 103(2): 197-206.

[96] Kang Y, Siegel PM, Shu W, Drobnjak M, Kakonen SM, Cordón-Cardo C, Guise TA, Massagué J. A multigenic program mediating breast cancer metastasis to bone. *Cancer Cell*. 2003; 3(6): 537-49.

[97] Blokzijl A, Dahlqvist C, Reissmann E, Falk A, Moliner A, Lendahl U, Ibáñez CF. Cross-talk between the Notch and TGF-β signaling pathways mediated by interaction of the Notch intracellular domain with Smad3. *J Cell Biol*. 2003; 163: 723–728.

[98] Zavadil J, Cermak L, Soto-Nieves N, Böttinger EP. Integration of TGF-beta/Smad and Jagged1/Notch signalling in epithelial-to-mesenchymal transition. *EMBO J*. 2004; 23(5): 1155-65.

[99] Qin JZ, Stennett L, Bacon P, Bodner B, Hendrix MJ, Seftor RE, Seftor EA, Margaryan NV, Pollock PM, Curtis A, Trent JM, Bennett F, Miele L, Nickoloff BJ. p53-independent NOXA induction overcomes apoptotic resistance of malignant melanomas. *Mol Cancer Ther*. 2004; 3(8): 895-902.

[100] Curry CL, Reed LL, Golde TE, Miele L, Nickoloff BJ, Foreman KE. Gamma secretase inhibitor blocks Notch activation and induces apoptosis in Kaposi's sarcoma tumor cells. *Oncogene*. 2005; 24: 6333–44.

[101] Hallahan AR, Pritchard JI, Hansen S, Benson M, Stoeck J, Hatton BA, Russell TL, Ellenbogen RG, Bernstein ID, Beachy PA, Olson JM. The SmoA1 mouse model reveals that notch signaling is critical for the growth and survival of sonic hedgehog-induced medulloblastomas. *Cancer Res*. 2004; 64: 7794–800.

[102] O'Neil J, Calvo J, McKenna K, Krishnamoorthy V, Aster JC, Bassing CH, Alt FW, Kelliher M, Look AT. Activating Notch1 mutations in mouse models of T-ALL. *Blood*. 2006; 107: 781–5.

[103] van Es JH, van Gijn ME, Riccio O, van den Born M, Vooijs M, Begthel H, Cozijnsen M, Robine S, Winton DJ, Radtke F, Clevers H. Notch/gamma-secretase inhibition turns proliferative cells in intestinal crypts and adenomas into goblet cells. *Nature*. 2005; 435: 959–63.

[104] Zeng Q, Li S, Chepeha DB, Giordano TJ, Li J, Zhang H, Polverini PJ, Nor J, Kitajewski J, Wang CY. Crosstalk between tumor and endothelial cells promotes tumor angiogenesis by MAPK activation of Notch signaling. *Cancer Cell*. 2005; 8: 13–23.

[105] Efferson CL, Elbi C, Tammam J, Carroll P, Kohl NE, Majumder PK. Inhibition of Notch by gamma-secretase inhibitors induces apoptosis through activated caspase-3 in LS-1034 colon cancer model. *FASEB J*. 2007 21:lb392 [Meeting Abstract].

[106] Rao SS, O'Neil J, Liberator CD, Hardwick JS, Dai X, Zhang T, Tyminski E, Yuan J, Kohl NE, Richon VM, Van der Ploeg LH, Carroll PM, Draetta GF, Look AT, Strack PR, Winter CG. Inhibition of NOTCH signaling by gamma-secretase inhibitor engages

the RB pathway and elicits cell cycle exit in T-cell acute lymphoblastic leukemia cells. *Cancer Res.* 2009; 69(7): 3060-8.

[107] Hoey T, Yen WC, Axelrod F, Basi J, Donigian L, Dylla S, Fitch-Bruhns M, Lazetic S, Park IK, Sato A, Satyal S, Wang X, Clarke MF, Lewicki J, Gurney A. DLL4 blockade inhibits tumor growth and reduces tumor-initiating cell frequency. *Cell Stem Cell.* 2009; 5:168-77.

[108] Zhen Y, Zhao S, Li Q, Li Y, Kawamoto K. Arsenic trioxide-mediated Notch pathway inhibition depletes the cancer stem-like cell population in gliomas. *Cancer Lett.* 2009 Dec. [Epub ahead of print]

[109] Eyler CE, Rich JN. Survival of the fittest: cancer stem cells in therapeutic resistance and angiogenesis. *J Clin Oncol.* 2008; 26(17): 2839-45.

[110] Hirose H, Ishii H, Mimori K, Ohta D, Ohkuma M, Tsujii H, Saito T, Sekimoto M, Doki Y, Mori M. Notch pathway as candidate therapeutic target in Her2/Neu/ErbB2 receptor-negative breast tumors. *Oncol Rep.* 2010; 23(1): 35-43.

[111] Bao S, Wu Q, Sathornsumetee S, Hao Y, Li Z, Hjelmeland AB, Shi Q, McLendon RE, Bigner DD, Rich JN. Stem cell-like glioma cells promote tumor angiogenesis through vascular endothelial growth factor. *Cancer Res.* 2006; 66: 7843-7848.

[112] Oka N, Soeda A, Inagaki A, Onodera M, Maruyama H, Hara A, Kunisada T, Mori H, Iwama T. VEGF promotes tumorigenesis and angiogenesis of human glioblastoma stem cells. *Biochem Biophys Res Commun.* 2007; 360: 553-559.

[113] Lee CW, Raskett CM, Prudovsky I, Altieri DC. Molecular dependence of estrogen receptor-negative breast cancer on a notch-survivin signaling axis. *Cancer Res.* 2008; 68(13): 5273-81.

In: Cancer Stem Cells
Editor: Melissa E. Jordan, pp. 125-140

ISBN: 978-1-61668-971-1
© 2010 Nova Science Publishers, Inc.

Chapter VII

CANCER STEM CELLS AND METASTASIS

*Benjamin Tiede and Yibin Kang**
Princeton University, Princeton, NJ 08544, USA.

ABSTRACT

Recent insights regarding the function of cancer stem cells are particularly intriguing when considered in the context of the metastatic cascade. As evidence for the direct involvement of cancer stem cells in initiating the growth of metastatic lesions is scant, this chapter will focus on known events in malignant transformation that are likely to involve or affect cancer stem cells, which may give rise to primary tumors of varying degrees of malignancy and metastatic potentials. The role of cancer stem cells in the later steps of the metastasis cascade will also be discussed. Finally, this chapter will explore potential characteristics vulnerabilities of cancer stem cells involved in metastasis, and speculate on how these weaknesses may be exploited to generate novel therapeutic and diagnostic approaches.

INTRODUCTION

The cancer stem cell (CSC) hypothesis, although proposed many years ago, has undergone a renaissance in the past few years as evident by the isolation and characterization of CSCs responsible for initiating tumorigenesis of a variety of solid and hematopoietic malignancies [1]. Part of the excitement surrounding this field has hinged on the fact that CSCs have been shown to be responsible for driving the recurrence of chemoresistant tumors [2]. As such, research into CSC function has sought to identify critical CSC vulnerabilities in order to improve cancer treatment. Ironically though, most CSC studies have focused on the role of CSCs during primary tumorigenesis, but not metastasis, which is responsible for 90%

---

* Correspondence concerning this article should be addressed to: Dr. Yibin Kang, Ph.D. Department of Molecular Biology, Princeton University, Princeton, NJ 08544, USA, Phone: +1 609 258 8834; Fax: +1 609 258 2340; ykang@princeton.edu.

of cancer related fatalities [3]. Therefore, the primary goals of this chapter are to speculate on what portions of the metastatic cascade are mediated by CSCs, identify critical research needed to validate these claims, and finally discuss how cancer treatment can shift to focus on the role of CSCs in metastasis.

Before proceeding with investigating the role of CSCs in metastasis, it is important to operationally define two different types of CSCs that play a role in two distinct steps in the tumorigenesis/metastasis cascade. The first population of CSCs (herein referred to as primary tumor CSCs, or pCSCs) are those that have been extensively studied for their role in primary tumorigenesis, and may give rise to highly or lowly metastatic tumors depending on early oncogenic events that drive their formation. The other population of CSCs (dubbed metastatic CSCs or mCSCs) are tumor cells that break off from the primary tumor, travel to the distant sites of metastasis and are responsible for the initiation and the propagation of metastatic lesions.

POOR PROGNOSIS, PRIMARY TUMORS AND pCSCs

For many years, tumor progression was believed to be the end result of a series of Darwinian natural selections that repeatedly enriched for cells that were fit to survive in the primary tumor microenvironment. While this idea undoubtedly holds a great deal of credence, it did leave one conceptual gap unanswered; how could metastatic cells that are adapted to travel through the circulation and survive at foreign tissues or organs be selected for at the site of the primary tumor? It would seem to be the case that mutations that favor metastasis but do not confer an advantage in primary tumor growth would not be enriched for in the primary tumor. One possible reconciliation to this puzzle is that metastasis potential is actually endowed early during tumorigenesis whereby initial oncogenic events produce distinct classes of tumors with distinct degrees of malignancy [4]. This speculation is likely to hold true when evaluating tumors which consist of subtypes that have a high degree of cellular and molecular heterogeneity (such as breast cancer and leukemia), compared to more homogeneous tumors such as colon and pancreatic cancers [5]. As such, this chapter will primarily focus on evidence from breast cancer and leukemia.

The early predetermination of malignancy hypothesis is supported by numerous studies which provided evidence that different prognoses, including risk of recurrence and distant metastasis, can be detected by profiling the bulk of the primary tumor. The fact that these phenotypes are shared by many of the primary tumor cells suggests that these cells share a common ancestor that was transformed and then expanded into the bulk of the tumor, rather than the entire tumor undergoing the same deregulation independently. For example, genomic analysis of breast tumors indicated at least five different subtypes for breast cancer based on their distinct gene expression profiles: a basal epithelial-like group, an ERBB2-overexpressing group, a normal breast-like group, a luminal A and a luminal B group [6,7]. Survival analyses showed significantly different outcomes for the patients belonging to the various groups, including a poor prognosis for the basal-like, ERBB2^{+} and luminal B subtypes [6]. Furthermore, it has been shown that expression profiling of primary tumor masses can identify poor prognosis signatures which can effectively predict metastasis formation [8,9,10,11]. Finally, expression profiling of a range of mouse breast cancer models revealed both a common tumorigenesis signature shared by all tumor types, and unique signatures that depended on the initial oncogenic events that correlated with subsequent tumor malignancy phenotypes [12].

The fact that the bulk of the tumor mass expresses a gene signature that can predict metastasis behavior suggests that metastasis potential is endowed early in tumorigenesis so that most cells express the poor prognosis signature, rather than later in tumorigenesis where a few highly metastatic variants would break off from the primary tumor. However, it should be kept in mind that these possibilities are not mutually exclusive; proof that poor prognosis signatures exist in certain tumors does not rule out the possibility for rare metastasis variants to arise late in tumorigenesis. Genomic profiling of primary tumors or metastases by nature will not be able to detect rare, metastatic variants which would not be populous enough to influence total tumor RNA levels [13]. Nevertheless, identifying the precise origin and characterizing the early activity of pCSCs remains a critical avenue of research to be explored to help explain tumor progression and metastasis.

pCSC Origins and Metastasis

Connecting the observations about tumor poor prognosis signatures with the CSC theory of carcinogenesis, a number of questions arise concerning how the origin and propagation of pCSCs could possibly account for the tumor-wide poor prognosis signatures that are observed. For instance, it is unknown whether the same pCSC population can give rise to tumors of varying degrees of malignancy if challenged by different transformation events (see Figure 1). Factors such as genomic instability, oncogenic stress, and microenvironment interactions could potentially alter the same pCSC population to produce tumors of different phenotypes. Early evidence in a leukemia model indicates this is the case as pre-pCSCs from a dendritic cell like leukemia can differentiate into both benign and malignant cell types depending on a variety of factors including the injection site and the immune background of the host [14]. Future studies should seek to expand these observations by testing different oncogenic stresses on the same population of pCSCs or pre-pCSCs to determine the precise role of early oncogenic events, before the majority of the tumor is formed, in predisposing tumors to metastasize.

It is also feasible that similar oncogenic stresses challenging two distinct cell populations, for instance a normal adult stem cell and a committed progenitor, could produce tumors of varying degrees of malignancy (see Figure 2). Preliminary evidence supporting this notion has come from studies which have sought to define the origin of pCSCs, where it has been suggested that both normal stem cells and committed progenitors could serve as the target for transformation. It is believed that normal stem cells or committed progenitors, rather than mature cell types, are the target for transformation because many mutational events rely on DNA replication and cell division: events which are restricted to stem/progenitor cells [5,15].

The inherent self-renewal capacity and long lifespan of normal adult stem cells presumably allows for a greater window of opportunity for their transformation by oncogenic events that may occur over a long period of time. The fact that normal adult stem cells often share surface marker expression profiles with their cancerous counterparts suggests, but does not prove, that normal stem cells may be the origin of pCSCs [1]. For instance, it could be the case that transformed progenitors re-adopt a stem cell surface profile as part of their oncogenesis (there is a precedent for normal epithelial cells to re-adopt a stem cell phenotype in a Wnt-dependent fashion in the hair follicle [16]). Additionally, there is a ~6 fold expansion of mammary stem cells in pre-neoplastic mouse mammary glands in a breast cancer model [17], but again, this does not prove that the normal stem cells are the origin of pCSCs. What has been lacking in the field is the observation or induction of transformation of adult stem cells into pCSCs as opposed to retrospective analyses. Part of the reason why this has been difficult lies in the fact that outside of the hematopoietic system true, adult tissue-specific stem cells have been difficult to identify and isolate. In contrast, it has been much easier to identify committed progenitors because of the less stringent criteria needed to characterize and isolate them, and their relative abundance compared to tissue-specific stem cells.

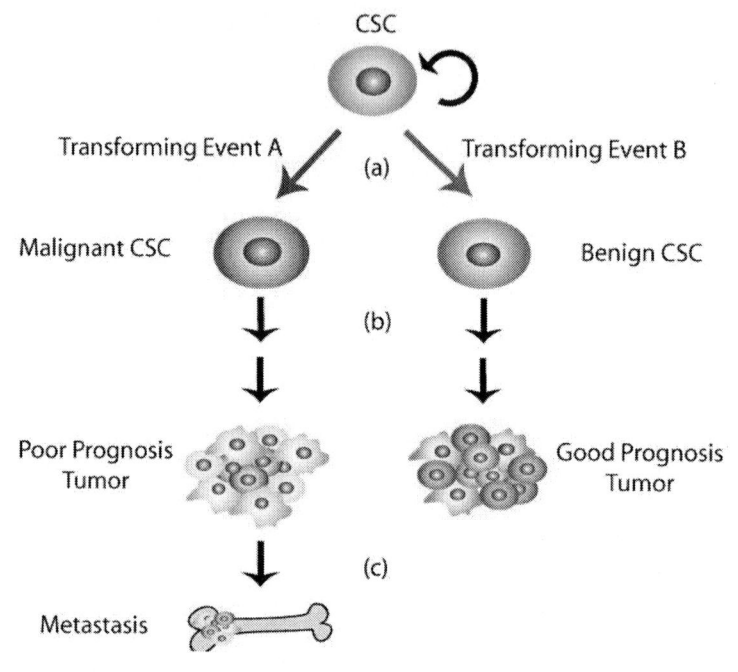

Figure 1. Single origin model of tumorigenesis. In this model, tumors of varying degrees of malignancy are the product of the same cellular origin because of different transformation events (a). These stresses result in the formation of distinct pCSCs (b) that divide and expand into good or poor prognosis tumors (c) that have a differential metastasis capacity.

The fact that committed progenitors are much more abundant than stem cells also suggests, based on probability, that they are more likely to be the target of oncogenic transformation. Given that committed progenitors are easier to isolate than true adult stem cells, it is not surprising that there is better evidence for committed progenitors serving as the origin of CSCs. For instance, committed myeloid progenitors have been shown to initiate leukemia development in mice when they are forced to overexpress Bcl-2 and BCR/ABL [18]. Furthermore, the 15:17 chromosome translocation associated with human acute promyelocytic leukemia (APL) is only found in committed progenitors, and not in hematopoietic stem cells [19]. Granulocyte-macrophage progenitors have also been shown to induce leukemia development, either when activating a self-renewal program through the upregulation of the Wnt/β-catenin pathway [20] or by the forced expression of the MLL-AF9 fusion protein [21]. Interestingly, expression profiling of the MLL-AF9 expressing cells revealed that they retained a progenitor gene expression profile, and not a hematopoietic stem cell profile. Similar evidence has also indicated that neural progenitors are likely to be the target of oncogenic transformations [22].

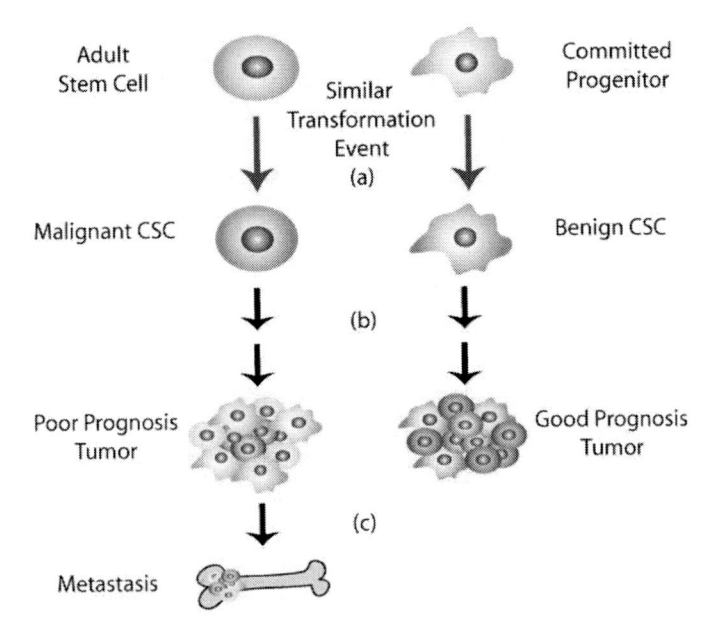

Figure 2. Multiple origin model of tumorigenesis. As opposed to Figure 1, in this scenario, differential metastasis ability is the result of a similar transformation event happening in different target populations (a, b). It is hypothesized, but not proven, that stresses initiated in normal adult stem cells will produce tumors that will metastasize more (c), because of their cellular plasticity and enhanced mobility.

Given that there is evidence for both normal adult stem cells and committed progenitors to serve as the origin of CSCs, and knowing that there are many different paths to tumorigenesis, it is likely to be the case that both stem cells and committed progenitors can serve as the targets for transformation. In fact, it has been shown that EGFR activation, combined with the loss of Arf and Ink4a is sufficient to drive the formation of high grade malignant gliomas in both transformed astrocytes and neural stem cells [23]. What is not clear however is if CSCs derived from different cell types can produce tumors with varying degrees of malignancy. Preliminary evidence has indicated that the same oncogenic stress can induce the formation of tumors with differential metastasis ability if induced in different starting populations. Forced expression of SV-40 large T antigen, hTERT and H-ras-v12 in two distinct human mammary epithelial cell types, derived from the same origin but cultured in different conditions, resulted in tumors with completely different metastasis capacity [24].

Further characterization of the initial oncogenic events that drive CSC formation, particularly with respect to endowing the pCSCs with the ability to metastasize may help to identify clinically relevant prognostic indicators for future tumor malignancy. For instance, it may be possible to isolate pCSCs from a given tumor and determine if they express a unique signature, the figurative "root" of the poor prognosis signature, which would provide stronger prognostic value over sampling of the entire tumor. It also should be kept in mind that most experimental manipulations to decipher the origin of pCSCs typically (by design) test one experimental variable at a time (i.e. whether the challenging stem cells and progenitors with an oncogenic stress results in tumor formation). While this aids in analysis of data, it unfortunately leads to oversimplification of complex *in vivo* interactions.

For instance, it may be the case that an initial transformation event *in vivo* may happen in a stem cell population which results in a pre-neoplastic cell that after differentiating into a progenitor is subject to a second transformation event that leads to typical tumor growth. There is strong observational evidence in leukemia and comparatively weaker evidence from breast cancer studies to suggest this progressive tumorigenesis model happens *in vivo*. Hallmark fusion proteins associated with chronic myelogenous leukemia (CML) as well as acute myelogenous leukemia (AML) (BCR-ABL and AML1-ETO, respectively) can be detected in human hematopoietic stem cells, however these cells are not tumorigenic [20,25]. Instead, further mutations that are only seen in downstream progeny are required to fully initiate tumorigenesis. In breast cancer, it has been shown that tumorigenic $CD44^+$ CSCs are clonally related to and share many genomic alterations with $CD24^+$ cells, but that $CD24^+$ cells express unique mutations [26]. This observation was interpreted to mean that $CD24^+$ cells are the progeny of $CD44^+$ cells that have undergone and initial transformation event. Experimentally testing scenarios such as these (and not just making retroactive conclusions based on tumor heterogeneity) will require a new wave of innovative research design strategies.

METASTATIC CANCER STEM CELLS

In addition to playing significant roles early during the tumorigenesis process that ultimately affect metastasis propensity, CSCs also play a significant role after tumor formation, during the formation of the actual metastatic lesion. Just as pCSCs are required for the initiation of the primary tumor, mCSCs are likely to be required for the formation of metastatic lesions. It has been known that a single cell is capable of initiating metastasis [27]. Thus, given the high number of cells found circulating in the blood of cancer patients and the comparatively low metastasis incidence, it seems likely that only rare CSCs could initiate metastatic lesions. These CSCs, termed metastatic CSCs or mCSCs, are a distinct entity from the pCSCs that gave rise to the primary tumor (although they may share many of the same properties, such as expression of critical tumor propagation factors). mCSCs must also express proteins that endow them with the ability to survive in the blood or lymphatic system as well to adapt to the different environments at the future site of metastasis. For instance, it has been shown that pancreatic mCSCs are a contained in a subset of $CD133^+$ CSCs that also express CXCR4 [28], which is known to be important in homing/anchorage of metastatic cells. Just as pCSCs are rare within a primary tumor, and are the only cells that can induce formation of a new tumor, mCSCs may be the only cells that can break off from the primary tumor and form a metastatic lesion. This could explain the observation that many cancer cells can be detected in the blood of patients with primary tumors, but they all do not form metastasis [29]. Only when a mCSC colonizes a foreign tissue or organ will a metastatic lesion form.

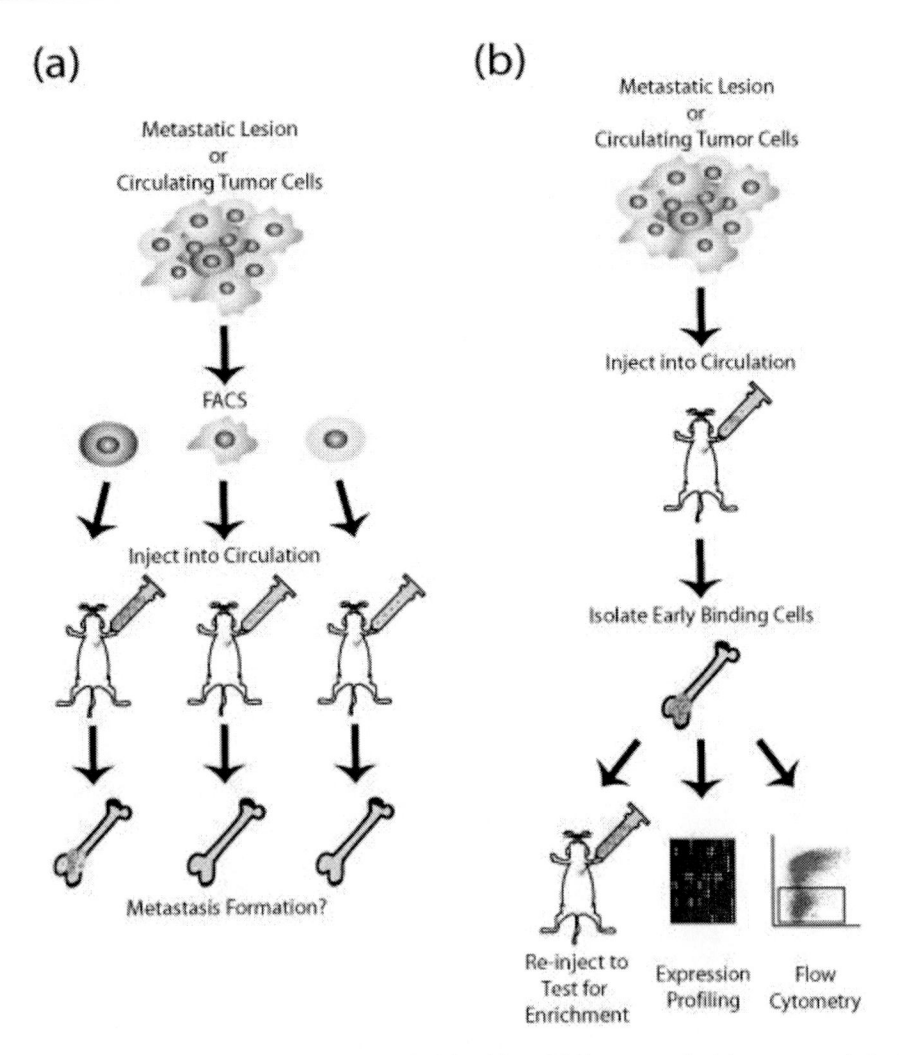

Figure 3. Two different strategies to prospectively identify mCSCs *in vivo*. In (a), a metastatic lesion or cancer cells isolated from the circulation of affected individuals are fractionated using FACS and then injected directly into the circulation of recipient mice. This allows for the direct determination of which cells are able to extravasate, colonize, and expand into a metastatic lesion, but requires the use of previously identified surface markers. As a complementary approach, (b) involves isolating similar tumor cells and injecting them directly into the circulation without fractionating them using FACS (labeling tumor cells with a drug selection marker or GFP would likely be critical before injecting). Soon after injection (~12hr to 2 days later), the cells which initially colonize the metastatic site are selected for, expanded in culture if needed, and reinjected to test for enriched tumorigenicity. These cells could be analyzed by expression profiling or flow cytometry to identify markers to enrich for these cells from other metastatic lesions to enable in further identification and characterization.

Despite speculation of their existence, the direct identification of mCSCs has only been accomplished in one experimental system [28], but could be done by similar xenograft transplantation assays that are used to identify pCSCs. Instead of fractioning a primary tumor and testing different cell populations for their ability to form primary tumors in subcutaneous or orthotopic transplantation models, metastatic lesions or tumor cells collected from the circulation of tumor bearing subjects need to be collected, fractionated based on different cell surface profiles, and tested *in vivo* using experimental metastasis assays (see Figure 3a).

These assays directly test the ability of cells to colonize the lung, bone, brain and other organs by injection into the blood circulation. If tumor cells were injected subcutaneously or orthotopically primary tumorigenesis would be a prerequisite of the cells in question, which may not be a property that mCSCs are endowed with. This approach understandably bypasses the initial intravasation step required for circulating tumor cells, but given the high numbers of circulating tumor cells that can be detected, this omission may not be a detrimental one. A complementary approach would involve isolating cells that initially lodge in the bone, lung or any metastatic site soon after injection in an experimental metastasis assay and testing to see if they have an enriched metastatic ability compared to the parental population that was initially injected (see Figure 3b). If this was the case, expression profiling could be used to identify relevant surface proteins that could be used to enrich for the mCSCs in the parental population which could then be characterized in subsequent testing.

It is interesting to note that in the identification of breast pCSCs, the majority of the tumor samples that were used to test pCSC function were pleural effusions, rather than primary tumors [30]. This could be the reason why the expression profiling of these cells identified a unique "invasiveness gene signature" that negatively correlated with metastasis free survival in breast and other cancer types [31]. Furthermore, cells with the breast CSC phenotype $CD44^+CD24^-$ [30] have been shown to be highly invasive *in vitro* [32], to overexpress motility and chemotaxis gene signatures [26], to be some of the first cells to metastasize to the bone in breast cancer patients [33], and when present in high numbers at the primary tumor to correlate clinically with distant metastasis [34]. These cells are also shown to contain a minority "side population", a group of cells known to have stem cell phenotypes and be chemoresistant [35]. These observations all suggest that breast pCSCs, in addition to forming primary tumors, may actually function as mCSCs as well.

Although the exact identity of mCSCs remains unknown, it is possible to study critical parts of the metastatic cascade that would affect their growth. For example, it has been shown that $CD133^+$ glioma CSCs are more adept at inducing angiogenesis, a critical early step in metastasis progression, during tumor formation compared to $CD133^-$ cells [36]. While this is clearly indicative of a role for CSCs in the early parts of the metastasis cascade, metastasis research relevant to the function of CSCs typically focuses on later steps in metastasis (i.e., determining tissue specificity, colonization and expansion).

Just as pCSCs are thought to share properties with normal stem cells, so too is the case with mCSCs. Connecting these stipulations, one of the most relevant avenues of research related to mCSCs concerns the role of the supportive niche, or microenvironment that metastatic cells reside in.

THE (PRE)-METASTATIC NICHE AND mCSCs

From drosophila through vertebrates, the protection, growth, and differentiation of normal adults stem cells have been shown in a variety of systems to be regulated by nearby niche cells that provide both a physical location for stem cells to reside in as well as secreting molecules to regulate stem cell function (reviewed in [37]). Interestingly, signaling molecules, such as Wnts and TGFβ, found to be secreted at normal stem cell niches are factors known to be important in tumor growth and metastasis [38]. Additionally, if mCSCs are similar to normal stem cells in that they have a high degree of cellular plasticity, they are likely to be better then other tumor cells at surviving in a foreign niche that is different than the microenvironment at the site of the primary tumor. It is possible that when mCSCs engraft in a tissue they may kick out resident stem cells from their niche. For instance, it is known that osteolytic bone metastasis results in the activation of endosteal osteoclasts [39] which can promote the mobilization of endosteal hematopoietic progenitor cells in the bone marrow [40]. In addition to invading already established niches, metastatic cells have also been shown to induce niche formation prior to leaving the primary tumor site.

In a seminal report in 2005, it was shown that metastatic lung and melanoma cells secrete factors including vascular endothelial growth factor (VEGF) and placental growth factor (PlGF) which induce the recruitment of bone marrow derived cells to the future sites of metastasis (dubbed the pre-metastasis niche) [41]. Blocking these factors was sufficient to reduce tumor metastasis, and interestingly, treating mice with conditioned media from one tumor type was sufficient to redirect the tissue tropisms of the other type. This suggested that once the pre-metastasis niche was initiated, factors were secreted by cells in the niche back to the primary tumor to help recruit metastatic cells. Two possible candidates to mediate this effect are the S100 cytokines S100A8 and S100A9. These cytokines, expressed by myeloid cells, were shown to be upregulated in the pre-metastatic lungs of tumor bearing mice, and when blocked reduced metastasis to the lung [42]. The molecular basis of this effect seems to be the induction of the p38 Map kinase pathway which enhanced tumor cell migration and invasion [42]. Once located in the niche, it is speculated that mCSCs may enter a period of dormancy, similar to that of normal adult stem cells, whereby some re-activation signal may trigger their expansion into a full blown metastatic lesion (see Figure 4) [1]. However, at this point, this idea remains purely speculation and lacks experimental validation.

Other microenvironment factors known to be important during tumorigenesis and metastasis may specifically be important in the regulation of mCSC growth and expansion. For example, when secreted by stromal cells, growth regulators such as Bmp and its inhibitor GREMLIN-1, which are known to regulate normal stem cell proliferation, have been shown to regulate basal cell carcinoma primary tumor growth [43]. Whether this is true in metastasis, and specifically in the regulation of mCSC behavior, remains to be determined. A number of other heterotypic examples between tumor cells and their microenvironment known to play a role in metastasis, such as hypoxia and immune surveillance (reviewed in [44,45]), may also specifically affect mCSCs. However, without their precise identity known, direct studies to characterize these interactions remain far off. Once identified, tests could be designed to determine whether or not circulating cancer cells from a patient contain a population of mCSCs which would predict future metastasis.

As the mCSC population that initially lodges in a metastatic niche is likely very small, profiling the aforementioned niche responses to tumor metastasis may provide an easier means to detect early metastatic lesions. Further research into mCSC behavior, both reliant and independent of niche interactions hopefully will lead to the development of the most clinically effective cancer therapeutics to date.

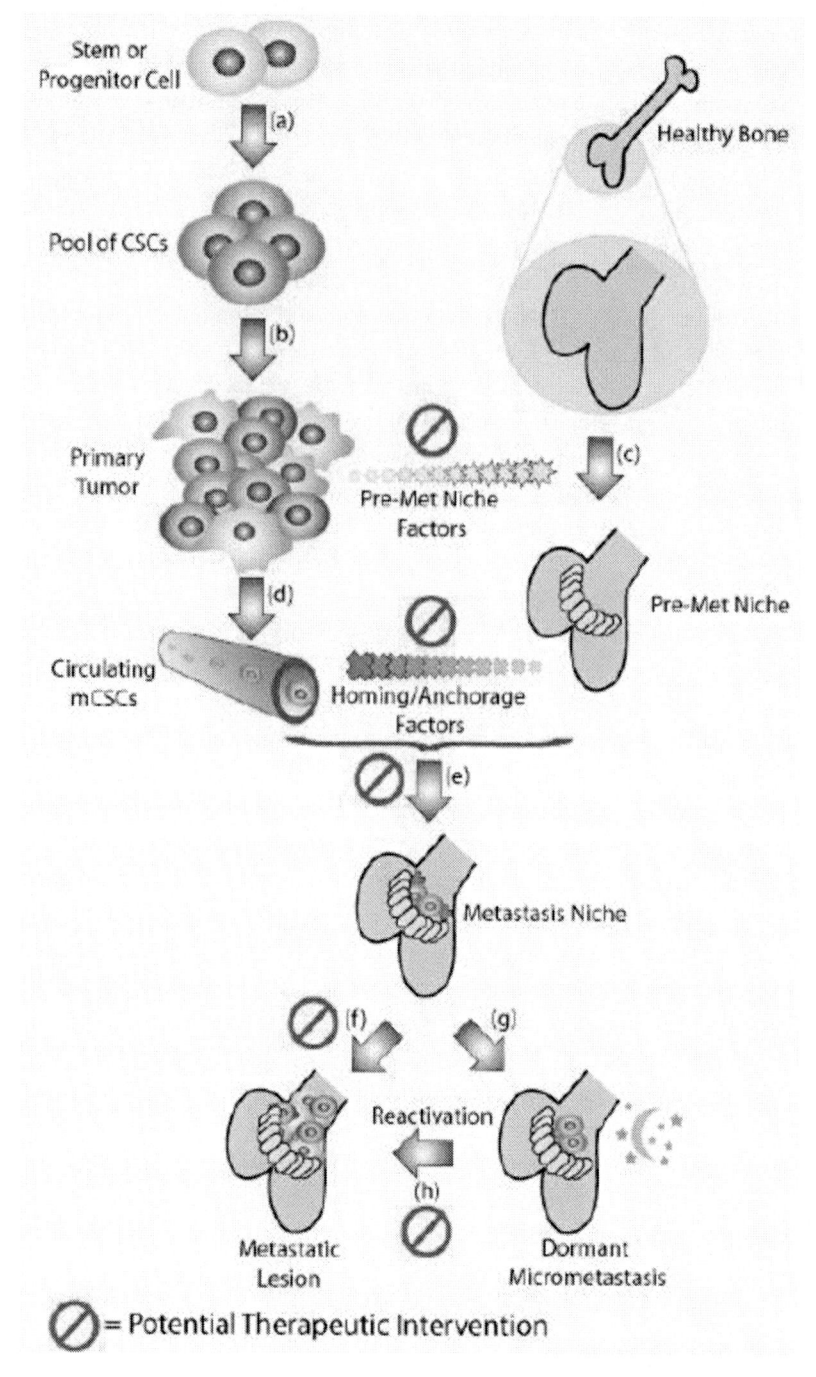

Figure 4. Critical stem cell-niche interactions in regulating metastasis (from [1]). Regardless of how it is derived (a), a pool of malignant pCSCs is formed which expands into a primary tumor (b). This primary tumor is capable of secreting pre-metastasis niche factors such as VEGF and PLGF (c) that induces the expression of homing and anchorage factors such as the S100 cytokines which guide circulating mCSCs (d). Once these mCSCs lodge in the niche (e), they can either proliferate into a metastatic lesion immediately (f) or enter into a period of dormancy (g) whereby reactivation signals induce their expansion (h). Ø = potential steps to target by therapeutic intervention.

METASTASIS, CSCs AND CHEMOTHERAPY

Much of the hype surrounding the CSC field has centered on the idea that by treating a small, typically chemoresistant population of cells responsible for initiating tumors, cancer treatment might finally deplete tumors of their lifeblood. However, the idea that these therapies might be designed to specifically ablate mCSCs has usually been little more than an afterthought. This fact should not be taken lightly as even if a CSC based therapy depletes all the tumor initiating cells from the primary tumor, mCSCs that have left the primary tumor and potentially have different molecular profiles than their primary tumor counterparts could be resistant to these therapies. It is also worth noting that many of these proposed therapies speculate on what the critical vulnerabilities of CSCs are, often times based on the known behavior of normal adult stem cells. However, before proceeding to discuss these approaches, it is important to think about the means of validating potential therapeutics, and about potential side effects of CSC based therapeutics.

The traditional standard of evaluating the effectiveness of a given anti-cancer drug is to determine the amount the drug can halt or shrink tumor growth. This is potentially problematic when considering CSC based therapeutics, since these cells are a minority population within a tumor. Treatment with CSC targeting agents in conjunction with traditional therapeutics may only result in a modest, if any, shrinking of the primary tumor compared to traditional drugs alone, but could have significant benefits when evaluating the recurrence- or metastasis-free survival. With respect to the potential side effects of CSC based therapy, there has been concern that if CSCs share properties with normal stem cells, then CSC based therapy may have deleterious side effects on these crucial cell types. This may not be much of a problem for breast cancer, where mastectomy is already an established acceptable treatment option but could be very serious for leukemia, where the normal stem cell and progenitor counterparts are essential for immune function. However, the increased proliferative potential of CSCs may provide a therapeutic window that could be exploited. This seems to be the case as leukemia initiating cells and normal hematopoietic stem cells have a differential dependence on the tumor suppressor PTEN [46].

Self-Renewal and Differentiation

Normal stem cells are known to possess the unique ability to self-renew to maintain a stem-cell pool and to differentiate into more committed progenitors. It is believed that either blocking CSC self-renewal ability or inducing differentiation may deplete these cells from the body. There are a variety of studies indicating this is the case in brain cancer. Treating glioblastoma derived neurospheres (cells dependent on stem cell function) with cyclopamine to block the Hedgehog pathway eliminated their ability to form new neurospheres. Additionally after cyclopamine treatment, glioblastoma cells were no longer able to form tumors *in vivo* [47]. Similar studies have demonstrated that using retinoic acid, a useful differentiation inducer in acute promyelocytic leukemia, also induces differentiation of glioblastoma cells [48]. Alternatively, using a γ-secretase inhibitor to block the Notch pathway resulted in differentiation of medulloblastoma cell lines, and a loss of colony- and tumor-forming ability. This effect appears to be due to a specific depletion of CD133[+] CSCs

[49]. Despite these significant findings, it remains to be determined whether mCSCS can be targeted by similar strategies or if they require unique therapeutic targeting.

Metastasis Niche

One therapeutic strategy unique to mCSCs involves targeting the critical mCSC/niche interactions that affect homing, engraftment and growth of tumor cells. It has been shown that blocking the pre-metastasis niche initiation using VEGF or PlGF antibodies was sufficient to reduce metastasis [41]. However, after the niche is initiated, other factors may be useful drug targets in blocking the binding of mCSCs to the niche. One possible factor is CXCR4, which is critical for leukemia cells binding to their niche [50], is important in breast cancer metastasis [51], and has been shown to enrich for mCSCs in pancreatic cancer [28]. Another factor is CD44, which positively selects for breast pCSCs. Blocking CD44 in a acute myelogenous leukemia model resulted in a significant deficiency in engraftment, even when the leukemia CSCs were injected directly into the bone marrow, indicating a specific defect in binding not homing [52]. Similar conclusions were also drawn regarding the essential nature of CD44 in chronic myelogenous leukemia [53]. Once mCSCs are identified and characterized extensively, it will be interesting to note determine what other factors are supplied by the niche to maintain their growth, and if these are potential therapeutic targets.

Reactivation

It is speculated, but remains to be proven, that mCSCs reside in niches in a state of dormancy before expanding into a full blow metastatic lesion. If this is the case, identifying the critical reactivation factors will certainly be of great interest. These potential therapies could have an advantage over drugs that target the homing or seeding of mCSCs because by the time of tumor diagnosis, mCSCs may have already left the primary tumor, migrated and lodged in metastatic niches. However, developing these therapeutics will not happen in the near future since the dormancy model first needs to be validated and characterized before creating drugs.

CSC Clearance

Cell surface marker profiling of CSCs may be useful beyond teasing out tumor initiating populations from the bulk of the tumor mass; the markers identified may be useful in creating cell specific clearance therapies, such as DNA vaccines or oncolytic viruses. When $CD44^+CD24^{-/low}$ pleural effusion cells are infected with capsid modified oncolytic adenoviruses, their tumor initiating capacity is abrogated [35]. Furthermore, these viruses when administered after tumor formation were able to significantly deplete the $CD44^+/CD24^{-/low}$ population within tumors. Since the surface markers used to identify CSCs are also shared by normal, non tumor cells, specific targeting of the viruses to the CSC population is likely to be a major hurdle to overcome in this line of research.

CONCLUSION

The unprecedented excitement surrounding the CSC field is certainly grounded in significant theoretical and experimental evidence. This excitement is particularly warranted when considering the role of CSCs in metastasis, since metastasis is responsible for the overwhelming majority of cancer deaths coupled with the fact that CSCs have been shown to be chemoresistant [2,3]. Characterizing the role of CSCs in metastasis involves two distinct portions of the metastatic cascade. First, the role of initial oncogenic events is important in deriving pCSCs that eventually produce tumors of varying degrees of malignancy. Understanding these events is likely to provide more prognostic, rather than therapeutic value. On the contrary, profiling the function of mCSCs, which are important for actually initiating and perpetuating metastatic lesion growth, may lead to novel therapeutic strategies. However, prudence dictates that scientists should acknowledge that while CSCs are a particularly intriguing line of research, at this juncture, we yet don't know if we will be successful in developing any new safe and effective therapeutics. Nevertheless, the future is filled with interesting avenues of research in the CSC field, many of which should shift to focus on the role of CSCs in metastasis and not just tumorigenesis. These studies may result in the development of the most powerful tools in prognostic and therapeutic oncology.

REFERENCES

[1] Li F, Tiede B, Massague J, Kang Y (2006) Beyond tumorigenesis: cancer stem cells in metastasis. *Cell Res.*

[2] Bao S, Wu Q, McLendon RE, Hao Y, Shi Q, et al. (2006) Glioma stem cells promote radioresistance by preferential activation of the DNA damage response. *Nature 444*: 756-760.

[3] Jemal A, Siegel R, Ward E, Murray T, Xu J, et al. (2007) Cancer statistics, 2007. CA *Cancer J. Clin. 57*: 43-66.

[4] Bernards R, Weinberg RA (2002) A progression puzzle. *Nature 418*: 823.

[5] Stingl J, Caldas C (2007) Molecular heterogeneity of breast carcinomas and the cancer stem cell hypothesis. *Nat. Rev. Cancer.*

[6] Sorlie T, Perou CM, Tibshirani R, Aas T, Geisler S, et al. (2001) Gene expression patterns of breast carcinomas distinguish tumor subclasses with clinical implications. *Proc. Natl. Acad. Sci. USA 98*: 10869-10874.

[7] Perou CM, Jeffrey SS, van de Rijn M, Rees CA, Eisen MB, et al. (1999) Distinctive gene expression patterns in human mammary epithelial cells and breast cancers. *Proc. Natl. Acad. Sci. USA 96*: 9212-9217.

[8] van de Vijver MJ, He YD, van't Veer LJ, Dai H, Hart AA, et al. (2002) A gene-expression signature as a predictor of survival in breast cancer. *N. Engl. J. Med. 347*: 1999-2009.

[9] van 't Veer LJ, Dai H, van de Vijver MJ, He YD, Hart AA, et al. (2002) Gene expression profiling predicts clinical outcome of breast cancer. *Nature 415*: 530-536.

[10] Wang Y, Klijn JG, Zhang Y, Sieuwerts AM, Look MP, et al. (2005) Gene-expression profiles to predict distant metastasis of lymph-node-negative primary breast cancer. *Lancet 365*: 671-679.

[11] Ramaswamy S, Ross KN, Lander ES, Golub TR (2003) A molecular signature of metastasis in primary solid tumors. *Nat. Genet. 33*: 49-54.

[12] Desai KV, Xiao N, Wang W, Gangi L, Greene J, et al. (2002) Initiating oncogenic event determines gene-expression patterns of human breast cancer models. *Proc. Natl. Acad. Sci. USA 99*: 6967-6972.

[13] Hynes RO (2003) Metastatic potential: generic predisposition of the primary tumor or rare, metastatic variants-or both? *Cell 113*: 821-823.

[14] Chen L, Shen R, Ye Y, Pu XA, Liu X, et al. (2007) Precancerous stem cells have the potential for both benign and malignant differentiation. *PLoS ONE 2*: e293.

[15] Cairns J (2002) Somatic stem cells and the kinetics of mutagenesis and carcinogenesis. *Proc. Natl. Acad. Sci. USA 99*: 10567-10570.

[16] Ito M, Yang Z, Andl T, Cui C, Kim N, et al. (2007) Wnt-dependent de novo hair follicle regeneration in adult mouse skin after wounding. *Nature 447*: 316-320.

[17] Shackleton M, Vaillant F, Simpson KJ, Stingl J, Smyth GK, et al. (2006) Generation of a functional mammary gland from a single stem cell. *Nature 439*: 84-88.

[18] Jaiswal S, Traver D, Miyamoto T, Akashi K, Lagasse E, et al. (2003) Expression of BCR/ABL and BCL-2 in myeloid progenitors leads to myeloid leukemias. *Proc. Natl. Acad. Sci. USA 100*: 10002-10007.

[19] Turhan AG, Lemoine FM, Debert C, Bonnet ML, Baillou C, et al. (1995) Highly purified primitive hematopoietic stem cells are PML-RARA negative and generate nonclonal progenitors in acute promyelocytic leukemia. *Blood 85*: 2154-2161.

[20] Jamieson CH, Ailles LE, Dylla SJ, Muijtjens M, Jones C, et al. (2004) Granulocyte-macrophage progenitors as candidate leukemic stem cells in blast-crisis CML. *N. Engl. J. Med. 351*: 657-667.

[21] Krivtsov AV, Twomey D, Feng Z, Stubbs MC, Wang Y, et al. (2006) Transformation from committed progenitor to leukaemia stem cell initiated by MLL-AF9. *Nature*.

[22] Vescovi AL, Galli R, Reynolds BA (2006) Brain tumour stem cells. *Nat. Rev. Cancer 6*: 425-436.

[23] Bachoo RM, Maher EA, Ligon KL, Sharpless NE, Chan SS, et al. (2002) Epidermal growth factor receptor and Ink4a/Arf: convergent mechanisms governing terminal differentiation and transformation along the neural stem cell to astrocyte axis. *Cancer Cell 1*: 269-277.

[24] Ince TA, Richardson AL, Bell GW, Saitoh M, Godar S, et al. (2007) Transformation of Different Human Breast Epithelial Cell Types Leads to Distinct Tumor Phenotypes. *Cancer Cell 12*: 160-170.

[25] Blair A, Hogge DE, Ailles LE, Lansdorp PM, Sutherland HJ (1997) Lack of expression of Thy-1 (CD90) on acute myeloid leukemia cells with long-term proliferative ability in vitro and in vivo. *Blood 89*: 3104-3112.

[26] Shipitsin M, Campbell LL, Argani P, Weremowicz S, Bloushtain-Qimron N, et al. (2007) Molecular definition of breast tumor heterogeneity. *Cancer Cell 11*: 259-273.

[27] Fidler IJ, Talmadge JE (1986) Evidence that intravenously derived murine pulmonary melanoma metastases can originate from the expansion of a single tumor cell. *Cancer Res. 46*: 5167-5171.

[28] Hermann P, Huber S, Herrler T, Aicher A, Ellwart J, et al. (2007) Distinct Populations of Cancer Stem Cells Determine Tumor Growth and Metastatic Activity in Human Pancreatic Cancer. *Cell Stem Cell 1*: 313-323.

[29] Fidler IJ (2003) The pathogenesis of cancer metastasis: the 'seed and soil' hypothesis revisited. *Nat. Rev. Cancer 3*: 453-458.

[30] Al-Hajj M, Wicha MS, Benito-Hernandez A, Morrison SJ, Clarke MF (2003) Prospective identification of tumorigenic breast cancer cells. *Proc. Natl. Acad. Sci. USA 100*: 3983-3988.

[31] Liu R, Wang X, Chen GY, Dalerba P, Gurney A, et al. (2007) The prognostic role of a gene signature from tumorigenic breast-cancer cells. *N. Engl. J. Med. 356*: 217-226.

[32] Sheridan C, Kishimoto H, Fuchs RK, Mehrotra S, Bhat-Nakshatri P, et al. (2006) CD44+/CD24- breast cancer cells exhibit enhanced invasive properties: an early step necessary for metastasis. *Breast Cancer Res. 8*: R59.

[33] Balic M, Lin H, Young L, Hawes D, Giuliano A, et al. (2006) Most early disseminated cancer cells detected in bone marrow of breast cancer patients have a putative breast cancer stem cell phenotype. *Clin. Cancer Res. 12*: 5615-5621.

[34] Abraham BK, Fritz P, McClellan M, Hauptvogel P, Athelogou M, et al. (2005) Prevalence of CD44+/CD24-/low cells in breast cancer may not be associated with clinical outcome but may favor distant metastasis. *Clin. Cancer Res. 11*: 1154-1159.

[35] Eriksson M, Guse K, Bauerschmitz G, Virkkunen P, Tarkkanen M, et al. (2007) Oncolytic Adenoviruses Kill Breast Cancer Initiating CD44(+)CD24(-/Low) Cells. *Mol. Ther.*

[36] Bao S, Wu Q, Sathornsumetee S, Hao Y, Li Z, et al. (2006) Stem Cell-like Glioma Cells Promote Tumor Angiogenesis through Vascular Endothelial Growth Factor. *Cancer Res. 66*: 7843-7848.

[37] Moore KA, Lemischka IR (2006) Stem cells and their niches. Science 311: 1880-1885.

[38] Li L, Neaves WB (2006) Normal stem cells and cancer stem cells: the niche matters. *Cancer Res. 66*: 4553-4557.

[39] Guise TA, Mohammad KS, Clines G, Stebbins EG, Wong DH, et al. (2006) Basic mechanisms responsible for osteolytic and osteoblastic bone metastases. *Clin. Cancer Res. 12*: 6213s-6216s.

[40] Kollet O, Dar A, Shivtiel S, Kalinkovich A, Lapid K, et al. (2006) Osteoclasts degrade endosteal components and promote mobilization of hematopoietic progenitor cells. *Nat. Med. 12*: 657-664.

[41] Kaplan RN, Riba RD, Zacharoulis S, Bramley AH, Vincent L, et al. (2005) VEGFR1-positive haematopoietic bone marrow progenitors initiate the pre-metastatic niche. *Nature 438*: 820-827.

[42] Hiratsuka S, Watanabe A, Aburatani H, Maru Y (2006) Tumour-mediated upregulation of chemoattractants and recruitment of myeloid cells predetermines lung metastasis. *Nat. Cell Biol. 8*: 1369-1375.

[43] Sneddon JB, Zhen HH, Montgomery K, van de Rijn M, Tward AD, et al. (2006) Bone morphogenetic protein antagonist gremlin 1 is widely expressed by cancer-associated stromal cells and can promote tumor cell proliferation. *Proc. Natl. Acad. Sci. USA 103*: 14842-14847.

[44] Barnhart BC, Simon MC (2007) Metastasis and stem cell pathways. *Cancer Metastasis Rev. 26*: 261-271.

[45] Gupta GP, Massague J (2006) Cancer metastasis: building a framework. *Cell 127*: 679-695.

[46] Yilmaz OH, Valdez R, Theisen BK, Guo W, Ferguson DO, et al. (2006) Pten dependence distinguishes haematopoietic stem cells from leukaemia-initiating cells. *Nature 441*: 475-482.

[47] Bar EE, Chaudhry A, Lin A, Fan X, Schreck K, et al. (2007) Cyclopamine-Mediated Hedgehog Pathway Inhibition Depletes Stem-Like Cancer Cells in Glioblastoma. *Stem Cells*.

[48] Park DM, Li J, Okamoto H, Akeju O, Kim SH, et al. (2007) N-CoR pathway targeting induces glioblastoma derived cancer stem cell differentiation. *Cell Cycle 6:* 467-470.

[49] Fan X, Matsui W, Khaki L, Stearns D, Chun J, et al. (2006) Notch pathway inhibition depletes stem-like cells and blocks engraftment in embryonal brain tumors. *Cancer Res. 66*: 7445-7452.

[50] Tavor S, Petit I, Porozov S, Avigdor A, Dar A, et al. (2004) CXCR4 regulates migration and development of human acute myelogenous leukemia stem cells in transplanted NOD/SCID mice. *Cancer Res. 64*: 2817-2824.

[51] Kang Y, Siegel PM, Shu W, Drobnjak M, Kakonen SM, et al. (2003) A multigenic program mediating breast cancer metastasis to bone. *Cancer Cell 3*: 537-549.

[52] Jin L, Hope KJ, Zhai Q, Smadja-Joffe F, Dick JE (2006) Targeting of CD44 eradicates human acute myeloid leukemic stem cells. *Nat. Med. 12*: 1167-1174.

[53] Krause DS, Lazarides K, von Andrian UH, Van Etten RA (2006) Requirement for CD44 in homing and engraftment of BCR-ABL-expressing leukemic stem cells. *Nat. Med. 12*: 1175-1180.

In: Cancer Stem Cells
Editor: Melissa E. Jordan, pp. 141-181

ISBN: 978-1-61668-971-1
© 2010 Nova Science Publishers, Inc.

Chapter VIII

HUMAN ADULT STEM CELLS AS TARGETS FOR CANCER STEM CELLS: EVOLUTION; OCT-4 GENE AND CELL-TO-CELL COMMUNICATION

James E. Trosko[*]

Michigan State University, East Lansing, Michigan, USA.

ABSTRACT

To examine the factors involving human carcinogenesis in order to design new strategies for prevention and treatment, a new approach from the current reductionalistic molecular oncological view will have to be made. In addition, this view must take into account both biological and cultural evolutionary factors that interact with the biology of the pathogenesis of cancer. An integrated hypothesist that links many incomplete hypotheses, such as the stem cell or de-differentiation theories of cancer, the multi-stage, multi-mechanism or "initiation/promotion/progression" theory, the mutation and epigenetic theories of carcinogenesis, and the "cancer stem cells" hypothesis, has been outlined. The emergence of somatic and germ-line stem cells during the biological evolution of the multi-cellular organism created new functions to regulate, homeostatically, phenotypes, such as growth control, differentiation, apoptosis, senescence and adaptive functions of terminally differentiated cells. The evidence supporting the stem cells as target cells for the initiation process was reviewed. The biological consequence of the initiation of an adult stem cell appears to be the inhibition of asymmetric cell division, or the blockage of "mortalization" of a normal "immortal" stem cell, not the "immortalization" of a normal, "mortal" cell. Promotion, functionally,

[*] Correspondence concerning this article should be addressed to: James E. Trosko, E-Mail: james.trosko@ht.msu.edu.

is the clonal expansion of initiated stem cells by both mitogenesis and the inhibition of apoptosis. These promoting conditions occur during wound healing, compensatory hyperplasia after cell death, chronic inflammation, growth factors and by many dietary and environmental, non-mutagenic chemicals. All of these promoting conditions inhibit cell-cell communication, either by disruption of gap junctions in progenitor cells or by interfering with secreted negative growth regulator-receptor signalling in cells not having functional gap junctions, thereby releasing initiated stem cells from mitotic inhibition. Tumor promoters are characterized by threshold levels, exposing the initiated cells for regular and long periods of time in the absence of anti-promoters and having species, gender, cell-type specificities. The normal stem cell appears to give rise to the initiated stem cell which ultimately can accrue all the phenotypes of an invasive, metastatic "cancer stem cell". As the tumor grows, some of these cancer stem cells can partially differentiate to become cancer "non-stem cells". Finally, to understand how cultural evolution affects the human cancer patterns, domestication of certain animals helped to change dietary habits which can influence the carcinogenic process. These dietary factors can influence the adult stem cells, in utero and postnatally, so as to either increase or decrease the risk to cancer by altering the stem cell pools and by increasing or decreasing the promotion of the initiated stem cells. This might provide a mechanistic basis for the "Barker hypothesis".

"Nothing in biology makes sense except in the light of evolution."
T. Dobzansky [1]

INTRODUCTION: THE COMPLEXICITY OF A COMPLICATED DISEASE; THE INTERACTION OF BIOLOGICAL AND CULTURAL EVOLUTIONARY FACTORS

The use of this quote by Theodosius Dobzhansky was done with a specific intent, namely, that in any attempt to understand carcinogenesis in human beings, outside the process of both biological and cultural evolution, will always come up with incomplete explanations. This review will attempt to provide some newer insights to this extremely complex disease. It should also be stated up front that "cancer" is not a single disease but multiple diseases that share several phenotypes or "hallmarks of cancer" [2]. Indeed, each cancer will be characterized by different phenotypes and genotypes within the tumor itself, due to alterations in the tumor micro-environment, causing both genetic and epigenetic instability as the tumor progresses.

Given this reality, one might wonder if any meaningful prevention and treatment strategies can be developed, not only for specific types of cancer (e.g., lung, prostate, colon), but, also, for different individuals with the same diagnosed cancer that shares the same 6 "hallmarks of cancer". This brings to mind a story of Albert Einstein's remark to a reporter who heard him gave a public lecture on his new theory of relativity. After his talk, this young reporter asked, "Professor Einstein, now that you physicists understand the workings of the universe, don't you think it's *complicated?* Einstein looked at the reporter and responded by saying, "Young man, if you *know nothing* of the universe, it is, indeed, *very complicated!* However, when you *begin to understand* it, it is *merely complex!*"

The goal of this overview *Commentary* is to try to integrate a number of well-known hypotheses of carcinogenesis (e.g., the stem cell versus the de-differentiation hypotheses, the multi-stage, multi-mechanism or "initiation, promotion, progression hypothesis; mutation versus epigenetic theories; and the oncogene- tumor suppression gene hypothesis of carcinogenesis). The attempt will, hopefully, demonstrate that this complicated carcinogenic process is "merely" complex. However, even with this incomplete understanding, new improved strategies can be made to prevent and treat the various cancers. Hopefully, unlike the old Indian fable of the six blind men who tried to describe the whole elephant, from which they only touched one part, medical science will at least try to integrate the different parts from various individual views in order to get a more realistic view of carcinogenesis.

NO ONE APPENDAGE DESCRIBES AN ELEPHANT, NOR DOES ONLY ONE THING CAUSE CANCER!

From early Greek observations to *Percival Pott's* observation on the relationship of soot to scrotal cancers in chimney sweepers and to the recent "discovery" of "cancer stem cells" [3], fundamental observations for hundreds of years have been made that give some insight into the factors influencing this whole animal/human biological process. However, the embryologists, pathologists, physiologists, biochemists, and molecular biologists saw cancers within the prisms of their reductionalistic training. The explosion of reductionalistic data being produced today, unfortunately, has no integrated framework on to which these data can be meaningfully interpreted. Because of the "success" of modern molecular oncology, with the discovery of oncogenes and tumor suppressor genes, many of the old observations and insights concerning the whole animal process of carcinogenesis have been ignored. The very idea that understanding the sequence of the human DNA will give us the "answer" to why we get cancer and how we can "cure" it, sounds much like the old fable of the 6 blind man.

In the field of embryology, Markert saw cancer as some developmental process that had been interfered with ("Cancer as a disease of differentiation") [4]. The following quote from one of his papers describes, beautifully, his perspective that has much relevance to our current understanding [5].

"Cells interact and communicate during embryonic development and through inductive stimuli mutually direct the divergent courses of their differentiation. Very little cell differentiation is truly autonomous in vertebrate organisms. The myriad cell phenotypes present in mammals, for example, must reflect a corresponding complexity in the timing, nature, and amount of inductive interactions. Whatever the nature of inductive stimuli may be, they emerge as a consequence of specific sequential interactions of cells during embryonic development.

The first embryonic cells, blastomeres, of mice and other mammals are all totipotent. During cleavage and early morphologenesis these cells come to occupy different positions in the three-dimensional embryo. Some cells are on the outside, some inside. The different environments of these cells cause the cells to express different patterns of metabolism in accordance with their own developing programs of gene function. These patterns of metabolism create new chemical environments for nearby cells and these changed environments induce yet new programs of gene function in responding cells. Thus a progressive series of reciprocal interactions is established between the cellular environment and the genome of each cell. These interactions drive the cell along a specific path of differentiation until a stable equilibrium is reached in the adult. Thereafter little change occurs in the specialized cells and they become remarkably refractory to changes in the environment. They seem stably locked into the terminal patterns of gene function characteristic of adult cells. The genome seems no longer responsible to the signals that were effective earlier in development.

Of course, changes can occur in adult cells that lead to renewed cell proliferation and altered differentiation as seen in neoplasms, both benign and malignant, but such changes are very rare indeed when one considers the number of cells potentially available for neoplastic transformation. Possibly, mutations in regulatory DNA of dividing adult cells can occasionally lead to new and highly effective programs gene function that we recognize as neoplastic or malignant. However, most genetic changes in adult cells can probably lead to cell death since random changes in patterns of gene activity are not likely to be beneficial."

Pierce, also, saw carcinogenesis as a defect in the differentiation of stem cells ("Cancer as a stem cell disease") [6]. After examining many hundreds of Morris hepatomas, Van R. Potter proposed the concept of "oncogeny as partially blocked ontogeny" [7]. It should be noted that while these scientists did not have individual stem cells on which to study the process of carcinogenesis, the concept of stem cells was sufficient to explain both the processes of development and carcinogenesis. It should be noted that the operational definition of an embryonic stem cell of today is that they will form teratomas when placed back into an adult animal. Ironically, both embryologists and stem cell researchers use this observation of the cancer field as a criterion of stemness.

When it was shown that all the cells within a tumor were clonally- derived, it provided even more experimental evidence of the role of stem cells and differentiation in carcinogenesis. It might seem a bit conflicting that, while all the cells within a tumor are genotyically and phenotypically unique [8], they were all derivatives of a single stem cell. The concept of genomic and epigenomic instability of the carcinogenic process was created to explain this apparent dilemma [9,10]. It must be pointed out, however, the idea that genomic and epigenomic stability is the "cause" of cancer has to be tempered with the possibility that these might be the consequence of a cell becoming a cancer cell, rather that the instability being the "cause" of cancer. Regardless of the ultimate resolution of this academic problem, this heterogeneity has been, and will continue to be, a major problem for prevention and treatment of cancer. That this is the case, for each tumor and each cell within that tumor, a different intracellular physiology, generated by different gene expressions and genetic abnormalities, poses a problem for treatment strategies.

From Single Cell Organisms to Multi-Cellular Organisms: Cancer as the "Faustian Bargain" We Paid for Our Survival

Until relatively recently, both the public and scientists wondered why the germ theory could not explain cancer as a disease. Even though clues that environmental agents, such as chimney soot, were associated with scrotal cancers by Percival Pott, it was difficult to put together a meaningful scientific hypothesis at that time. Although the clue that genetic factors might play a role came when Boveri [11] noticed abnormalities in chromosomes in cancer cells, until more direct evidence, such as the lack of the ability to repair ultraviolet light-induced DNA lesions in a cancer prone skin cancer syndrome, xeroderma pigmentosum [12], did a new perspective emerge. The role of the inability to repair UV-induced DNA lesions was associated with the production of mutations [13,14] and the molecular basis of specific UV mutations in the p53 tumor suppressor gene of skin cancer cells [15]. The new paradigm was generated, "cancers as mutagen" [16], that took hold and from that time until just recently, carcinogenesis research became very reductionalistic with the new focus on the specific genes in cells, when mutated, "proto-oncogenes" and "tumor suppressor" were thought to provide the ultimate understanding of the carcinogenic process.

There is no doubt today, that the production of mutations does play a role in the complex carcinogenic process, as evidenced by (a) the inherited germ line mutations that led to cancer predispositions, such as the xeroderma pigmentosum, retinoblastoma, Down's, Fanconi's anemia, etc [17]; (b) agents associated with the induction of cancer inducing mutations in various short term in vitro assays; (c) mutations found in the oncogenes or tumor suppressor genes of cancer cells; and (d) DNA lesions found in cells of the cancer prone organs treated with various carcinogens. However, as will be discussed later, this view was too narrow, for it now has been shown that epigenetic alterations in the nuclear genome (defined here as the alteration in the expression of the genome at the transcriptional, translational or posttranslational levels) could also give rise to a component of the carcinogenic process.

However, to continue the focus on the role of evolution and cancer, one must realize that without mutations (as well as epigenetic changes) in the genome, that first living single cell organism would not have survived as a species. Clearly, if that early organism did not form any new genetic sequences, when the environment changes, as it inevitably has changed, and will continue to change, the genes that coded for those proteins and enzymes would be useless in the new challenging environment. The species could not survive in new harsh environments. Therefore, without the ability to protect DNA from having DNA lesions and from repairing, perfectly, the DNA lesions being formed by the errors of DNA repair or by errors of DNA replication, mutations could be generated in a population. In such cases, possibly one of those mutations could code for a protein that allows the organism to survive and reproduce, and, thus, saving the species. However, we must view the two extremes in mutation production. No mutations clearly lead to species failure in a changing environment. Too many mutations would also complicate survival. This is especially true in a multi-cellular organism.

Therefore, obviously, during the course of evolution, a balance was made between (a) protecting the DNA from any external damage that might lead to mutations and the perfect repair and replicating of DNA (which would lead to the extinction of the species) and (b) the lack of excessive DNA protection and the excessive production of errors of DNA repair and replication (which would also lead to the extinction of the species). While single cell organisms survive by unrestricted or immortalized ability to reproduce, in a population that is large enough, the population will have a few individuals that had accrued a mutation that allowed it to survive and reproduce when its sibs could not. Only temperature, nutrient depletion, pH changes, gravity and radiation would have environmental limiting influence on these single cell organisms' ability to proliferate.

When during the course of biological evolution that the first multi-cellular organism appeared, several new phenotypes had to accompany this new society of cells. Clearly, the aggregation of cells into a closed system would not have survived environmental changes had there not been some evolutionary advantage. One advantage would have been the appearance of specialized cells within the closed system that would enhance the survivability of the group as a whole. The appearance of the ability to form these specialized cells or *to differentiate* from a very primitive state to a very high "differentiated" cell, which could perform "higher order" functions, such as touch, sight, thermal regulation, muscle movement, etc., added to the single cell organism's ability to proliferate in, basically, an uncontrolled manner.

However, if a social colony of cells, which could form cooperating, but specialized functions, had no growth control, the colony would, in effect, become a tumor. Therefore, a second new phenotype had to be a new form of *growth control* in a closed system. In a society of single cell organisms, there are methods of "communicating" with each other via secreted factors. During the transition from the single cell to the multi-cell organism, this communication mechanism was not lost, but it was supplemented by the appearance of the gap junction, a membrane-associated protein channel that allows direct transfer of ions and small regulatory substrates to be transferred between the coupled cells [18]. Today, twenty connexin genes, those coding the proteins that are assembled into hexamers that comprise the hemi-channel of the cell which couples with the neighboring hemi-channel, are evolutionarily conserved, thus implying their importance in the survival of the metazoan [19]. These different connexin genes appear to serve the function of providing differential signalling mechanisms to regulate various cellular functions, including allowing for differential differentiation within an organism [20]. Equally important, these new means of communication between neighboring cells in direct contact with each other seem to be involved in growth control via "contact inhibition" [21].

Another new phenotype also appeared during this transition in evolution. It was the function of *programmed cell death* or *apoptosis*. If, in fact, a multi-cellular organism was to be successful in maintaining its species, it could also "improve" its ability to survive by changing its phenotype to add new survival functions, such as the transition from an insect larva to a flying butterfly. However to make this extraordinary advance, those specialized cells of the larva had to give way to new cells that would be needed for pigmentation, flight muscles, wings and other new sensory organs. This could only happen if whole battery of genes in those cells, needed for the larval function, is replaced with new differentiated cells having new battery of genes expressed for the new functions of a flying butterfly. The original fertilized egg of that butterfly had both sets of genes but they were expressed only when needed for that particular stage of development.

Equally important during this transition of the single to multi-cell organism was the "Faustian" bargain. That is, in return for higher order functions that differentiation of highly specials cells could give to the species' survival, was the "mortality" or senescence of the whole organism. Clearly, if *all* the cells of the multi-cellular organism senesced or became mortal, the species would not survive. With the appearance of the ability to form specialized *"immortal" germ cells,* the "Faustian" bargain, then, excluded the germ cells from the curse of "mortality". Moreover, if the multi-cell organ was to have additional adaptive functions, such as continued growth of the non-germ line cells, tissue replacement of damaged or diseased tissue, and for extended life span, not only was the germ-line cells privileged with the characteristic of "immortality", but also, some somatic or non-germ cells were selected that had this feature. These germ line and somatic "immortal cells" are the so-called adult "stem" cells.

If we now view these new phenotypes that emerged during multi-cellular development, and if we view what happens in a multi- celled organism when it has a cancer, we note that cancers (a) no longer have growth control; (b) can not terminally differentiate; (c) do not apoptose normally; and (d) have the ability to be immortal. In effect, they have "de-evolved" to a single-cell organism-like state. It is interesting to note that the appearance of the connexin gene appeared early in the evolution of the multi-cellular organism [22]. It is also interesting that cancer cells have no functional gap junctional intercellular communication [23], either because the connexin genes were never expressed or that they were expressed but rendered non-functional by activated oncogenes or mutations [24]. Whether this association of the loss of function of the gap junction with the loss of growth control, differentiation, abnormal apoptosis and the appearance of immortality in the cancer cell was just coincidence or causal, has to be resolved.

STEM CELLS, CELL COMMUNICATION AND DEVELOPMENT

During the development of a human being from a single fertilized egg, the zygote or "toti-potent" stem cell, approximately 100 trillion cells are produced. In order that development of the embryo, fetus, neonate, adolescent, mature and geriatric individual be normal, a very delicate orchestration of communication processes (extra-, intra, and gap junctional inter-cellular communication mechanisms) must be integrated, in order that the hierarchy of different cell types (embryonic, pluri-potent, multi-potent, bi-polar stem cells; progenitor stems, and terminally-differentiated cells) be done in a sequential, concatenated manner to allow the total genome to be specifically regulated in each cell type (Figure 1).

Genes for "stemness", such as Oct-4, nanog, Sox-2 [25], must be expressed in the embryonic and adult stem cells (multi-potent, bi-polar). Other genes must be expressed in order that specific differentiation genes might be regulated during development, growth and in cell replacement in tissues, and during wound-healing. Gap junctions genes, the 20 connexin genes [19], do seem to be required for the specific differentiation of cells within and between tissues of different organs [20]. Temporal expressions of genes are needed for the normal process of apoptosis or programmed cell death and even for removal of damaged cells [26]. For cells in solid tissues, gap junction function seems to be required for apoptosis to occur [27].

This extremely complex communication between the adult stem cells in their niches [28], their committed progenitor or "transit" cells [29], and the terminally- differentiated daughter cells must exist. Since it seems that the early blastocyte cells do not have function gap junctions [30], and that several adult human stem cells also do not express their connexin genes or have functional gap junctional intercellular communication (GJIC) [31], communication between the stem cells and the surrounding committed progenitor cells, that do seem to have gap junctions, and the terminally differentiated cells, that might or might not have gap junctions during their whole life time, must be mediated by secreted factors [32-33]. The progenitor cells, both epithelial, endothelial, and fibroblasts, do have contact-inhibitory means to regulate proliferation [34]. Gap junctions have been associated with growth control [35], differentiation [36] and apoptosis [27].

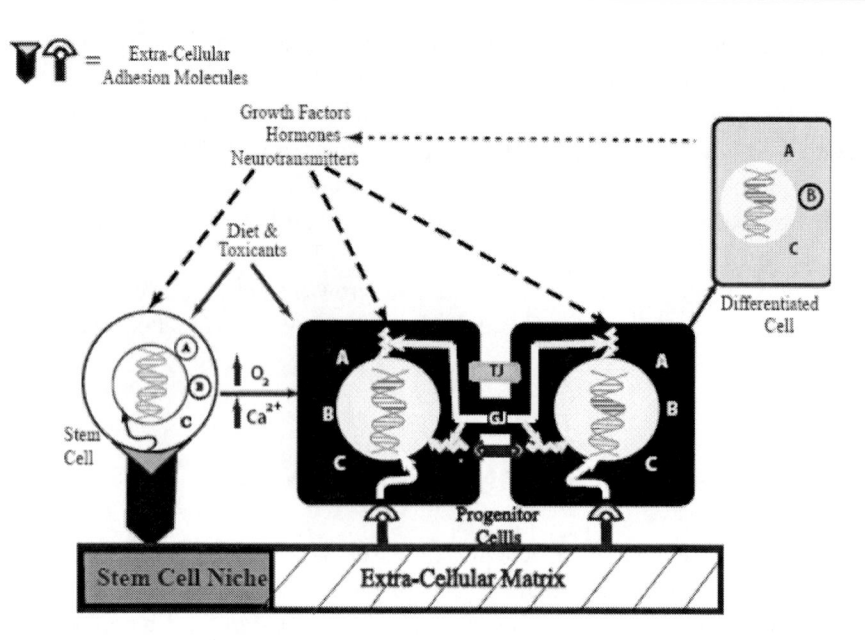

Figure 1. Gap junctions in cellular homeostasis. Extracellular signals, such as growth factors, toxicants, extra-cellular matrices and cell adhesion molecules that vary for each cell type (adult stem cell, progenitor and terminally-differentiated), interact with membrane receptors, which then activate intracellular signal transduction pathways that induce the transcription of genes (A,B,C) through activated transcription factors. These specific intracellular pathways operate under cascading systems that cross communicate with each other in controlling the expression of genes that direct the proliferation, differentiation and apoptosis of cells within a tissue. These multiple intracellular signalling check points are further modulated by intercellular signals traversing gap junctions, thereby maintaining the homeostatic state of a tissue. Abnormal interruption of these integrated signalling pathways by food-related and environmental toxicants results in diseased states, such as the tumor promotion phase of carcinogenesis, teratogenesis during early development, atherogenesis, immunotoxicity, reproductive- and neuro-toxicities.

The stem cell is defined as a cell that has the ability to divide either symmetrically to form two identical daughter stem cells (if it divides to commit both daughter to terminal differentiation, that would be the end of that stem cell's contribution to the organism's life) or asymmetrically to form one daughter cell (a progenitor) that is now committed to form a lineage of differentiated cells and one daughter that remains capable of self-renewal or stemness. To view stem cells, in this light, is to realize that a stem cell is naturally an "immortal" cell and it becomes "mortal" when it is induced to form a terminally-differentiated or "mortal" cell. Therefore, this decision point in a multi-cellular organism's evolutionary advance over single cell organism, namely, the control of symmetric versus asymmetric cell division will be of critical importance during normal development and during carcinogenesis.

Exactly how a stem cell determines whether it should divide symmetrically or asymmetrically is not currently known. However, from a conceptual standpoint, the stem cell must receive a number of signalling mechanisms. The first is signalling the stem cell receives from its anchored niche-substrate extra-cellular molecules. In the case of non-anchored stem cells, extra-cellular secreted signalling ions and molecules probably provide the same signal. Together with the secreted factors such as a hormone, growth factor, cytokine, chemokine, or ions, such as calcium, that might trigger some specific intra-cellular signalling, the net-effect of these signals would be result of the "cross-talk" of these extra- cellar signalling triggered intra-cellular signal pathways. Together with an important environmental factor, oxygen [37], the net effect of the interactive signals determine which genes are going to be transcribed and which existing proteins will be posttranslationally-modified for activity, inaction or ubquitization. That will lead to the molecular decision mechanism for symmetric or asymmetric cell division.

A Symmetrical Division

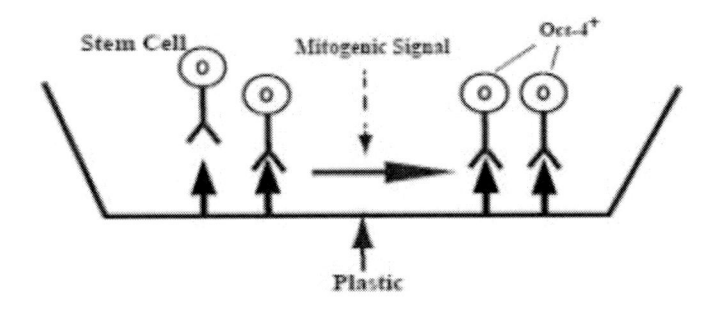

B Asymmetrical Division

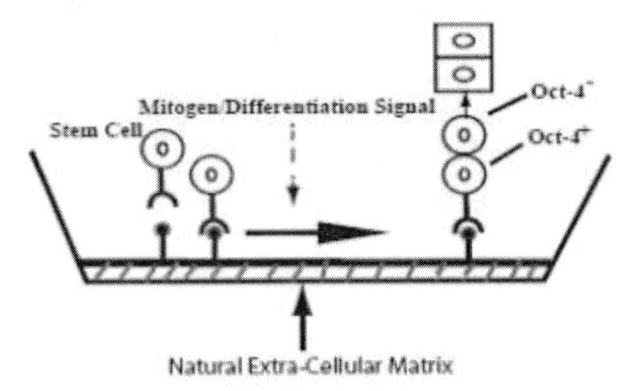

Figure 2. These diagrams illustrate two possible means by which stem cells (Oct-4+) decide to divide by symmetrical or asymmetrical division. In panel A, if a stem cell binds to a specific extracellular matrix, as symbolized by attaching to a coated plastic dish, the signal received combines with signals in the medium (growth factors, Ca++, nutrients, oxygen, etc.) to stimulate genes and gene products to bring about the division plane to be perpendicular to the attachment plane. As a result, both daughter cells continue to have identical signalling as did the maternal stem cell (symmerical cell division or expansion of the stem cell population). In panel B, the stem cell binds to a different substrate molecule, as represented by a natural extra-cellular molecule, such as laminin or collagen type 4. In this case, the signal this substrate molecule induces a different intracellular signal that interacts with the same signals from the medium, Ca++, oxygen, etc. to stimulate different genes and gene products to cause a division plane within the stem cell to be formed parallel to the attachment plane. In this case, the daughter cell on the bottom will mimic the same intracellular signalling as its maternal stem cell. Important to note that if these stem cells do not have functional gap junctional intercellular communication, then these signals are not transmitted to the other daughter cell because that daughter cell does not interact with the substrate signal. As a result, these daughter cells receive a different set of combined signals that trigger a commitment to become a progenitor and ultimately terminally differentiated progeny.

Conceptually, one model that might help to explain how the role of gap junctions might come into play in this process of symmetric and asymmetrical stem cell division. In Figure 2, it is speculated that, depending on the mix of signals a stem cell gets in its niche, the stem cell anchored to the niche extra-cellar matrix might form a mitotic division plane that is parallel to the plane of the stem cell niche extra-cellular matrix. In this case, the new daughter that is still attached to the niche extra-cellular matrix will continue to receive the same signal as did its stem cell mother.

On the other hand, because the other daughter is not attached to the extra-cellular niche matrix and does not communicate directly via gap junctions to its sister cell (a stem cell), its new mix of signals coul d induce the expression of connexin genes and form functional gap junctions. This cell is now a progenitor cell and is growth inhibited every time it is stimulated to proliferate by these gap junctions and it can differentiate via these gap junctions.

On the other hand, if the mix of signals the anchored stem cell gets triggers genes that cause the mitotic division plane to be vertical to the stem cell niche plane, then both new daughter cells would still be anchored to the same extra-cellular matrix molecule that helped to determine stemness. Since neither sister stem cell has gap junctions, they do not differentiate.

THE STEM CELL OR DE-DIFFERENTIATION HYPOTHESIS OF CARCINOGENESIS

One of the oldest theories of cancer is that a cancer cell started as a stem cell but was blocked in its ability to terminally differentiate or to become "mortal". That is the essence of Markert's quote and led to his view that cancer was a disease of differentiation [4]. In addition, the views of Pierce ("Cancer as a stem cell disease") [6], Potter's concept of "oncogeny as partially blocked ontogeny" [7], together with the experimental demonstrations of the clonal origin of all the cells within a tumor [37-38] and the immortally of tumor cells, contribute to a hypothesis that the normal immortal stem cell was the target cell for the ultimate cancer cell.

Yet this hypothesis has not gone unchallenged, as there are those who feel any cell, save those terminally-differentiated cells with no nuclei (red blood cells or lens cells), can de-differentiate to the "embryonic-stem" cell state and then progress to the carcinogenic process. In more modern terms, this "de-differentiation" might be re-named, "re-programmed" [39]. In deed, with some evidence being presented, adult differentiated mouse fibroblasts have been interpreted to be re-programmed after being genetically modified to over express copies of the Oct-4 gene [40-42]. Yet, these data also can be challenged in that the original adult mouse skin fibroblast culture probably contained some normal adult skin stem cells expressing Oct-4. The transfected recovered cells might have been a transfected normal skin adult stem cell. More experiments will be needed to resolve this possibility.

The de-differentiation hypothesis does challenge the basic tenet in science, namely, *Ocham's Razor*. Whenever multiple hypotheses are offered to explain an observation, one should first stick with the simplest explanation for it is the easiest to disprove. In the case of the de-differentiation hypothesis, one needs to re-program the genome, such that, at least those genes that limited the life span of the progenitor or terminally differentiate cell would need to be repressed and the stemness or Oct.4 gene be expressed. Basically, while in principle, this is logical, it does add another step in an otherwise, already complex carcinogenic process.

Probably another concept that has to be considered, in the context of the stem cell theory, is the current paradigm in the cancer field, namely, that the first step in the carcinogenic process must be the induction of "immortalization" in a normal, "mortal" cell [43]. In this paradigm, cancer is thought to arise from a normal, mortal cell, such as a primary culture of mammalian tissue. Since these primary cells, primarily fibroblasts, were characterized as having a finite life span in vitro, the "Hayflick limit" [44], any induced neoplastic cell derived from this population was assumed to be "mortal". Therefore, the first step in the carcinogenic process was to induce "immortality" in a mortal, normal cell. This allowed the immortalized cell to live long enough to accrue additional genetic and epigenetic changes needed for complete neoplastic transformation. However, if the target cell for carcinogenesis is the stem cell, then one can see the current paradigm is exactly backwards. If the stem cell, which is naturally "immortal" until it is induced to differentiate or to become "mortal", is the stem cell, then the new paradigm should be that the first step in the carcinogenetic process must be to block "mortalization" of an immortal normal stem cell. This now sets up the discussion of the next hypothesis of carcinogenesis.

Stem Cells, the Multi-Step, Multi-Mechanism Carcinogenic Process of Initiation, Promotion and Progression

With the possible exception of the formation of teratomas, all other cancers appear to require multiple distinct events from each other, in order that a single, normal cell becomes an invasive, metastatic cancer cell, having all those "Hallmarks" associated with all cancer cells. With the early demonstration using mouse skin and rabbit ears [45,46], it was shown that a one" hit" hypothesis of carcinogenesis was inappropriate to explain the multiple treatments an organism must get in order that a tumor appear.

Even with later studies on human genetic predisposing cancer syndromes, such as retinoblastoma [47], it was clearly evident that, just because all the cells of a person's body contained the cancer-predisposing gene, only a very few gave rise to a cancer.

In these early animal experiments, the concepts of "initiation", "promotion" and "progression" were coined, as "operation" terms.

Initiation was the event that occurred in only a few cells of organism, was basically *irreversible*. If the initiator was known to be associated with the induction of the target organ when given at high concentrations or doses, then at a low, non-cancer- inducing concentration or dose, the animal will not form any tumors. However, if followed by the next step (promotion), one can surmise that an irreversible event had occurred in a few cells of that organism. In the case of the mouse skin or rat liver, the initiated cell could remain quiescent in the animal for months, only to be stimulated later to start the carcinogenic process. The initiated cell did not die or was not "restored" to the normal state during this period. *Operationally,* initiation is only the production of a stable cell that can not terminally differentiate or apoptose easily. Consequently, initiation is that fundamental event that affects a stem cell's ability to divide, asymmetrically. This is probably the most accurate operational definition of initiation. While few studies have given us an insight as to what might be the gene or genes involved in this critical biological process of stem cells, Ko and associates have identified a gene, CoAA, that could be involved in this process [48]. A conceptual manner of viewing this initiation process in an adult stem cell is seen in Figure 4.

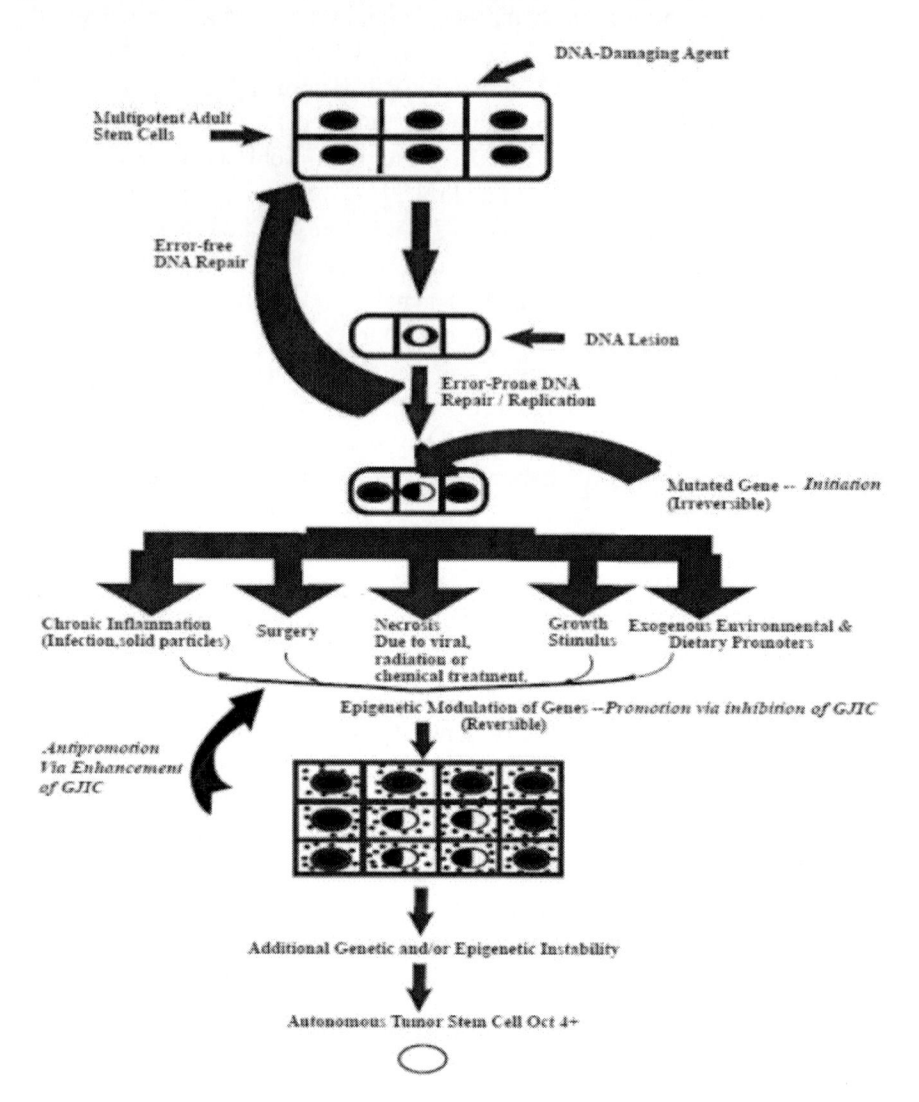

Figure 3. A diagrammatic heuristic scheme to depict the postulated mechanisms of the initiation and promotion phase of carcinogenesis. DNA lesions, induced by physical mutagens or by errors in DNA replication, are substrates in adult stem cells (Oct-4+) that can be fixed if they are not removed in an error-free manner prior to DNA replication. Promotion includes those conditions (i.e., chronic inflammation induced by infectious agents, solid particles; surgery or wounding; necrotic cell death; normal growth stimuli caused by growth factors, hormones; and exogenous epigenetic natural and synthethic epigenetic molecules), in which a pluripotent, but surviving, initiated adult stem cell (Oct-4+), can escape the nonproliferative state. The build up of initiated cells allows them to "resist" the anti-mitotic influence of neighboring non-initiated cells. In addition, the changing micro-environment within the growing benign tumor will cause some of the initiated adult stem cells to partially differentiate into cancer non-stem cells. This, together with either addition mutations or stable epigenetic changes, might allow a given initiated adult stem cell to have autonomous, invasive properties of a malignant cell.

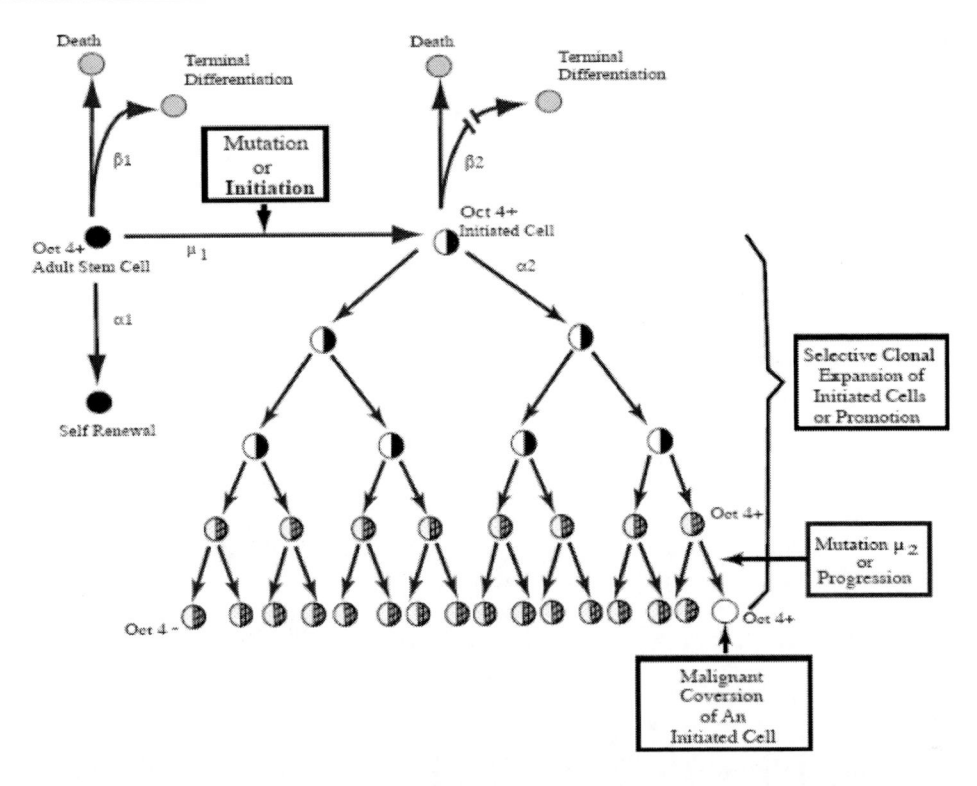

Figure 4. In this diagram, a normal adult stem cell is shown dividing asymmetrically to form one daughter that is committed to ultimately terminally differentiate. The other daughter is designated to be identical to its mother adult stem cell (Oct-4+). If that adult stem cell is exposed to some condition that prevents asymmetrical cell division, but does not suppress the Oct-4 expression, it is operationally an initiated cell. That is, if mitotically stimulated to divide, it divides symmetrically to form two initiated, non-terminally differentiated cell. Initiation is, then, defined as the process that prevents an "immortal" normal adult stem cell to terminally differentiate or become "mortal". These adult initiated stem cells are still Oct-4 positive or benign cancer stem cells. As these initiated Oct-4+ cells are stimulated to proliferate and resist apoptosis, the growing benign tumor micro-environment changes, some of these initiated Oct-4 + cells can partially differentiate into "cancer non-stem cells"[Oct-4 negative]. Evening, additional stable mutational or epigenetic events occur, providing the benign Oct-4+ cancer stem cells to become invasive, metastatic "cancer stem cells".

Promotion, on the other hand, was that process that occurred only after the animal was initiated (or as will be seen later, it could also occur on cells that were "spontaneously" initiated). In fact, especially in the case of a long-lived species, such as the human being, all individuals have spontaneously-initiated cells, and the longer one lives, the greater that number of initiated stem cells. The process of tumor promotion is when the initiated animal is exposed on a regular basis, for a long period of time, at threshold and above concentrations and in the absence of "anti-promoters", causing the single initiated cell to form a tumor. In the absence of this promotion process, no tumors appear [49]. Clearly, if the promotion process is stopped or interrupted, or given together with anti-promoters, then no initiated cell can accrue the necessary characteristics needed to have all the "hallmarks" of cancer. *Operationally,* the promotion process, one that is interruptible or even reversible [50], is one where the single "initiated" cell can be clonally expanded to reach a mass of cells, in which one cell can now acquire an addition stable change to give it a more selective advance to acquire more changes. It was also noted that promotion, which leads to the expansion of initiated cells, also involves the acquisition of a resistance to apoptosis. Therefore, the increased accumulation of initiated cells by promotion could be the result of mitogenesis and an inhibition of apoptosis.

Promotion appears to be able to allow an initiated cell to escape mitotic suppression by surrounding normal cells. The literature has shown that (a) wound healing after removal of tissue by surgery, (b) chronic inflammation, (c) cell death due to burns, viruses, or non-genotoxic toxicants, such as alcohol or carbon tetrachloride, (d) growth factors and hormones, and (e) exogenous non-genotoxic chemicals, such as Phenobarbital or polybrominated biphenols, can be tumor promoters. Promotion has been shown to be induced in initiated rodent skin, ears, mammary tissue, bladder, and liver. Physical agents, such as asbestos fibers, carbon particles, and solid metal objects, such as nanoparticles, can induce chronic inflammation to act as promoters [51]. There are species and strain specific promoters [52].

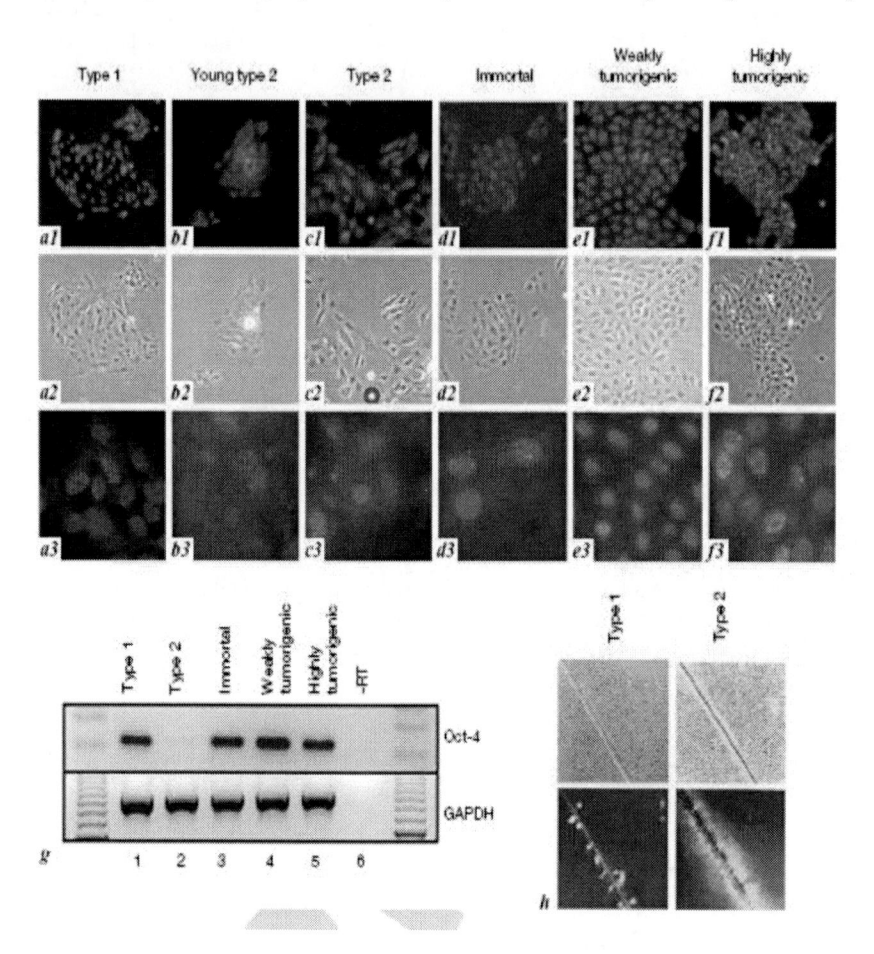

Figure 5. The composite of these three figures illustrated that (a) the clonally-derived normal human adult breast stem cells expressed Oct-4 (Figure 5.A panel) via immunohistochemical use of fluorescent antibodies to Oct-4 in the normal breast stem cells, but not in the differentiated breast cells (Figure 5.C panel), still expressed in SV40 "immortalized" normal breast stem cells which were not tumorigenic (Figure 5.D panel), still expressed in the irradiated and weakly tumorigenic breast stem cells (Figure 5.E panel) and expressed in the neu/ErB-2 highly transformed clone (Figure 5.F panel). In Figure 5.G, the RT-PCR data correlated with the immunohistochemical data of Oct-4 in this series of human breast adult stem cells. In Figure 5.H, the data clearly show that the normal breast adult stem cells have no functional gap junctional intercellular communication as measured by the fluorescent.

Although it was postulated in 1979 that tumor promoters worked, mechanistically, by inhibiting gap junctional intercellular communication [53], it still has not been integrated into the cancer field, as evidenced by the lack of references to this insight by the molecular oncologists. Most, if not all, chemical tumor promoters have been shown to inhibit, reversibly, GJIC at threshold and above concentrations which are non-cytotoxic [54]. In fact, the role of gap junctions has further been strengthened by the fact that many chemopreventive and anti-carcinogenic agents, such as green tea, [55], resveratrol [56,57], caffeic acid phenylester [58], or chemotherapeutic agents, such as lovastatin [59], kaempherol [60], SAHA [61], and beta-sitosterol [62], restore GJIC in cancer cells, Even various oncogenes, such as ras, src, neu, mos, have been shown to inhibit, stably, GJIC [63]. Genetic transfection of connexin genes in non-GJIC functioning cancer cells restores GJIC and normal cell growth with reduced tumorigenicity [63]. On the other hand, anti-sense connexin genes in normal cells triggered the tumorigenic phenotype of these cells [63]. Collectively, the role of GJIC must play some role, as Lowenstein and Kanno predicted in 1966 [64], in the carcinogenic process.

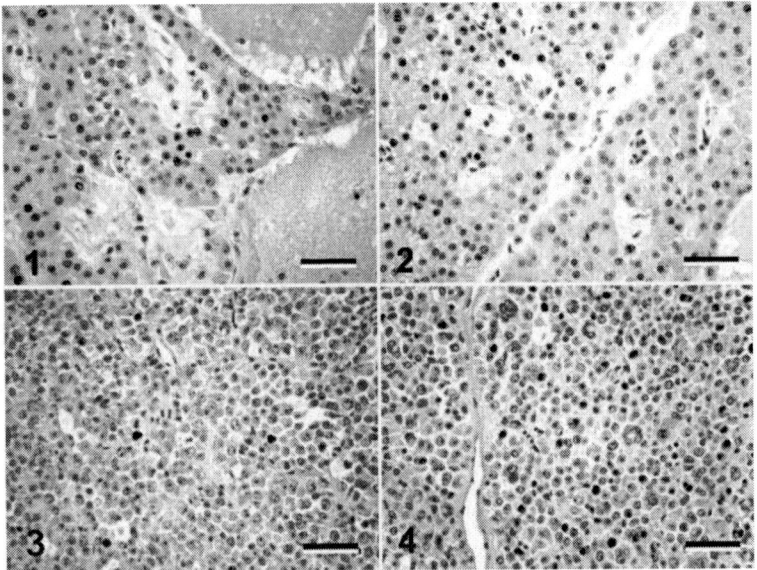

Figure 6. These photographs of Oct4 expression in spontaneous canine tumors reflect the intertumor and intratumor variation. Low (Figures 1, 3) and High (Figures 2, 4) frequencies of Oct-4 expressing cells in canine hepatocellular carcinomas (Figures 1, 2) and seminomas (Figures 3, 4 , respectively. Variation in the relative proportion of the Oct-4 –positive cells (brown nuclear precipitate) was seen in both between and within different types of spontaneous canine tumors. Immunohistochemical staining with mouse anti-human Oct-4 monoclonal antibody was visualized with the substrate 3,3'-diaminobenzidine with hematoxylin counterstain. Bar= 80 μm. Permission granted by American Society of Veterinary Pathology, Allen Press, Lawrence, Kansas, USA.

Progression is the final complex step (probably involving multi-events) that, *operationally*, converts one single initiated cell in the heterogeneous clone produced by promotion (e.g., a skin papilloma, liver enzyme foci, a colon polyp or a nodule in the breast). This step, also, appears to be irreversible and leads, ultimately, to an invasive, metastatic cell with all the "hallmarks of cancer".

To try to integrate the stem cell theory into this "initiation/ promotion/progression" hypothesis, it should be obvious that, if initiation occurs in an adult normal immortal stem cell, the initiation event must be the process that inhibits asymmetric cell division, but not the symmetric cell division of an immortal adult stem cell. This could, then, induce signalling in some of the "pre-cancer stem cells" so that they "partially" differentiate into " cancer non-stem cells", cancer cells which are no longer able to sustain the growth of the tumor.

THE MUTATION OR EPIGENETIC THEORIES OF CARCINOGENESIS

Since inherited genes that predispose cancer in patients, such as xeroderma pigmentosum or retinoblastoma, carry a germ line mutation. In the case of cells of the skin-cancer predisposed xeroderma pigmentosum, which do not repair their DNA after ultraviolet light-induced DNA damage [65], their cells have a higher mutation frequency than their normal counterparts [13,14]. From this, it is clear that mutations must play some role in carcinogenesis. In deed, when one examines oncogenes and tumor suppressor genes in various tumor cells, one frequently finds mutations in these genes. Especially, in the case of the mutations of the p53 gene in skin cancer patients, the mutations found correspond to that expected type if formed from unrepaired UV lesions of these cells [15]. Even in the cancer prone multi-cancer syndrome, Bloom's syndrome, the spontaneous mutation rates were found to be higher than from cells of normal patients [66].

These kinds of examples provide strong evidence that mutations, being basically an irreversible event, could be the mechanistic basis for the "initiation" event that starts the multi-stage process. This assumption has been carried over to the prominent paradigm of today's cancer research field, namely, "carcinogen as mutagen" [67]. However, the uncritical interpretation of results from in vitro studies to test if "carcinogens" are mutagens, as well as from ill-design bioassays on rodents [68], has brought massive confusion to the cancer-risk assessment field, as well as to practice assessment of new drugs and chemicals. While this does not imply that mutations do not play a role in carcinogenesis, it does question if *chemicals* (not radiation) cause mutations found in the oncogenes and tumor suppressor genes of the tumors associated with that exposure. With the demonstration that the mutation spectrum of an oncogene found in tumor cells of cigarette smokers being essentially the same as the spectrum for mutations found in the oncogenes of lung tumors of non-smokers [69], the question is raised whether the chemicals in cigarette smoke acted as promoters, rather than as initiators [68]. Animal experiments, as well as epidemiological evidence from smokers who quit smoking, suggest, strongly, that these chemicals acted more like promoters than initiators. Stopping smoking acted as stopping phorbol esters or phenobarbital on the interruption of promotion of skin and liver cancers, respectively. Must recently, Upham and co-workers [70-72] showed that the predominant chemicals in cigarette smoke performed, mechanistically, like tumor promoters, at non-cytotoxic concentrations. Promoters, by blocking intercellular communication, either by interfering with secreted growth inhibitors or their receptor-signaling, or by reversibly blocking GJIC, could block the cellular functions of "contact-inhibition", differentiation, or apoptosis. All three of these cellular phenotypes are affected by the carcinogenic process.

The important point to be made here, in trying to resolve the issue of finding DNA lesions in cells after an animal or cells in culture are exposed to chemicals associated with the appearance of tumors or neoplastic transformed cells, is that there are two sources of DNA which could be targets for DNA damage caused by electrophiles or free radicals. The first is the mitochondrial DNA where oxidative metabolism is occurring and the second is the nuclear DNA, which is sequestered away from oxidative damaging free radicals and electrophiles (except during ionizing radiation). In addition, there are three types of cells in which these two DNA targets are found, the few stem cells, the many progenitor cells with a limited life span and the terminally differentiated cells, which do not proliferate or give rise to cancers. Since very few of the studies demonstrating the existence of DNA lesions after chemical exposures separate the two sources of DNA before analysis, one can not rigorously state these lesions are those that led to mutations found in the oncogenes of tumor cells found after the chemical exposure. If one does find these DNA lesions in the nuclear DNA then, in all likelihood, the cell would have died from such massive production of electrophiles and free radicals that exceeded the cellular defence mechanisms, and traversed from the cytoplasm to the nuclear membrane. Under those conditions, the plasma membrane would be destroyed and the cell would die by necrosis. The death of these cells (usually the terminal differentiated cells, which express large amounts of metabolizing enzymes) could act as "indirect" tumor promoters by stimulating the stem cells to proliferate. If the stem cell was previously initiated by errors in replication or by UV radiation induced mutations, then the chemical could give the appearance of causing the DNA damage and mutations. In brief, while a statement suggesting that chemicals do not induce mutations that cause cancer is clearly heretical, the evidence suggesting otherwise is yet to be rigorously demonstrated. These so-called "mutagenic carcinogens" are more likely tumor promoters rather than initiators. These cancer-associated chemicals selectively promote spontaneously initiated stem cells [68].

If mutations might be the mechanistic basis for the initiation and the progression stages, one should not ignore the possibility that a stable epigenetic event could also bring about an initiation event. In the case of teratomas, it has been shown that a metastatic teratocarcinoma cell, when placed back into a blastocyst of a genetically-marked mouse, could participate in the normal development of a mosaic mouse, whereby, the teracarcimoa cells helped to generate normal tissues [73]. This could not have happened if the original teratocarcinoma cell was generated by an irreversible mutational event. The example also re-enforces the stem cell theory of cancer. The normal definition of an embryonic stem cell is that it forms a teratoma when injected into an adult animal. That implies the embryonic stem cell, when placed in a strange micro-environment, will modulate its gene expression patterns in bizarre ways, so as to differentiate but in an unorganized fashion. If a mutated cancer cell is transplanted into an adult host, it might partially differentiate or even partly apoptose, but will continue to form a tumor.

ONCOGENES, TUMOR SUPPRESSOR GENES, AND CANCER CELLS

The success of modern molecular oncology, with the discovery of oncogenes and tumor suppressor genes, easily diverted the cancer community from the classic whole animal studies to that of mutated DNA sequences in certain genes associated with a cell becoming a cancer. The emergence of the Human Genome project, with its promise to cure human diseases, such as cancer, simply by comparing sequences of cancer and non cancer patients, as well as providing new strategies for prevention or "cures", turns out not to be able to deliver on many of those promises. In fact, the insights, gained by the classic studies on carcinogenesis, as well as some of the ignored "hallmarks" of cancer [74], have already provided new insights without the need for all that Human Genomic information.

Harris has reviewed hundreds of studies on the most common tumor suppressor gene found in human cancers (but it should be noted, not all human cancers), the p53 gene [75]. Multiple oncogenes have been identified and are still being reported [48]. In brief, the functional roles, albeit each works by different molecular/biochemical mechanisms, of these two classes of cancer-related genes is to stimulate the growth of pre-malignant (initiated) and malignant cells and to inhibit the growth of these pre-malignant cells, respectively. *Operationally*, stimulation of the increase of initiated cells can occur by either or both inhibiting "contact-inhibition" and apoptosis and by stimulating mitogenesis. In addition, this includes the fact that initiation, operationally, *prevents asymmetric cell division of the initiated adult stem cell under normal conditions*, the oncogene or tumor suppressor genes might affect the regulation of symmetric and asymmetric cell division. Few in the cancer field have addressed this as a fundamental problem to be solved. Since oncogene and tumor suppression genes affect cell proliferation and cell cycle regulation of the single cell, the molecular oncologists have ignored the fact that cell proliferation also involves cell-cell interactions, either heterogeneous, such as stromal- epithelial interactions [76,77] by secreted factors (extra-cellular communication) or by gap junctional intercellular communication between heterologous and homologous cells within a tissue [78]. In other words, there are other genes working at a higher systems level, which transcends the reductionalists' thinking that predominates the cancer field today.

The fact that gap junction genes have been shown to be tumor suppressor genes, and the function of the these connexin genes is to affect intercellular regulation of single cell's cycle cycle control, to differentiate by receiving signals from without the cell or to apoptose by reaching signals from outside the cell, a different manner of viewing carcinogens must be gained than just from molecular or in vitro studies. As the late V.R. Potter had stated [79]:

> "The cancer problem is not merely a cell problem; it is a problem of cell interaction, not only within tissues, but also with distal cells in other tissues. But in stressing the whole organism, we must also remember that the integration of normal cells with the welfare of the whole organism is brought about by molecular messages acting on molecular receptors."

ADULT STEM CELLS AS THE TARGETS FOR CARCINOGENIC INITIATION

Given the previous experiments that demonstrated cancer cells were "immortal", that they resisted terminal differentiation but could partially differentiate under certain conditions, that they were monoclonally derived and that they could invade and metastasize, as well as induce angiogenesis, one is struck by the similarities of these "hallmarks" of cancer with the normal properties of stem cells. Two "hallmarks" that were not identified were the stem-like nature of the cancer cell and the lack of functional cell-cell communication [74].

Conceptually, however, the initiation/promotion/progression hypothesis seems, best, to support the idea that the single cell that is initiated is a normal adult stem cell. In the case of teratomas, the single cell might be an embryonic stem cell. However, in adult cancers, since stem cells do exists for most, if not all, organs, these cells, being either multi-potent or bi-potent, could after initiation, depending on the genes affected and the micro-environment, in which the cell finds itself, cause partially differentiation of the initiated stem cell into the identifiable tumor types of that particular organ (e.g., hepatocellular carcinomas or cholangiocellular carcinomas in the liver). In other words, for some initiated adult stem cells, these new changes in the micro-environment can induced these cells to have asymmetric cell division in order to partially differentiate.

Initiation is that operational step to cause a cell, presumably an adult stem cell, to start the complex evolutionary process for all tumors. If this cell is a normal, immortal adult stem cell, and if it is assumed that the initiation process is one that inhibits the stem cell to asymmetrically divide (i.e., it cannot normally terminally differentiate), then, "Are initiated stem cells those that give rise to the so-called newly discovered *cancer stem cells*" which have the potential to perpetuate the growth of a tumor?" [80]. Clearly, in a tumor, there are *"cancer non-stem cells"*, those that appear to be partially differentiated and can not perpetuate the growth of the tumor [81]. Of course, it has not been rigorously ruled out that some differentiated progenitor cell could be "re-programmed" to de-differentiate to become "immortal" again and then start the carcinogenic process. In this case, the "initiation" step would be the so-called "immortalization" of a normal, mortal progenitor cell as the prevailing hypothesis would suggest [43].

However, there are times when "Ocham's Razor" comes in handy in trying to resolve multiple scientific interpretations of observations. In the case of the "de-differentiation" or "re-programming" hypothesis of the origin of cancer cells, if an adult or somatic differentiated cell is "initiated", it must involve at least one additional step before it can utilize its new-found "immortality", compared to the normal adult step cell which is naturally immortal" at the time of initiation. Recent claims that an adult mouse skin fibroblast cell could be "re-programmed" when genetically transfected with "stemness" genes, such as oct-4, nanog, etc, would seem, at least, to keep open the possibility that "initiation" of an adult differentiated cell might happen [40-42]. However, in this case, "initiation" is operationally very different than "initiation" of a normal immortal adult stem cell. It must include two steps; one to reprogram whole sets of genes that determine the differentiation of a mature, differentiated skin fibroblast cell, which had its Oct-4 (and other "stemness" genes) transcriptionally suppressed and its senescence genes transcriptionally, operational. It, then, had to start where the normal adult get was when it was "initiated", namely already immortal but now blocked in its ability to divide asymmetrically under normal conditions.

However, there is another interpretation of these results of "re-programming" of an adult somatic, differentiated skin fibroblast cell. That is, if the original rescued genetically-engineered cell, done with a drug-resistance gene that presumably turned on the stemness genes, was originally a normal adult stem cell with it's already expressed Oct-4 and other stemness genes, then, in fact, those rescued cells were hardly highly differentiated somatic differentiated skin fibroblasts. The point being made is that adult stem cells do exist in most, if not all, adult organs, especially the skin. Many adult stem cells have been isolated from adult tissues that express Oct4 and did not express the connexin genes or have functional gap junctions [82-88]. These are real multi-potential stem or bi-potential stem cells. They are not simply pluri-potential embryonic stem cells migrating throughout the body of adult organisms.

Since adult stem cells have been isolated for many years, "Is there evidence that these adult stem cells can give rise to cancer?" The answer is "yes". When human adult breast stem cells were isolated and reported in 1995 [83], it was, then, subsequently shown that SV40 could block their ability to terminally differentiate (an operational definition of initiation) [89]. These cells were unable to form tumors in an appropriated animal model. While SV40 and other viruses (i.e. human papilloma virus) have been termed, "immortalizing viruses", it appears that this might be a major misnomer. It is well known that when primary human cell cultures are infected with these viruses, the majority of the cells eventually go through "crises", while a few rare cells survive and are characterized as "immortal". The idea is that either some rare insertional mutational event had occurred in these few surviving cells or that the virus genome somehow affected the senescence genes to be re-programmed" and the immortalization process started. There is a simpler explanation, supported by the experiments with human adult breast stem cells [31]. That is, the infecting SV40 or papilloma viruses, while infecting all the cells of the primary culture, only affected the few adult stem cells of that culture. These viruses did not induce "immortalization" but, in fact, blocked "mortalization" of an already normal, immortal adult stem cell. Chang and associates showed that these cells were able to perpetuate themselves in vitro and, upon, radiation and oncogene transfection become tumorigenic, whereas, no normal, differentiated human adult breast epithelial cell became "immortal" or neoplastically transformed [89].

It's important to discuss how the original adult human kidney stem cell was isolated and reported in 1987 [82]. The idea that stem cells might be the target cell for initiating the carcinogenic process came from studies to determine the extreme variability of inducing neoplastic transformed Syrian hamster cells in vitro. Nakano and T'so were trying to discern why cultures of Syrian hamster embryo cells could be exposed to some carcinogen on one day in the lab and formed many neoplastic transformed clones, but in the same cultures, on another day or in another lab, no transformants were induced [90]. To make a long story short, they noticed that, only in those cultures with "contact-insensitive" populations of cells, could one obtain neoplastic transformed clones. Our lab speculated these "contact insensitive", normal embryonic cells in these cultures might be stem cells. We further reasoned that their "contact-insensitivity" was the result of not expressing connexin genes or having functional gap junctional intercellular communication. We, therefore, assumed, in all adult tissues, there existed a few adult stem cells that did not have functional GJIC. By designing an in vitro assay with lethally-irradiated human fibroblast cells, which have functional GJIC, we disassociated normal kidney tissue into single cells. This mixture of normal kidney cells contained the many progenitor cells, which have functional GJIC, the terminally differentiated cells which can not proliferate and the few adult stem cells, which we assumed had no functional GJIC. After putting these cells on the lethally irradiated monolayer of human fibroblasts, we obtained a few clones of cells, which were later shown to be the adult stem cells of the human kidney (They expressed no connexin genes or had functional GJIC but they expressed Oct-4). As controls in this experiment, 8 human carcinoma cell lines, which had no GJIC, also could be recovered on this assay system. The rationale for the selection system was that if a normal cell had functional GJIC, it would couple with the dying x ray lethally-irradiated cells and die. Only those cells with no functional GJIC would proliferate on this monolayer. All of the human adult stem cells that have been reported appear not to express any connexion genes or have functional GJIC [82-88].

The reality is that in an adult animal, including the human being, adult committed stem cells exists normally for tissue replacement and growth. These stem cells are not merely pluripotent or multi-potent stem cells floating around only to differentiate when needed in particular micro-environments. Each tissue contains these stem cells. It is these adult organ-specific stem cells that are the suspected targets for the initiation of the carcinogenic process.

CANCER STEM CELLS:
A RE-DISCOVERY OF AN OLD IDEA

One of the recent paradigm-changing observations that has occurred in the cancer field happened when Al Hajj et al [80] reported that they identified a presumptive unique class of breast cancer cells within the breast tumor that had the ability to perpetuate the growth of the tumor, i.e., a breast *"cancer stem cell"*, whereas the other cancer cells within that tumor did not have this ability. These might be referred to as *cancer non-stem cells*. They are partially differentiated and ultimately senesce or apoptose. Later, Ponti et al [91] were able to show that these breast cancer stem cells to perpetuate the growth of the tumor. However, much earlier, Chang and his associates had already identified and partially characterized the normal human breast stem cell and showed that these stem cells could be "initiated" and neoplastically transformed [92]. In effect, he produced, in vitro, the human breast cancer stem cell that gave rise to a tumor when the cells were placed into an immune-compromised mouse.

Historically, when it was shown that the embryonic stem cell expressed a few unique "embryonic stem cell markers" (e.g., Oct-4, Sox 2, nanog genes) [93], Oct-4 seemed to have been correctly identified, early in the characterization of expressed genes in embryonic stem cells, as a critical "stemness-determining gene" [94]. Later, observations showed that when these cells differentiated, the oct-4 gene was transcriptionally suppressed [95]. There were others that claimed that no Oct-4 expression could be found in normal differentiated tissues. Then, when a few reports saw Oct-4 expression in a few cells of some types of tumors [96,97], it was suggested that Oct-4 must have been re-expressed or re-programmed during the neoplastic transformation process. It has been used to confirm the accepted paradigm [43] that the normal differentiated progenitor cells do not express immortalizing potential that the Oct-4 gene seems to possess.

Because our group, believers in the stem cell theory of cancer, knew the adult differentiated tissues must have a few adult stem cells, which were probably overlooked in these previous reports, we decided to examine the many isolated human adult stem cells we had in our lab (kidney, breast, liver, pancreas, mesenchyme) for the expression of Oct-4. We also assumed that these few normal adult stem cells were the target cells for the cancers seen in human organs. In addition to testing for Oct-4, we also tested for the expression of the major connexins and for functional GJIC which is required for these stem cells to differentiate. In brief, we showed that all of these normal adult stem cells expressed Oct-4 and when the stem cells differentiated, Oct-4 was repressed.

In a classic set of experiments, Dr. Chang's group obtained a series of clonally-derived cells from the normal adult breast stem cells which (a) could be differentiated into normal epithelial cells (no expression of Oct-4, but they expressed Cx43 and had functional GJIC); (b) were SV-40 transfected but non-tumorigenic and unable to terminally differentiate, had Oct-4 expressed but no GJIC; (c) after x-rayed irradiated produced a weakly tumorigenic clone with Oct-4 expressed; and (d) which, after a neu/Erb2 transfection, a highly tumorigenic derivative of the weakly tumorigenic clone was obtained, which still expressed Oct-4 [98]. In essence, we showed that Oct-4 was expressed in the normal adult stem cell, stayed expressed when SV40 prevented asymmetric cell division, remained expressed during the induction of tumorigenesis by X rays and oncogene transfection. It was transcriptionally suppressed only during differentiation of the normal adult stem cells [98]. These differentiated breast epithelial cells were unable to re-program the Oct-4 gene or become immortal or tumorigenic under the conditions where the normal adult stem cell was easily blocked from differentiating and neoplastically transformed. These experiments clearly support the stem cell theory and are harder to explain using the "de-differentiation" or "re-programming" hypothesis of carcinogenesis.

It is important to note that these normal breast adult stem cells expressed the estrogen receptor, a marker found in a majority of human breast cancers. In addition, since the commonly used human breast carcinoma cell line in breast cancer studies, MCF-7, expresses the estrogen receptor, but not the connexin43 gene [99], but does express the Oct-4 in vitro [98], one might speculate that MCF-7 was originally derived from a normal adult breast stem cell similar to our normal human isolated adult breast stem cell.

It is also important to note that MCF-7 is not a homogeneous cell population [98]. It is an immortal cell line because it contains some "cancer stem cells" that help to perpetuate the cell line indefinitely. *In vitro, as in vivo, the cells create different micro-environments for these cancer stem cells, causing some of them to partially differentiate into cancer non-stem cells or to regain some asymmetric cell division potential.* The implication from these observations is that, all tumors during their growth will be a mixture of cancer stem cells and cancer non-stem cells. The ratio of these two types of cancer cells is probably influenced by some stromal-epithelial interactions, as has been demonstrated in vivo and in vitro [76,77,100].

To illustrate this, we were the first to detect in vivo that 100% of 83 canine tumors from 21 different organ sites expressed Oct-4 in the tumors (the "cancer stem cells", but the ratio of the cancer stem cell to the cancer non-stem cells varied from tumor to tumor. [81] Later it was shown that 34/35 human bladder tumors expressed Oct-4, and the ratio of the two types varied widely between tumors [101]. At this point, one can only speculate that the differences in the ratio of the two types of cancer cells might be due to genetic, environmental or dietary factors that influences symmetric and asymmetric cell division of the cancer stem cell.

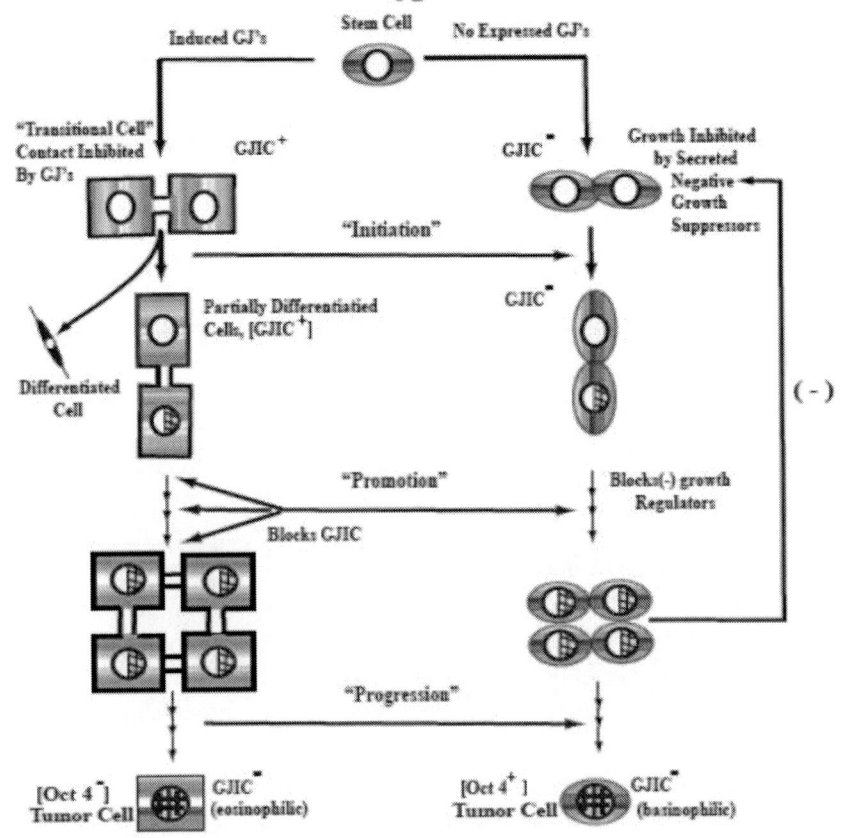

Figure 7. This figure illustrates a hypothesis to explain the existence of two types of cancer cells, namely, those that lack GJIC communication because (a) the connexin genes were never transcribed, as in HeLa or MCF-7 cancer cell lines, or (b) the expressed connexion genes could not form functional gap junctions due to oncogenes or mutations that render the connexin proteins forming functional gap junction, as in ras, raf, neu, src or mos-activated oncogene-transformed cancer cells. In other words, all cancer cells seem to be dysfunctional with regard to having GJIC, either because the connexin genes were never transcribed or if the transcribed proteins were not functional. There are several possible explanations, one being that the original stem cell, lacking expressed connexins, got initiated and subsequently promoted by agents that inhibited secreted negative growth regulators of stem cells. These might be the origin of the "cancer stem" cells. Now the cancer cells with activated oncogenes might inactivate functional GJIC by modifying, posttranslationally, the connexin proteins and gap junctions. There could be at least two explanations for this. One is that if the very early committed progenitor cells of the adult stem cell was initiated while it still expressed Oct-4 and telomerase, then its growth inhibition via gap junctions had to be inhibited by promoters that reversibly blocked GJIC, until late in promotion, when activated oncogenes stably and irreversibly inhibited gap junction proteins, such as via hyper-phosphorylation of connexins by ras, src and neu. Alternatively, these non-functional GJIC tumor cells might be derived from "cancer stem cells" but which were partially differentiated by the developing and changing microenvironments of all tumors to become "cancer non-stem cells".

In a recent cautionary note, it was stated that "tumor growth need not be driven by rare cancer stem cells" [102]. The authors drew their conclusion, based on showing that isolated primary pre-B7B lymphoma cells from 3 independent Eu-myc transgenic mice could give rise to tumors in congenic mice, independent of the cells injected. Their conclusion, based on everyone's assumption was that, in all tumors, the "cancer stem cells" were "rare". In the study on canine tumors, and on human bladders [81,101], the numbers of Oct-4 "cancer stem cells" varied widely. Therefore, this cautionary note might be very misleading.

The excitement seen after the reports of the existence of various "cancer stem cells" has given new insights to the reasons why past cancer therapies have failed, i.e., they failed to target the "cancer stem cells" in the tumors. In addition, one of the explanations why these various therapeutic treatments failed was because the treatments, themselves, induced drug resistance genes that allowed these drug resistant cells to re-emerge. It now seems that a more plausible explanation exists for "induced drug resistance". The normal adult stem cell and its derived "cancer stem cell" might be naturally resistant to toxic chemotherapeutic agents. Again, the quote, "Nothing in biology makes sense except in the light of evolution", seems appropriate here.

From an evolutionary standpoint, if, during the emergence of the multi-cellular organism and the development of both germ line stem cells and adult somatic stem cells, both the stem cells and their differentiate lineage progeny were equally sensitive to environmental toxicant, the individual, hence, species, would never have survived. Therefore, it was imperative that the stem cells evolved with some mechanism(s) to protect itself from the exposure to these toxic agents. One means was to develop mechanisms to pump out foreign chemicals before they could damage the cell. Therefore, if an organism is exposed to some toxic agent, the differentiated cells might die; however, if the adult stem cell survived, it could replace the dead, specialized, differentiated cells and the organism and species would survive.

Evidence has been reported that, when tumor cells are exposure to some toxic fluorescent agent and then passed through a cell sorter, two populations of cells are recovered. One that contains the fluorescent compound and the other, the "side population", cells are non-fluorescent. It is these "side population" cells that seem to have stem-like properties, in that they can differentiate into the cell-lineage from which the tumor is derived [103]. One of these factors that rendered these cells to be drug resistant is because they naturally expressed various drug resistant genes, such as ABCG-2 [104].

In brief, drug resistance was not induced by the cancer chemotherapy, but it was the result of "cancer stem cells", which are naturally, expressing drug resistance genes, were selected from the mixed population of cancer cells.

A new perspective for cancer prevention and therapy is now obvious. The real target cell for prevention and treatment should be the "cancer stem cells". Oct-4 expression appears to by a critical gene to maintain "stemness" of both the normal stem cell and "cancer stem" cell. The ultimate goal in cancer prevention and therapy will be to render, transcriptionally or posttranslationally, the Oct-4 gene inoperative.

This goal still has the same current intractable problem that has been plaguing the old therapeutic approaches. Since Oct-4 is expressed in both the normal and cancer stem cells, one must be able to target only the cancer stem cell, in order from preventing the therapy from reducing the normal stem cell pool. In addition, since the tumor contains both the cancer stem and cancer non-stem cells, which could inhibit the therapy designed to target the cancer stem cells, a dual approach might be implemented.

First, apply some therapy that can "easily" remove these cancer non-stem cells. After these are reduced, if the cancer stem cells, which express oct-4 and drug resistance genes, inhibiting the pump activity at the functional or enzymatic level, then treating with a toxic chemical, used to kill the cancer non-stem cells, would render these cancer stem cells to behave as functional cancer non-stem cells.

This approach has been tried in the past without our current knowledge of the cancer stem cell concept. Another strategy would be to target the Oct-4 gene with transcriptionally-modifying potential to block its expression, using targeting strategies that identify the organ markers for the adult stem cells, such as the estrogen receptor for adult human breast cancer stem cells and some other "cancer stem cell" marker not expressed in the normal adult stem cell.

DIETARY MODULATION OF NORMAL AND CANCER STEM CELL POOLS: A VIEW OF HOW DIET, SYSTEMS VIEW OF CELL BIOLOGY, AND THE RISK TO CANCER INTERACT

It is well known that genetic predispositions, gender, developmental state, caloric balance (gluttony or caloric restriction), exercise, life style, cultural, environmental, medical, or pharmacological treatments can influence the multi-stage, multi-mechanism process of carcinogenesis. What is clearly emerging is the powerful role that dietary factors play in experimental, as well as epidemiological studies, to either increase or decrease one's risk to various cancers. What has not been clearly demonstrated is, the interaction of these dietary factors and the adult normal and cancer stem cells. In fact, a new view is emerging that takes us away from only thinking, reductionalistically, about what might happen in a single adult stem cell that eventually could give rise to an initiated cancer stem cell, but how diet can involve the stem cell pool to affect the risk to increase or decrease the risk to cancer from a *systems* vantage point. In deed, this new view also will take our attention away from only viewing the cancer stem cell role as only a biological problem, but one that involves many cultural evolutionary changes.

Because of cultural evolution, which affects our dietary intake of the quantity and quality of food much more rapidly than the biological evolution needed to adapt to these changes, the long biological evolutionary adaptive balance with the diet of early humanoids, the new dietary behaviours are creating many new health problems [105-109]. Transmigration studies of humans have shown in several cases that the patterns of cancer frequencies of various ethnic groups conform to the new cultural (presumably) dietary behaviour compared to their country of origin.

Because of modern methods of altering native cultural diets to global diets, cancer patterns are changing. In fact, for a number of reasons, these new dietary habits are shaped by economic costs, availability of certain foods (depletion of tuna for sushi and sashimi), substitution of red meats for fish, agricultural genetic breeding of foods that sell or are needed for "fast food industries", and the psychological selling via mass marketing. The complexity of "diets" (calories, vitamins, nutrients, food components, processing and preparation of foods, etc.) makes epidemiological studies difficult to interpret since these studies are but a small snapshot in a dynamic time and place experience in an ever-changing dietary climate probably within every 20 years. These studies are now compounded in complexity by increasing uses of food supplements, pharmaceutical drugs, changing life styles and individual behaviours. The World Health Organization's estimation that there might be more over weight individuals than under weight in the world today suggests that global chronic (as well as acute) diseases are being affected by, on one hand, too many calories (not necessarily too many nutrients) or too few calories and nutrients [110]. Therefore, the next question has to be asked: "Which of the three stages of carcinogenesis seem to be most affected by diet modification?"

One can speculate that, since the initiation stage must take place in a single cell in a limited number of critical cancer-related genes, either by a mutational or stable epigenetic event, it will be impossible to reduce the risk to zero in the body of 100 trillion cells, most of which are not the target or adult stem cells. Initiation can occur when DNA damage is not repaired correctly (errors in DNA repair), such as in the xeroderma pigmentosum example. We can, of course, prevent the risk from being higher, such as not exposing ourselves to too much sunlight. In addition, we must recognize that mutations can be produced every time a cell replicates (errors in replication). We can never prevent this source of mutations that might initiate an adult stem cell. Cells are replicating day and night, 7 days a week and for our whole lives. Therefore, it is would seem that we will never reduce to zero the initiating event. *In fact, this source of spontaneously-originating errors in replication of DNA in stem cells might be the main source of initiated cells of the body, except for the UV-light induced initiation of skin stem cells.*

Promotion, on the other hand, takes decades, in most cases (except in children), to reach the progression stage. From a practical standpoint of designing an intervention chemoprevention strategy that would be the most efficacious, to decrease the risk to carcinogenesis, at least from the view that we, as individuals, might have some control of this process, the promotion phase would be a *life-long* process. Since the progression phase appears to occur in a single promoted initiated cell (a "pre-cancer stem cell"), that requires the phenotypes needed for invasion, metastasis and induction of angiogenesis, it might also be impossible to modify, appreciably, this phase of carcinogenesis because one might not know when to intervene. *By intervening during the promotion phase (during one's adult lifespan), diet can make a difference on the progression, hence carcinogenic transition.*

There is no question, that using the initiation, promotion and progression models of carcinogenesis, one can increase or decrease the cancer frequencies. Even using surrogate in vitro models, (transformation assays; gap junction modulation assays, etc.), one can identify dietary, as well as environmental factors, that can either increase or decrease endpoints in these models that correspond to the experimental or epidemiological evidence [111]. Of course, while there hasn't been perfect correspondence of the in vitro assay results with the experimental or epidemiological data, it should not be surprising, given the shortcomings of in vitro and in vivo animal data [68], let alone epidemiological data [112]. Most of these studies are lacking the mechanistic basis of either the assays used or the understanding of the biology of the carcinogenic process in the design or interpretation of the epidemiological studies.. The failure of the CARET study is a perfect example of this point [113]. The original design ignored previous studies on the mechanism of action of this class of natural chemicals on GJIC [114]. In addition, studies have shown that anti-oxidants can become pro-oxidants [115]. It has even been shown that some of the same class of molecules could become tumor promoters [116]. By the same interesting challenge to our understanding, many tumor promoters have been shown to be anti- carcinogens [117-119]. The conflicting and non-reproducible epidemiological studies are also not surprising, because human populations can not be controlled like rats in a laboratory. Genetic differences, exposures to unreported factors that might be additive, antagonistic or even synergistic to the factor that is under study, critical threshold concentrations, anti-oxidant proficiencies or deficiencies of the individuals, time and duration of exposures, etc., can modify the results of one study compared to another.

The critical importance of understanding the underlying mechanisms of promotion and the role of stem cells in carcinogenesis have not yet entered the cancer prevention or treatment area. A case in point is the recent TASK FORCE REPORT to suggest new approaches to identify potential cancer chemo-preventive compounds [120]. No mention was made of the mechanistically-based in vitro (and in vivo) assay, based on the prevention of tumor promoting agents from down-regulating gap junctional intercellular communication. Many agents that can, reversibly, down regulate GJIC have been shown to be potential tumor promoters by various biochemical mechanisms [121]. The consequence of inhibiting GJIC by any biochemical mechanism in normal tissues is dis-regulation of homeostasis of cell proliferation and differentiation of stem cells, progenitor and differentiated cells. Classic tumor promoters, such as phorbol esters and phenobarbital, have shown correspondence of the in vitro results with the in vivo results [52]. In deed, even the opposite case to support the role of GJIC in chemoprevention, and even chemotherapy, has been made in vitro, as well as in vivo., with a large number of dietary factors, such as green tea [55], resveratrol [56,57], caffeic acid ethyl ester [58], beta-sitosterol [62]and lovastatin [59], SAHA [61].

WHY DOGS AND COWS CAUSED HUMAN PROSTATE AND BREAST CANCERS: THE INTERACTION OF BIOLOGICAL AND CULTURAL EVOLUTION, DIET, ADULT STEM CELLS AND CANCER

To bring this *Commentary* to full circle, the quote made by D. Coffey should serve to provide a "systems view" of the human cancer problem. In his article comparing the similarities of breast and prostate cancers, he stated:

"Certainly, looking for simple relation will not be sufficient, but delineating the exact mechanisms of cell cycle control and stem cell development in prostate cancer should be helpful in understanding these early preneoplastic lesions and their relations to diet." [122].

Up until now, the focus for trying to understand the complex carcinogenic process has been through the "light of biological evolution". The formation of a multi-cellular organism created a need to coordinate cell proliferation, differentiation, apoptosis, senescence and adaptive responses of adult stem cells, progenitor and terminally-differentiated cells. The need to have both somatic and germ-line stem cells served both the individual and species The fact that the DNA is not immune to DNA damage, errors in repair or in DNA replication was selected for a the production of mutations at a rate that would ensure survival of the species in an ever changing physical environment, yet not so high as to jeopardize either the individual or species' survival. Neither the somatic adult stem cells nor the germ-line stem cells were immune to these mutations.

In the case of the human species, the individual was served by these somatic adult stem cells to provide growth, differentiation of highly specialized cells, and wound-healing. These were needed to allow the individual to live long enough to reach sexual maturation, to leave offspring, and to take care of the offspring until they were able to repeat this process. This ensured the survival of the species. After that period of life span (approximately mid-fourties), the individual's contribution to evolution was essentially finished. At which time, sufficient mutations had occurred in both the germ line and somatic stem cells. The geriatric individual, save for some accumulated experiences ("wisdom"), was basically a drain on limited resources for the survival of the young. As pointed out above, the adult stem cell is most likely the target cell for cancer. However, the multi-stage, multi-mechanism carcinogenic process, probably played little role as a negative selection factor for evolution, as most cancers would appear long after the median life span of most individuals in early pre- and real human biological evolutionary history.

Clues to the roles of both biological and cultural evolution, diet and breast and prostate cancers have been noted before [122,123]. Unlike the roles that biological evolution, changing physical environment and diets of non-human animals played in their evolution, human's brought with them the emergence of 4 critical new phenotypes [to consciously create symbols; to communicate with those symbols; to create new technologies using those symbols and communication skills; and to value or make choices on which technology to use or not use [124]. Unlike non-human animals, their "detritus" disappears in short time. However, as it has been stated by a philosopher, "Men build walls and walls build men". The point being that what we do to our physical and cultural environments has lasting and major impacts on future generations of both the non-human animal and the human animal.

Human beings have created a cultural environment which, among many other things, shapes both our physical environment and our diet. As noted in the subtitle of this section, early humans learned a few things that helped to rescue them from hunting and gathering and a "feast-fast"- type of dietary behaviour that shaped our biological evolution. That is, we had to have those molecular, cellular and physiological adaptive features, stored in the genome of our germ and somatic stem cells, that allowed us to survive under these "feast and fast"- conditions. We inherited these from our pre-human and non-human animal ancestors. With the domestication of the cow, which provided work, food, and clothing, and of the dog, which aided human's hunting abilities; we find clues as to how these cultural evolutionary facts have impacted on human stem cells and cancer. In both of these cases, these two animals have helped to "cause" breast, colon and prostate cancers in humans. In the case of the bovine, one might note there seems not to be any significant mammary cancers associated with its existence, so why is there a link to human breast cancer? In the case of the canine, this animal seems to have a significant prostate cancer problem similar to human beings [122,123]. Can comparative oncology provide some answers or will a simple "systems" view do?

To first view how diet might affect the multi-stage, multi-mechanism process of carcinogenesis, we need to view the shared general concepts of the aforementioned integrated hypothesis, and how prostate and breast carcinogenesis might have a "higher order" or cultural component in their dietary risk factors.

When one views the current studies on the cancers found in the atomic bomb survivals of Hiroshima and Nagasaki, breast cancers seem to be one of the highest solid tumors to which could be attributed to the exposures to radiation [125]. One of the reasons it was noted is because the background frequency of breast cancers of those Japanese women was extremely low, such that any attributed increase by radiation was noted to be statistically significant. While the main focus of the interpretation of these data has been the radiation exposures, little attention has been given to why the attributed increase was the level seen. In the first place, one interpretation has been that soy products which has been for generations a major component of the Japanese women's diet might have been the reason for (a) small breasts and (b) low breast cancer frequencies. Because soy contains many anti-cancer nutritional components, genistein and Bowen-Birks Inhibitor [126,127], it has been speculated that these dietary components contributed to lowering the breast cancer frequencies of both the control and a bomb survivors. From a mechanistic perspective and our theme that adult stem cells are the target cells for carcinogenic initiation, the next question is: "How do these soy products work on the multi-stage, multi-mechanism process of breast carcinogenesis."

In the first place, human adult breast stem cells have been isolated from normal human breast tissue [83]. These breast stem cells can be neoplastically transformed in vitro.[89] Moreover, while there is no existing evidence that genistein could lower or increase the ionizing radiation genetic damage in human breast stem cells, there is compelling evidence that genistein can induce differentiation of the adult human breast stem cells. [128] Therefore, if either the mother of the daughter, exposed to the a bomb radiation, eat lots of soy products during pregnancy, the female embryo and fetus would have few breast stem cells because the breast stem cell would have been induced to asymmetrically divide rather that symmetrically divide to produce many adult breast stem cells. Further, after birth and during adolescent development, the daughter also consumed lots of soy products. Therefore, from these facts of diet on stem cells during development and adolescent growth, this dietary habit could be a chemo-preventive factor by reducing the breast stem cell pool. This alone would reduce the risk to breast cancer by reducing the number of possible initiated breast stem cells, all other factors being the same. This could be a mechanistic basis of the Barker hypothesis [129]. The hypothesis basically states that whatever might happen in utero to the embryo/fetus could affect the risk or resistance or sensitivity to diseases later in the life of the offspring.

While radiation is assumed to be the initiators of the exposed breast stem cells, could the soy products affect the promotion of cancer? The evidence, on the whole, seems to indicate that these soy components can be chemo-preventive by their ability to interfere with the promotion process, although there is some rodent evidence it could act as a tumor promoter [130]. Again, this points out the need for better understanding of the underlying mechanisms, especially when using either animal bioassays or epidemiological studies. It should now be pointed out that, with the introduction of dairy products into the Japanese diet and the transmigration studies of Japanese, who move to Western countries, soon changed their dietary habits and frequencies of breast cancers to match to of the host country. In addition, it should also be noted that the Japanese women, who contribute to the longest median life span also pay a heavy price for their past dietary practices, namely the high frequency of osteoporosis. Could it be that the soy products which induced differentiation and asymmetrical cell division of the breast stem cell also did the same for the osteoblast precursor stem cells? This then opens up another health aspect of stem cell pool modulation, namely the reduction of stem cells via either diet or environmental agents could affect the aging process itself, as well as the diseases of aging [131,132].

To further analyze how diet can influence breast cancer and getting back to the bovine, milk, cheese, red meat, all factors associated with both breast and colon cancer, were introduced during the domestication of the bovine. Many of the components of these bovine products, aside from the caloric content, is the introduction of dietary components that are known tumor promoters in animal model systems, in vitro model systems, such as those that detect their ability to reversibly inhibit gap junctional intercellular communication [111]. Unsaturated fatty acids, insulin, insulin –like growth factors, among others factors, could cause both the symmetrical cell division in adult breast stem cells (increasing the risk to initiation) and act as tumor promoters of initiated breast stem cells. Note that, prior to the Second World War, few dairy products (cheese, meat, milk) were in the Japanese diet. Today, it is becoming a major component.

Back to the human prostate, when the early humans domesticated the canine, the hunter became more successful. The canine and the human started to share the same diet of red meat that was now grilled. While early humans did not survive long enough to manifest prostate cancers, today with the median life span in developed countries having been significantly increased over the last century, so too has the prostate cancer frequency.

An example of how both an environmental factor and the soy dietary factors play a role in prostate cancer has recently been reported. Ho et al [133] showed that pregnant rodents fed a diet contaminated with bisphenol A gave rise to male offspring that had a high incidence of prostate cancers, even though the male offspring were not exposed to the environmental non-genotoxic chemical after birth. On the other hand, if these pregnant rodents were fed both soy products and the bisphenol-A, the risk to prostate cancer in the male offspring was dramatically reduced. Clearly, if one assumes that the stem cells of the prostate are the target cells for prostate cancers, and that the effects seen occur in utero during fetal development, one can speculate that the bisphenol-A caused the prostate stem cells to symmetrical division, increasing the prostate stem cell pool. This alone, all other factors being the same, would increase the risk to cancer. On the other hand, if during fetal development the components of the soy diet cause the prostate stem cell to divide asymmetrically and to differentiate, then the stem cell pool would decrease, lowering the risk to prostate cancer.

It must be pointed out the bisphenol A is an epigenetic, not genotoxic, toxicant. Dietary chemicals, such as genistein and environmental toxicants, such as bisphenol A, TCDD, PBB, PCB, DDT, can effect, epigenetically gene expression of the offspring when agents are applied in utero. The studies by the Jirtle group showed that the genetic strain of agouti mice could have their coat color modulated by epigenetic agents [134]. The molecular alterations in methylation and histone acetylation suggest that they are associated with the altered phenotypes. However, there is another interpretation. The altered gene expression might be due to altered stem cell pools (recall that the gene patterns of particular adult stem cells will always be different from their differentiated daughter lineage cells that contribute to the agouti phenotype).

In a brief analysis of how dietary nutrients, contaminants and process of preparation, such as frying or grilling, diets, that affect either or both breast and prostate cancer (or any other kind), probably affect the promotion, rather that the initiation process. They could affect initiation, indirectly, by altering the stem cell pool that is exposed to an initiator. Most, if not all, promoters reversibly inhibit cell-cell communication to affect proliferation, differentiation and apoptosis. Promotion is the stage that would most likely be impacted by dietary factors and intervention practices to lower cancer frequencies. Several promoters and anti-promoters come to mind with the advent of cultural evolutionary changes, contributed by the bovine and canine. The animal fats, the excessive calories, the cholesterol, hormones, such as estrogens, insulin, pyrolytic polyaromatic hydrocarbons [68], which both the bovine and canine gave humans (and to the canine by us in return for its hunting and companionship attributes), we can attribute, in part, both the rise in breast cancer and prostate cancers. In the case of breast cancers, the cultural practice, now, of postponing of early marriage and children only raises the breast cancer risk.

It is interesting to note that β-sitosterol, a component of fibers of vegetables and fruits, can lower cholesterol levels [135] and inhibit the ras oncogene effect on cell-cell communication in tumor cells. [62]. It is also, a major component of olive oil [136] and this has been suggested as a possible risk reducer of both cardiovascular and prostate cancer frequencies in the Mediterranean diet. Bovine animals with large mammary glands, unlike the canine with prostate cancers due to its companionship with the humans and their diets, eats lots of plant products containing β-sitosterol (of course, they do not live long enough to develop cancers; however, it they did, it is unlikely they would have a high frequency of mammary cancers).

CONCLUSION

The implications of understanding the mechanisms of carcinogenesis are immense. Currently, the many known factors that must influence the mechanism of forming a tumor (e.g., genetics, developmental stage, gender, environmental agents, calories, exercise, diet, life-style and cultural behaviours, etc.) appear to prevent the generation of a coherent integrated hypothesis. However, many old ideas, such as the multi-stage, multi-mechanism hypothesis, the stem cell theory, and newer observations in molecular oncology, toxicology of chemical "carcinogens", stem cell biology, oncogene / tumor suppression gene functions, plus the re-discovery of "cancer stem cells", have made it possible to gain a new insight.

While a tumor consists of billions of genotypically- and phenotypically-heterogeneous cells, we do know they all had a single common origin. While still debated, that single normal cell, which was altered during the "initiation" phase of carcinogens, appears to have been a normal, immortal adult stem cell. "Initiation" appears to be a process that blocks that normal stem cell's ability to divide, asymmetrically, under normal conditions of proliferation; in other words, it can not terminally differentiate senesce or apoptose. While the risk to the initiation phase, caused by either mutations or stable epigenetic mechanisms, can be minimized, it can never be reduced to zero. However, the promotion phase, which brings about the clonal expansion of these initiated stem cells or "pre-cancer stem cells", can take decades to generate an invasive and metastatic "cancer stem cell". The promotion of these initiated stem cells can be interrupted or accelerated by environmental-, dietary-, hormone-, inflammatory-, cytokine-, and growth- factors, as well as caloric restriction or gluttony. Cell-cell communication, by either secreted or gap junction-mediated factors, triggers redox-intracellular signalling to alter gene expression, can be either decreased (tumor promotion) or increased (chemo-prevention or anti-tumor promotion). The discovery that the Oct-4 gene can be a marker for both maintaining "stemness" in the normal embryonic and adult stem cells, as well as a marker for the pre-malignant and malignant " cancer stem cells", makes it possible to target these cells with new strategies for chemo-prevention and chemotherapy. Evidence supporting the adult stem cell as the target cell or the cell of origin of the "cancer stem cell" , while supported by experiments with human adult breast stem cells, is also supported by evidence of the existence of adult stem cells in higher plants that can give rise to callas and ultimately a whole plant (137). This gave the authors of that study to state: "...callus resembles the tip of a root meristem, even if it is derived from aerial organs such as petals, which clearly hows that callus formation is not a simple reprogramming process backward to an undifferentiated state as widely believed."

From this new integration of observations and hypotheses, comes another new important implication, namely, one's risk to cancer might be influenced during pregnancy when the mother's dietary or medical treatments could either increase or decrease the adult stem cell pools in various organs. Keeping all other cancer-influencing factors equal, just increasing or decreasing the adult stem cell pool would alter the risk to cancer in adulthood, based on the adult stem cell being the "target" for the initiation phase. On the other hand, what we as inheritors of these adult stem cells from our mothers do to any "initiated" stem cell in our body can either increase or decrease the risk to the promotion phase of carcinogenesis. In other words, *"What our mother's ate or didn't eat (or get exposed to) can influence the number of our adult stem cells; what we eat or do to these initiated stem cells can modulate our risk to cancer."*

REFERENCES

[1]   Dobzhansky, T. (1975) Nothing in Biology makes sense except in the light of evolution. *Am.Biol. Teachers, 35*, 125-129.

[2]   Hanahan, D. and Weinberg, R.A. (2000). Hallmarks of cancer. *Cell, 100*, 57-70.

[3]   Al Hajj, M., Wicha, M.S., Benito-Hernandez, A., Morrison, S.J., and Clarke, M.F. (2003). Prospective identification of tumorigenic breast cancer cells. *Proc. Nat. Acad. Sci. USA, 100*, 3983-3988.

[4]   Markert, C.L. (1968). Neoplasia: A disease of differentiation. *Cancer Res., 28*, 1908-1914.

[5]   Markert, C. L. (1984). Genetic control of cell interactions in chimeras. *Develop Genet., 4*, 267-279.

[6]   Pierce, B. (1974). Neoplasms, differentiation and mutations. *Am. J. Pathol., 77*, 103-118.

[7]   Potter, V.R. (1978). Phenotypic diversity in experimental hepatomas: Concept of partially blocked ontogeny. *Br. J. Cancer, 38*, 1-23.

[8]   Kerbel, R.S., Frost, P., Liteplo,R., Carlow, D.A., and Elliot, B.E. (1984). Possible epigenetic mechanisms of tumor progression: Induction of high frequency heritable but phenotypically unstable changes in the tumorigenic and metastatic properties of tumor cell populations by 5-azacytidine treatment. *J. Cell Physiol., 3*, 87-97.

[9] Tlsty, T.D., Briot, A., Gualberto, A., Hall, I., Hess, S., Hixon, M., Kuppuswamy, D., Romanov, D., Sage, M., and White, A. (1995). Genomic instability and cancer. *Mutation Res.*, 337, 1-7.

[10] P.W.Laird. (2005). Cancer epigenetics. *Hum. Mol. Genet., 14*, R65-R76.

[11] Boveri, T. (1914). *Zurfrage der Entstehung Maligner Tumoren.* Jena: Gustav Fisher.

[12] Cleaver, J.E. and Trosko, J.E. (1970). Absence of excision of ultraviolet-induced cyclobutane dimers in Xeroderma pigmentosum. *Photochem. Photobiol., 11*, 547-550.

[13] Maher, V.M. and McCormick, J.J. (1976). Effect of DNA repair on the cytotoxicity and mutagenicity of UV irradiation and of chemical carcinogens in normal and xeroderma pigmentosum cells. In: J.M. Yuhas, R.W. Tennant and J.D. Regan (Eds.), *Biology of Radiation Carcinogenesis* (pp. 129-145). New York: Raven Press.

[14] Warren, S., R.A. Schultz, C.C. Chang, M.H. Wade and Trosko, J.E. (1981). Elevated spontaneous mutation rate in Bloom syndrome fibroblasts. *Proc. Natl. Acad. Science USA, 78*, 3133-3137.

[15] Brash, D. E., Rudolph, J.A., Simon, X., Lin, A. and McKenna, G.J. (1991). A role for sunlight in skin cancer: UV-induced p53 mutations in squamous cell carcinomas. *Proc. Natl. Acad. Sci. USA, 88*, 10124-10128.

[16] Ames,B.N., Durston,W. E., Yamasaki, E. and Lee, F. D. (1973). Carcinogens are mutagens a simple test system combining liver homogenates for activation and bacteria for detection. *Proc. Natl. Acad. Sci. USA, 70*, 2281-2285.

[17] Marsh, D.J. and Zori, R.T. (2002). Genetic insights into famial cancers-update and recent discoveries. *Cancer Letters, 181*, 125-164.

[18] Evans, W.H. and Martin, P.E.M. (2002).Gap junctions: Structure and Function. *Molec. Membr. Biol., 19*, 121-136.

[19] Cruciani, V. and Mikalsen, S.-O. (2005). The connexin gene family in mammals. *Biol Chem., 386*, 325-332.

[20] Willecke, K., Eiberger, J., Degen, J., Eckhardt, D., Romauldi, A., Guldenagel, M., Duetsch, U. and Sohl, G. (2002). Structural and functional diversity of connexion genes in the mouse and human genome. *Biol. Chem., 383*, 725-737.

[21] Eagle, H. (1965). Growth inhibitor effects of cellular interactions. *Isreal J. Med. Sci., 1*, 1220-1228.

[22] Revel, J.P. (1988). The oldest multicellular animal and its junctions. In: Hertzberg, E.L. and Johnson, R. (Eds.), *Gap Junction* (pp 135-149). N.Y.: Alan Liss, Inc.

[23] Loewenstein, W.R. (1966). Permeability of membrane junctions. *Ann. N.Y. Acad. Sci., 137*, 441-472.

[24] Trosko, J.E. (2007). Stem cells and cell-cell communication in the understanding of the role of diet and nutrients in human diseases. *J. Fd. Hyg. Safety, 22*, 1-14.

[25] Takahashi, K. and Yamanaka, S. (2006). Induction of pluripotent stem cells from mouse embryonic and adult fibroblasts cultures by defined factors. *Cell, 126*, 663-676.

[26] Shi, Y. (2004). Caspase activation, inhibition, and reactivation: A mechanistic view. *Protein Science, 13*,1979-1987

[27] Wilson, M.R., Close, T.W. and Trosko, J.E. (2000). Cell population dynamics (apoptosis, mitosis and cell-cell communication) during disruption of homeostasis. *Exp. Cell Res., 254*, 257-268.

[28] Tumbar, T., Guasch, G., Greco, V., Blanpain, C., Lowry, W.E., Rendl, M. and Fuchs, E. (2004). Defining the epithelial stem cell niche in skin. *Science, 303*, 359-363.

[29] Juckett D. A. (1987). Cellular aging (the Hayflick limit) and species longevity: a unification model based on clonal succession. *Mech Ageing Devel., 38,* 49–71.

[30] Kalimi and Lo blastocyte lack og GJ Lo, C.W. (1996). The role of gap junction membrane channels in development. *J. Bioenerget. Biomembr., 28,* 379-385.

[31] Trosko, J.E., Chang, C.C., Wilson, M.R., Upham, B.L., Hayashi, T. and wade, M. (2000). Gap junctions and the regulation of cellular functions of stem cells during development and differentiation. *Methods, 20,* 245-264.

[32] de Rooij, D. G., Lok, D., Wennk, D. (1985). Feedback regulation of the proliferation of the undifferentiated spermatogonia in the Chinese hamster by differentiating spermatogonia. *Cell Tissue Kinet, 18,* 71–81.

[33] Kimchi, A., Wang, X. F., Weinberg, R. A., Cheifetz, S. and Massague, J. (1988). Absence of TGF-b receptors and growth: Inhibitory responses in retinoblastoma cells. *Science, 290,* 196–198.

[34] Borek, C. and Sachs, L. (1966). The difference in contact inhibition of cell replication between normal cells and cells transformed by different carcinogens. *Proc. Natl. Acad. Sci. USA, 56,* 1705-1711.

[35] Yamasaki, H. and Naus, C.C.G. (1996). Role of connexion genes in growth control. *Carcinogenesis, 17,* 1199-1213.

[36] Csete, M. (2005). Oxygen in the cultivation of stem cells. *Ann. N.Y. Acad. Sci., 1049,* 1-8.

[37] Fialkow, P. J. (1979). Clonal origin of human tumors. *Am. Rev. Med., 30,* 135-176.

[38] Nowell, P.C. (1976). The clonal evolution of tumour cell populations. *Science, 194,* 23-28.

[39] Sell, S. (1993). Cellular origin of cancer: De-differentiation or stem cell maturation arrest? *Environ. Health Perspect., 101,* 15-26.

[40] Wernig, M., Meissner, A., Foreman, R., Brambrink, T., Ku, M., Hochedlinger, K., Berstein, B.E., and Jaenisch, R. (2007). In vitro reprogramming of fibroblasats into a pluripotent ES-cell-like state. *Nature, 448,* 318-323.

[41] Macerali N., Sriharan, R., Xie, W., Utikal, J., Eminli, S., Arnold, K., Stadfeld, M.,Yachechko, R., Tchieu, J. Jaenisch, R., Plath, K. and Hochedlinger, K. (2007). Directly reprogrammed fibroblast show global epigenetic remodelling and widespread tissue contribution. *Cell Stem Cell, 1,* 55-70.

[42] Okita, K., Ichisak, T. and Yamanaka, S. (2007) Generation of germline-competent induced pluripotent stem cells. *Nature, 488,* 313-319.

[43] Land, H., Parada, I.E. and Weinberg, R.A. (1983). Tumorigenic conversion of primary embryo fibroblasts requires at least two cooperating oncogenes. *Nature, 304,* 596-602.

[44] Hayflick, L. (1965). The limited in vitro lifespan of human diploid cell strains. *Exp. Cell Res., 37,* 614-636.

[45] Berenblum, P.M. (1954). A speculative review: The probable nature of promoting action and its significance in the understanding of the mechanisms of carcinogenesis. *Cancer Res., 14,* 471-477.

[46] Yamagiwa, K. and Ichikawa, K. (1977). Experimental study of the pathogenesis of carcinoma. *CA Cancer J. Clin., 27,* 174-181.

[47] Knudson, A.G. (1971). Mutations and cancer: statistical study of retinoblastoma. *Proc. Natl. Acad. Sci. USA, 68,* 820-823.

[48] Yang, Z., Sui, Y., Xiong, S., Liour, S.S., Phillips, A.C. and Ko, L. (2007). Switched alternative splicing of oncogene CoAA during embryonal carcinoma stem cell differentiation. *Nucleic Acid Res., 35*(6),1919-1932.

[49] Trosko, J.E. (2001). Is the concept of tumor promotion a useful paradigm? *Molec. Carcinogen., 39,* 131-137.

[50] Goodman, J.A. (2001). Operational reversibility is a key aspect of carcinogenesis. *Toxicol. Sci., 64,* 147-148.

[51] Trosko, J.E. and Tai, M.-H. (2006). Adult stem cell theory of the multi-stage, multi-mechanism theory of carcinogenesis: Role of inflammation on the promotion of initiated cells. In Dittmar, T., Zaeker, K.S. and Schmidt, XXX (Eds.), *Infections and Inflammation: Impacts on Oncogenesis* (Contributions to *Microbiology,* Vol. *13,* pp. 45-65). K. Karger AG.

[52] Klaunig, J. and Ruch, R.J. (1987). Strain and species effects on the inhibition of hepatocyte intercellular communication by liver tumor promoters. *Cancer Letters, 36,* 161-168.

[53] Yotti, L.P., Chang, C.C. and Trosko, J.E. (1979). Elimination of metabolic cooperation in Chinese hamster cells by a tumor promoter. *Science, 206,* 1089-1091.

[54] Trosko, J.E. and Chang, C.C. (1988). Nongenotoxic Mechanisms in carcinogenesis: role of inhibited intercellular communication. In: Hart, R.W. and Hoerger, F.D. (Eds), *Banbury Report 31: Carcinogen Risk Assessment: New Directions in the Qualitative and Quantitative Aspects (pp. 139-170).* Cold Spring Harbor, N.Y.: Cold Spring Harbor Laboratory.

[55] Sai, K., Kanno, J., Hasegawa, R., Trosko, J.E., and Inoue, T. (2000). Prevention of the down regulation of gap junctional intercellular communication by green tea in the liver of mice fed pentachlorophenol. *Carcinogenesis, 21,* 1671-1676.

[56] Nielson, M., Ruch, R.J., and Vang, O. (2000). Reservatrol reverses tumor-promoter-induced inhibition of gap junctional intercellular communication. *Biochem. Biophys. Res. Commun., 275,* 804-809.

[57] Upham, B.L. Gu˘zvic, M., Scott, J., Carbone, J.M., Blaha, L., Coe, C.Li, L. L., Rummel, A.M., and Trosko, J.E. (2007). Inhibition of Gap Junctional Intercellular Communication and Activation of Mitogen-Activated Protein Kinase by Tumor-Promoting Organic Peroxides and Protection by Resveratrol. *Nutrition and Cancer, 57*(1), 38–47.

[58] Na, H.-K., Wilson, M.R., Kang, K.S., Chang, C.C., Grunberger, D. and Trosko, J.E. (2000). Restoration of gap junctional intercellular communication by caffeic acid phenethyl ester (CAPE) in a ras-transformed rat liver epithelial cell line. *Cancer Letters, 157,* 31-38.

[59] Ruch, R.J., Madhukar, B.V., Trosko, J.E., and Klaunig, J.E. (1993). Reversal of ras-induced inhibition of gap junctional intercellular communication, transformation and tumorigenesis by lovastatin. *Molec. Carcinogen., 7,* 50-59.

[60] Nakamura, Y., Chang, C.C., Mori, T., Sato, K., Ohtsuki, K., Upham, B.L., and Trosko, J.E. (2005). Augmentation of differentiation and gap junction fubction by kaempferol in partially-differentiation colon cancer cells. *Carcinogenesis, 26,* 665-671.

[61] Ogawa, T., Hayashi, T., Tokunou, M., Nakachi, K., Trosko, J.E., Chang, C.C., and Yorioka, N., (2005). Suberoylanilide hydroxamic acid enhances gap junctional

intercellular communication via acetylation of histone containing connexin43 gene locus. *Cancer Res.*, *65*, 9771-9778.

[62] Nakamura, Y., Yoshikawa, N., Hiroki, I., Sato, K., Ohtsuki,K., Chang, C.C., Upham, B.L., and Trosko, J.E. (2005). β- Sitosterol, From Psyllium Seed Husk (Plantago ovata Forsk), Restores Gap Junctional Intercellular Communication in Ha-ras Transfected Rat Liver Cells. *Nutrition Cancer, 5*, 218-225.

[63] Trosko, J.E. and Ruch, R.J. (1998). Cell-cell communication in carcinogenesis. *Front. Biosci., 3,* 208-236.

[64] Loewenstein, W.R and Kanno, Y. (1966). Intercellular communication and the control of tissue growth: Lack of communication between cancer cells. *Nature, 209,* 1248-1249.

[65] Cleaver, J.E. (1978). Xeroderma pigmentosum: genetic and environmental influences in skin carcinogenesis. *International Journa of Dermatology, 17,* 435-444.

[66] Warren, S., Schultz, R.A., Chang, C.C., Wade, M.H. and Trosko, J.E. (1981). Elevated spontaneous mutation rate in Bloom syndrome fibroblasts. *Proc. Natl. Acad. Science USA, 78,* 3133-3137.

[67] Ames, B.N., Lois, Swirsky, Gold, L.S., and Shigenaga, M.K. (1996). *Cancer Prevention, Rodent High-Dose Cancer Tests, And Risk AssessmentRisk Analysis, 16,* 613-617.

[68] Trosko, J.E. and Upham, B.L. (2005). The emperor wears no clothes in the field of carcinogen risk assessment: Ignored concepts in cancer risk assessment. *Mutagenesis, 20,* 81-92.

[69] Thilly, W.G. (2003). Have environmental mutagens caused oncomutations in people? *Nat. Genet., 34,* 255- 259.

[70] Upham, B.L., Weis, L.M. and Trosko, J.E. (1998). Modulated gap junctional intercellular communication as a biomarker of PAH epigenetic toxicity: structure--function relationship. *Environ. Health Perspect. 106*(Suppl 4), 975--981.

[71] Weis,L.M., Rummel,A.M., Masten,S.J., Trosko,J.E. and Upham,B.L.(1998). Bay or baylike regions of polycyclic aromatic hydrocarbons were potent inhibitors of gap junctional intercellular communication. *Environ.Health Perspect., 106,* 17--22.

[72] Tai, M.H., Upham, B.L., Olson, L.K., Tsao, M.S., Reed, D.N., and Trosko, J.E. (2007). Cigarette smoke condensate inhibited intercellular communication and differentiation in human pancreatic ductal epithelial cells. *Int. J. Cancer, 120,* 1855-1862.

[73] Minsk, B. and Illensee, K. (1975). Normal genetically mosaic mice produced from malignant teratocarcinoma cells. *Proc. Natl. Acad. Sci. USA, 72,* 3585-3589.

[74] Trosko, J. E. (2006). From adult stem cells to cancer stem cells: Oct-4 gene, cell-cell communication and hormones during tumor promotion. *Ann. N.Y. Acad. Sci., 1089,* 36-58.

[75] Wang X. and Harris, C. (1997). p53 tumor- suppressor gene: clues to molecular carcinogenesis. *J. Cell Physiol., 173,* 247-255.

[76] Barcellos-Hoff, M.H. (2001). Three down and counting: The transformation of human mammary cells from normal to malignant in three steps. *Trends Molec. Med., 7,* 142-143.

[77] Bissell, M.J. and Radisky, D. (2001). Putting tumors in context. *Nature Rev. Cancer, 1,* 46-54.

[78] Trosko, J.E., Chang, C.C., Upham, B. and Wilson, M. (1998). Epigenetic toxicology as toxicant-induced changes in intracellular signalling leading to altered gap junctional intercellular communication. *Toxicol. Lett., 102-103*, 71--78.

[79] Potter, V.R. (1973). Biochemistry of cancer. In Holland, J. and Frei, E (Eds.), *Cancer Medicine* (pp. 178-192). Philadelphia: Lea, E. and Febiger.

[80] Al Hajj, M., Wicha, M.S., Benito-Hernandez, A., Morrison, S.I. and Clarke, M.F. (2003). Prospective identification of tumorigenic breast cancer cells. *Proc. Natl. Acad. Sci. USA, 100*, 3983-3988.

[81] Webster, J.D., Yusbasiyan-Gurkan, V., Trosko, J.E., Chang, C.C., and Kiupel, M. (2007). Expression of the embryonic transcription factor Oct4 in Canine neoplasms: A potential marker for stem cell subpopulations in neoplasia. *Vet. Pathol., 44*, in press.

[82] Chang, C.C., Trosko, J.E., El-Fouly, M.H., Gibson, D.R. and D'Ambrosio, S.M. (1987). Contact insensitivity of a subpopulation of normal human fetal kidney epithelial cells and of human carcinoma cell lines. *Cancer Res., 47*, 1634-1645.

[83] Kao, C.Y., Nomata, K., Okley, C.S., Welsch, C.W. and Chang, C.C. (1995). Two types of normal human breast epithelial cells derived from reduction mammoplasty: Phenotypic characterization and response to SV40 transfection. *Carcinogenesis, 16*, 531-538.

[84] Linning, K.D., Tai, M.H., Madhukar, B.V., Chang, C.C., Reed, D.N., Ferber, S., Trosko, J.E., and Olson, L.K. (2004). Redox-mediated enrichment of self-renewing adult human pancreatic cells which possess endocrine differentiation potential. *Pancreas, 29*, e64-e76.

[85] Lin, T.-M., Tsai, J.-L., Lin, S.-D., Lai, C.-S., and Chang, C-C. (2005). Accelerated Growth and prolonged lifespan of adipose tissue-derived human mesenchymal stem cells in a medium using reduced calcium and antioxidants. *Stem Cells Devel., 14*, 92–102.

[86] Yang, Y.C., S.W. Wang, H. Y.Hung, C.C. Chang, I.C. Wu, Y.L. Huang, T. M. Lin, J. L. Tsai, A. Chen, F.C. Kuo, W.M. Wang and D.C. Wu. (2007). Isolation and characterization of human gastric cell lines with stem cell phenotypes. *J. Gastroenterology Hepatology,* doi:1111/j.1440-1746.2007.05031.x.

[87] Matic, M., Evans, W.H., Brink, P.R. and Simon, M. (2002). Epidermal cells do not communicate through gap junctions. *J. Invest. Dermat., 118*, 110-116.

[88] Matic, M., Petrov, I.N., Chen, S., Wang, C., Dimitrijevich, S.D., and Wolosin, J.M. (1997). Stem cells of the corneal epithelium lack connexins and metabolic transfer capacity. *Different., 61*, 251-260.

[89] Kang, K.S., Sun, W., Nomata, K., Morita, I., Cruz, A., Liu, C.J., Trosko, J.E. and Chang, C.C. (1998). Involvement of tyrosine phosphorylation of p185 c-erB2/neu in tumorigenicity by X rays and neu-oncogene in human breast epithelial cells. *Molec. Carcinogen., 21*, 225-233.

[90] Nakano, S., Ueo, H., Bruce, S.A. and Ts'o, P.O.P. (1985). A contact-insensitive subpopulation in Syrian hamster cell cultures with a greater susceptibility to chemically induced neoplastic transformation. *Proc. Natl. Acad. Sci. USA, 82*, 5005-5009.

[91] Ponti, D., Costa, A., Zaffaroni, N., Pratesi, G., Petrangolini, G., Coradini, D., Pilotti, S., Pierotti, M.A. and Daidone, M.A. (2005). Isolation and In vitro propagation of tumorigenic breast cancer cells with stem/progenitor cell properties. *Cancer Res., 65*, 5506-5511.

[92]   Chang, C.C., Sun, W., Cruz, A., Saitoh, M., Tai, M.H. and Trosko, J.E. (2001). A human breast epithelial cell type with stem cell characteristics as targets for carcinogenesis. *Radiat. Res., 155*, 201-207.

[93]   Takahashi, K. and Yamanaka, S. (2006). Induction of pluripotent stem cells from mouse embryonic and adult fibroblast cultures by defined factors. *Cell, 126*, 663-676.

[94]   Okamoto, K., Okazawa, H., Okuda, A., Sakai, M., Muramatsu, M. and Hamada, H. (1990). A novel octamer binding transcription factor is differentially expressed in mouse embryonic cells. *Cell, 60*, 461-472.

[95]   Niwa, H., Miyazaki, J. and Smith, A.G. (2000). Quantitative expression of 0ct3/4 defines differentiation, de-differentiation or self-renewal of ES cells. *Nat. Genet. 24*, 372-376.

[96]   Rosner, M.H., Vigano, M.A., Ozato, K., Timmons, P.M., Poirier, F., Rigby, P.W. and Staudt, L.M. (1990). A POU-domain transcription factor in early stem cells and germ cells of the mammalian embryo. *Nature, 345*, 686-692.

[97]   Monk, M and Holding, C. (2001). Human embryonic genes re-expressed in cancer cells. *Oncogene, 20*(20), 8085-8091.

[98]   Tai, M.H., Chang, C.C., Kiupel, M., Webster, J.D. and Trosko, J.E. (2005). Oct-4 expression in adult stem cells: Evidence in support of the stem cell theory of carcinogenesis. *Carcinogenesis, 26*, 495-502.

[99]   Momiyama, M., Omori, Y., Isizaki, Y., Nishikawa, Y., Tokairin, T., Ogawa, J. and Enomoto, E. (2003). Connexin 26 mediated gap junctional communication reverses the malignant phenotype of MCF-7 breast cancer cells. *Cancer Sci., 94*: 501-507.

[100] Barcellos-Hoff, M.H. (2001). It takes a tissue to make a tumor: epigenetics, cancer and the microenvironment. *J. Mammary Gland Neoplasm, 6*, 213-221.

[101] Atlasi, Y., Mowla, S.T., Ziaee, S.A. and Bahrami, A.R. (2007). Oct-4, an embryonic stem cell maker is highly expressed in bladder cancer. *Internatl. J. Cancer, 120*, 1598-1602.

[102] Kelly, P.N., Dakic, A., Adams, J.M., Nutt, S.L. and Strasser, A. (2007). Tumor growth need not be driven by rare cancer stem cells. *Science, 317*, 337.

[103] Umemoto, T. Yamato, M., Nishida, K., Yang, J., Tano, Y. and Okano, T. (2005). Limbal epithelial side-population cells have stem cell-like properties, including quiescent state. *Stem Cells, 24*, 86-94.

[104] Kim; M., Turnquist, H., Jackson, J., Sgaglas, M., Yan, Y., Gong, M., Dean, M., Sharp, J.G., and Cowan, K. (2002). The multidrug resistance transporter ABCG2 (Breast cancer resistance protein 1) effluxes Hoechst 33342 and is overexpressed in hematopoietic stem cells. *Clinical Cancer Res., 8*, 22-28.

[105] Trosko, J.E. (2007). Stem cells and cell-cell communication in the understanding of the role of diet and nutrients in human diseases. *J. Fd. Hyg. Safety,* 1-14.

[106] Milton, K. (2000). Back to basics: Why foods of wild primates have relevance for modern human health. *Nutrition, 16*, 480-483.

[107] Kiple, K.F. (Ed). (2000). *The Cambridge World History of Food.* Cambridge University Press.

[108] Teaford, M.F. and Ungar, P.S. (2000). Diet and the evolution of the earliest human ancestors. *Proc. Natl. Acad. Sci. USA, 97*, 13506-13511.

[109] Mariani-Constantini, A. (2000). Natural and cultural influences on the evolution of the human diet: Background of the multifactorial processes that shaped the eating habits of Western societies. *Nutrition, 16*, 483-486.

[110] Popkin, B.M. (2007). The world is fat. *Sci. Amer., 297*, 88-95

[111] Trosko, J.E. and Ruch, R. J. (2002). Gap junctions as therapeutic targets. *Curr. Drug Targets, 3*, 465-482.

[112] Franco,E.L., Correa,P., Santella,R.M., Wu,X., Goodman,S.N. and Petersen,G.M. (2004). Role and limitations of epidemiology in establishing a casual association. *Semin. Cancer Biol., 14*, 413--426.

[113] Goodman G.E., Thornquist, M.D., Balmes, J., Cullen, R.M., Meysken, F.L., Omenn, G.S., Valanis, G.S. and Williams, J.H. (2004). The beta-carotene and retinol efficacy trial: Incidence of lung cancer and cardiovascular disease mortality during 6 year follow-up after stopping beta-carotene and retinol supplements. *J. Natl. Cancer Instit., 96*, 1743-1750.

[114] Shuin, T., Nishimura, R., Noda, K., Umeda, M., and Ono, T. (1983) Concentration-dependent differential effect of retinoid acid on intercellular metabolic cooperation. *Gann, 74*, 100-105.

[115] He,K., Nukada, H., Urakami, T. and Murphy, M.P. (2003). Antioxidant and pro-oxidant properties of pyrroloquinoline quinine (PQQ): Implications for its function in biological systems. *Biochem.Pharmocol., 65*, 67-74.

[116] Henning, H., Wenk, M.L., Dohahoe, R. (1982). Retinoic acid promotion of papilloma formation in mouse skin. *Cancer Letters, 16*, 1-5.

[117] Cohen, G.M., Bracken, W.H., Iyer, R.P., Berry, D.L., Selkirk, J.K., and Slaga, T. J. Anticarcinogenic effects of 2,3,7,8-tetrachlorodibenzo –p-dioxin on benzo(a) pyrene and 7,12-dimethylbenz (a) anthrcene tumor initiation and its relationship to DNA binding. *Cancer Res., 39*, 4027-4033.

[118] Kushida, M., Sukata, T., Uwagawa, S., Ozaki, K., Kinoshita, A., Wanibusbuchi, H., Morimura, K., Okuno, Y. and Fukushima, S. (2005). Low dose DDT inhibition of hepatocarcinogenesis by diethylnitrosamine in male rats: Possible mechanisms. *Toxicol. Appl. Pharmacol., 208*, 285-294.

[119] Lee, G.H. (2000). Paradoxical effects of Phenobarbital on mouse hepatocarcinogenesis. *Toxicol. Pathol., 28*, 215-225.

[120] Kelloff,G.J., Lippman,S.M., Dannenberg, A.J., Sigman, C.C.H.L., Reid, B.J., Szabo, E., Jordan, V.C., Spitz, M.R., Mills,G.B., Papadimitrakopoulou, V.A., Lotan,R., Aggarwal,B.B., Bresalier, R.S., Banu Arun, J.K., Lu,K.H., Thomas, M.E., Rhodes, H.E., Brewer, M.A., Follen, M., Shin,D.M., Parnes, H.L., Siegfried, J.M., Evans, A.A., Blot, W.J., Chow, W.-H., Blount, P.L., Maley, C.C., Wang, K.K., Lam, S., Lee, J.J., Dubinett, S.M., Engstrom, P.F., Meyskens, Jr. F.L., O'Shaughnessy, J., Hawk, E.T., Levin, B., Nelson, W.G., Hong, W. K. (2006). Progress in Chemoprevention Drug Development: The Promise of Molecular Biomarkers for Prevention of Intraepithelial Neoplasia and Cancer—A Plan to Move Forward. *Clin. Cancer Res., 12*, 3661-3697.

[121] Upham, B.L., K.-S. Kang, H.-Y Cho, J.E. Trosko (1997). Hydrogen peroxide inhibits gap junction intercellular communication in glutathione sufficient but not glutathione deficient cells. *Carcinogenesis., 18*, 37-42.

[122] Coffey, D.S. (2001). Similarities of prostate and breast cancer: Evolution, diet and estrogens. *Urology, 57*, 31-38.

[123] Grover, P.L. and Martin, F.L. (2002). The initiation of breast and prostate cancer. *Carcinogenesis, 23*, 1095-1102.

[124] Trosko, J.E. (1984). Scientific views of human nature: Implications for the ethics of technological intervention. In D. H. Brock (Ed). *The Culture of Biomedicine (*Vol. *1.*, pp. 70-97) Newark: University of Delaware Press.

[125] Thompson, D.E., Mabuchi, K., Ron, E., Soda, M., Tokunaga, M., Ochikubo, S., Sugimoto, S., Ikeda, T., Terasaki, M., Preston, D.L. (1994). Cancer incidence in atom bomb survivors. Part II: Solid tumors 1958-1987. *Radiat. Res., 137*, S17-S67.

[126] Murrill, W. B., Brown, N., Zhang, J.X., Manzolillo, A., Barnes, S. and Lamartiniere, C.A. (1996). Prepubertal genistein exposure suppresses mammary cancer and enhances gland differentiation in rats. *Carcinogenesis, 17*, 1451-1457.

[127] Kennedy, A.R. (1998). The Bowman-Birk inhibitor from soy beans as an anticarcinogenic agent. Am. *J. Clin. Nutr., 68*,1406s-1412s.

[128] Hsieh C.Y. and Chang, C.C. (1999) Stem cell differentiation and reduction as a potential mechanism for chemoprevention of breast cancer. *Chinese Pharm. J., 51*, 15-30.

[129] . Barker, D.J. P., Mothers, Babies, And Health Later In Life. (2nd ed.). Churchill Livingstone. New York

[130] Ju, Y. H., Allred, C.D., Allred, K.F., Karko, K.L., Doerge, D.R. and Helferich, W.G. (2001). Physiological concentrations of dietary genistein dose-dependently stimulate growth of estrogen-dependent human breast cancer (MCF-7) tumors implanted in athymic mice. *J. Nutr., 131*, 2957-2962.

[131] Trosko, J.E. (2003) Human stem cells as targets for the aging and diseases of aging processes. *Medical Hypo., 60*, 439-447.

[132] Trosko, J.E. (2007). Aging as the 'System's' Breakdown of Communication between the Quality and Quantity of Stem Cells. In *The "Manifesto" For a Long Life.* In Press.

[133] Ho, S.M., Tang, W.Y., de Frauto, J.B., and Prins, G.S. (2006). Developmental exposures to estradiol and bisphenol A increases susceptibility to prostate carcinogenesis and epigenetically regulates phosphodiesterase Type 4 Variant 4. *Cancer Res., 66*, 5624-5632.

[134] Dolinoy, D.C., Weidman, J.R., Waterland, R.A. and Jirtle, R. I. (2006). Maternal genistein alters coat color and protects AVY mouse offspring from obesity by modifying the fetal epigenome. *Environ. Health Perspect. 114*, 567-572.

[135] Moghadasian, M.H. and Frohlich, J.J. (1999). Effects of dietary phytoterols on cholesterol metabolism and atherosclerosis: Clinical and experimental evidence. *American J. Med., 107*, 588-94.

[136] De la Puerta, R., Martinez-Dominguez, E., and Riuz-Gutierrez, V. (2000). Effect of minor componbents of virgin olive oil on topical antiinflammatory sassays. *Z. Naturforsch. C., 55*, 814-819.

[137] Sugimoto, K., Jiao, Y., Meyerowitz, E.M. (2010). Arabidopsis regeneration from multiple tissues occurs via a root development pathway. Devel. Cell 18, 463-471.

INDEX

D

E

N

Q

R

S

T

U